ANNALS OF
THE NEW YORK ACADEMY
OF SCIENCES

Volume 459

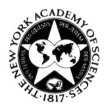

EDITORIAL STAFF

Executive Editor
BILL BOLAND

Managing Editor
JOYCE HITCHCOCK

Associate Editor
RANDI E. SCHOLNICK

The New York Academy of Sciences
2 East 63rd Street
New York, New York 10021

HEMATOPOIETIC CELLULAR PROLIFERATION

AN INTERNATIONAL CONFERENCE IN HONOR OF EUGENE P. CRONKITE

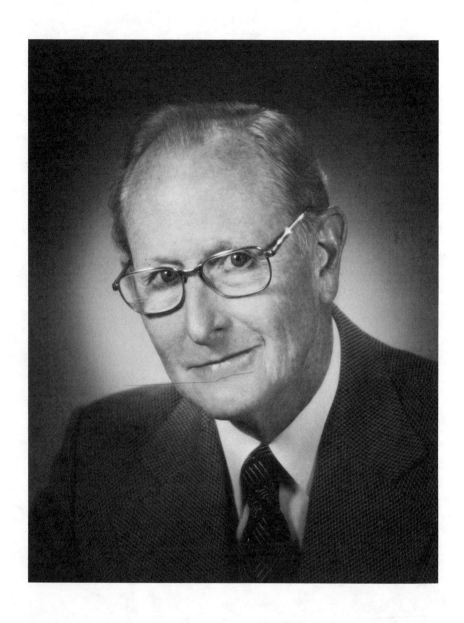

Eugene P. Cronkite

ANNALS OF THE NEW YORK ACADEMY OF SCIENCES
Volume 459

HEMATOPOIETIC CELLULAR PROLIFERATION

AN INTERNATIONAL CONFERENCE IN HONOR OF EUGENE P. CRONKITE

Edited by Victor P. Bond, Pradeep Chandra, and Kanti R. Rai

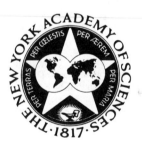

The New York Academy of Sciences
New York, New York
1985

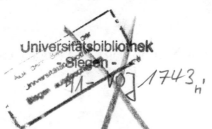

Library of Congress Cataloging-in-Publication Data
Main entry under title:

Hematopoietic cellular proliferation.

(Annals of the New York Academy of Sciences, ISSN
0077-8923; v. 459)
Based on a conference sponsored by the U.S. Dept.
of Energy, Brookhaven National Laboratory, and Associated
Universities, Inc., held Oct. 6-7, 1983 at Brookhaven
National Laboratory in Upton, N.Y.
Includes bibliographies and index.
1. Hematopoiesis—Congresses.   2. Transplantation
immunology—Congresses.   3. Carcinogenesis—Congresses.
4. Tumors, Radiation-induced—Congresses.   5. Leukemia—
Congresses.   6. Cronkite, Eugene P.—Congresses.
I. Cronkite, Eugene P.   II. Bond, Victor P.   III. Chandra,
Pradeep.   IV. Rai, Kanti R.   V. United States, Dept. of
Energy.   VI. Brookhaven National Laboratory.
VII. Associated Universities, Inc.   VIII. Series.
[DNLM: 1. Cell Division—congresses.   2. Hematopoietic
Stem Cells—cytology—congresses. W1 AB626YL v.459/
WH 380 H4868 1983]
Q11.N5 vol. 459   500 s   85-31929
[QP92]   [599'.01'13]
ISBN 0-89766-313-6
ISBN 0-89766-314-4 (pbk.)

PCP
Printed in the United States of America
ISBN 0-89766-313-6 (cloth)
ISBN 0-89766-314-4 (paper)
ISSN 0077-8923

ANNALS OF THE NEW YORK ACADEMY OF SCIENCES
Volume 459
December 31, 1985

HEMATOPOIETIC CELLULAR PROLIFERATION
AN INTERNATIONAL CONFERENCE IN HONOR OF EUGENE P. CRONKITE[a]

Editors
VICTOR P. BOND, PRADEEP CHANDRA, AND KANTI R. RAI

Conference Organizers
VICTOR P. BOND, ARJUN D. CHANANA, PRADEEP CHANDRA,
MICHAEL GREENBERG, KANTI R. RAI, AND LEWIS M. SCHIFFER[b]

CONTENTS

[a]This volume is the result of a conference sponsored by the U.S. Department of Energy, Brookhaven National Laboratory, and Associated Universities, Inc. entitled Hematopoietic Cellular Proliferation: An International Conference in Honor of Eugene P. Cronkite. It was held October 6-7, 1983 at Brookhaven National Laboratory in Upton, New York.

[b]Deceased August 16, 1985.

Financial assistance was received from:
- U.S. DEPARTMENT OF ENERGY
- ASSOCIATED UNIVERSITIES, INC.
- THE BILL BERNBACH FOUNDATION
- DOYLE DANE BERNBACH, INC.
- BURROUGHS WELLCOME COMPANY
- COULTER ELECTRONICS, INC.
- MR. NED DOYLE
- U.S. ENVIRONMENTAL PROTECTION AGENCY
- THE ROSENSTIEL FOUNDATION
- SMITH KLINE BECKMAN CORPORATION
- HENRY M. AND LILLIAN STRATTON FOUNDATION, INC.
- MR. JESSE WOLFF

Foreword

A student of medicine or biology today readily accepts and uses certain terms and concepts which, just a generation ago, were either unknown or considered as abstract and unproven notions. The concepts of pluripotent stem cell, radiation oncogenesis from small exposures, cell-cycle specificity, and T and B lineages of lymphocytes and their respective subpopulations are but a few examples of what was little appreciated just 35 years ago. It is largely because of Dr. Eugene P. Cronkite's contributions as a researcher, as a thinker, and as a guide and counsel for innumerable young scientists that hematopoietic cellular proliferation has become the foundation for studies in cancer research, radiation biology, and immunology of transplantation. This conference was planned to celebrate the thirty-fifth anniversary of his scientific leadership in these areas of research. It brought together distinguished investigators from all parts of the globe, a cross section of scientists whose work set the pioneering pace a few decades ago and those whose work currently in progress may very well be blazing new trails for future scientists to follow. An additional prerequisite for their participation was that they be either collaborators, colleagues, or students of Dr. Cronkite.

VICTOR P. BOND
PRADEEP CHANDRA
KANTI R. RAI

The Development of Immunological Reactivity in Fetal Lambs

BEDE MORRIS AND M. W. SIMPSON-MORGAN

Department of Immunology
The John Curtin School of Medical Research
Australian National University
Canberra, Australia

The capability of an animal to respond immunologically to foreign substances depends on the development of a range of discriminatory functions that enable non-self materials to be identified, phagocytosed, and processed by those cells of the lymphoreticular system that are responsible for the production of specific antibodies and specific cell-mediated reactions.

While these outcomes are the generally accepted phenotypes of the immune response, their measurement tells us very little about the physiological basis on which the immune response is founded and gives us no idea at all of the complexities of the interacting systems that initiate the immune response and regulate it. However, it has been the measurement of specific features of the immune response that has largely determined the emphasis of research into immune phenomena. This is because methods for studying the immune response depend principally on techniques that measure only the specificity of antigen-antibody reactions or cell-mediated responses.

General aspects of the immune response by and large cannot be measured in conventional experimental animal models for their lymphoid systems have invariably been modified by previous antigenic experiences. These changes confound the analysis of the outcome of any intentional challenge. Once an animal is born and exposed to the environment it is probably no longer possible to study in that animal an authentic primary response to any foreign substance.

Certain animal species such as sheep and cattle have a particular type of placentation that effectively removes the fetus from contact with maternal or environmental antigens throughout its uterine development. It is possible to investigate both specific and general aspects of primary immune responses in these species because, during *in utero* life, the fetal lamb and calf acquire immunological competence in the absence of extraneous antigenic stimulation. These fetal animals are essentially agammaglobulinemic up until the time they are born.

THE ONTOGENY OF THE LYMPHOID APPARATUS IN THE FETAL LAMB

Immune responses depend on the reactivities of cells of the reticuloendothelial system and they take place within the anatomical framework of the lymphoid apparatus. Immunological competence, as manifest by specific antibody production, cannot be acquired until all the cellular participants in the humoral response are present in an appropriate environment where the various inductive and modulating stimuli that determine their development can operate on them. Because the individual components of the lymphoid apparatus develop at different times during fetal life it is possible to study the involvement of these components in the immune response in the fetus separately from one another.

Thymus

The thymus is the first organ to contain lymphocytes and these cells are present around 40-45 days of age. At this time the lymphocytes are scattered throughout the gland and there is no histological distinction between the cortex and the medulla. The cortex and medulla are clearly differentiated in the thymus of 60-day fetuses, the cortex being distinguished by its greatly increased content of lymphocytes. Hassall's corpuscles first appear around 65-70 days and from this time on, the thymus has most of its mature histological features. Lymphopoiesis is very active in the thymus from the outset. Many cells in the gland become labeled following a single intravenous injection of [³H]thymidine (FIGURE 1A). Removal of the thymus at around 55-65 days gestation prevents the normal complement of lymphocytes from developing and at birth thymectomized lambs have only 10-20% of the normal number of lymphocytes.[1, 2]

Spleen

The spleen is visible macroscopically at around 60 days gestation and at first it is comprised mostly of hemopoietic tissue. In fetuses of 70 days gestation clusters of lymphocytes are present, many adjacent to the splenic blood vessels. Larger aggregations of lymphocytes develop around the sheathed arteries. Lymphoid follicles are present in the spleen by 120 days gestation but germinal centers are not normally found in the white pulp until after birth. Lymphopoiesis in the spleen is much less active than that in the thymus and only relatively small numbers of cells become labeled following the intravenous injection of [³H]thymidine (FIGURE 1B).

Lymph Nodes

Lymph nodes are first found in fetuses around 55-60 days gestation. The mesenteric nodes are visible some 5-10 days before nodes elsewhere in the body are large enough to be seen and dissected out. The nodes at first are made up of a loose connective tissue interspersed with a few lymphocytes. By 100 days gestation the cortex has differentiated from the medulla and the number of lymphocytes has increased. The structural differentiation of the lymph nodes, however, is not completed during *in utero* life. Vestigial primary follicles develop in the lymph nodes of fetuses near to

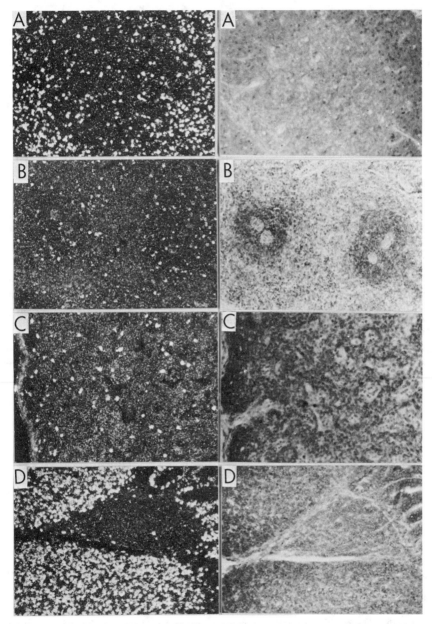

FIGURE 1. Lymphopoiesis in the lymphoid tissues of the fetal lamb. Dark (left side) and bright (right side) field views of the same area are shown. (A) Autoradiograph of the thymus of a fetus of 100 days gestation 1 hr after an intravenous injection of [³H]thymidine. (B) Autoradiograph of the spleen of a fetus of 140 days gestation 1 hr after an intravenous injection of [³H]thymidine. (C) Autoradiograph of the mesenteric lymph node of a fetus of 140 days gestation 1 hr after an intravenous injection of [³H]thymidine. (D) Autoradiograph of the Peyer's patches of a fetus of 140 days gestation 1 hr after an intravenous injection of [³H]thymidine. (Original magnification of parts (A)-(D), ×125; all reduced to 72% of original size.) Courtesy of Dr. J. D. Reynolds.

term but normally no germinal centers appear during fetal life. Lymph nodes in fetuses older than 100 days have well-developed medullary cords and sinuses which contain free-floating lymphocytes. Lymphopoiesis is not active in fetal lymph nodes. Following intravenous injection of [³H]thymidine, labeled cells appear in the primary follicles and throughout both the cortex and the medulla but they are relatively few in number (FIGURE 1C). There are significant numbers of lymphocytes leaving fetal lymph nodes in the lymph from at least 90 days gestation onward. The cell output from the prescapular node between 100 and 150 days gestation is of the order of 20-50 $\times$ 10⁶ cells per hour.

Peyer's Patches

Accumulations of lymphoid cells which are the precursors of Peyer's patches can be identified histologically in the lamina propria of the jejunum and the ileum adjacent to domes of gut epithelium in fetal lambs as early as 70 days gestation. The Peyer's patches of the terminal ileum develop somewhat later at around 120 days gestation; they grow rapidly and reach a mature histological structure before birth. The ileal Peyer's patch at birth extends some 2 m or more along the gut. The estimated mass of lymphoid tissue in the Peyer's patches of lambs at term is around 3 g (Reference 3). The follicles of the Peyer's patches are sites of intense lymphopoiesis throughout *in utero* life; essentially all cells in the follicles become labeled following an intravenous injection of [³H]thymidine (FIGURE 1D). The Peyer's patches are the principal source of Ig-bearing lymphocytes in the fetal lamb and removal of the ileum prior to birth prevents the development of this population of cells. Lambs that have been ileectomized *in utero* have less than 5% of their total lymphocytes with surface Ig at birth; unlike that in normal lambs, this population of cells in ileectomized lambs does not develop further.[4]

THE ONTOGENY OF THE CELLULAR COMPONENTS OF THE IMMUNE RESPONSE

Macrophages

Macrophages and fixed phagocytic cells are present in the circulating blood and in the endothelium of the hepatic sinuses of fetal lambs as early as 24 days gestation, some 15 days before lymphocytes are present in the circulating blood and some 35-40 days before the fetus is able to respond to antigenic challenge by producing specific antibody. These cells are full of fragments of extruded red cell nuclei and other hemopoietic cellular detritus from the outset. The free-floating and fixed macrophages can recognize and engulf foreign material such as bacteria and carbon particles injected intravenously in the absence of opsonins such as immunoglobulins and these cells represent the earliest cellular defense system in the fetus (FIGURE 2). The population of free-floating macrophages is present in the blood of the fetal lamb for the first

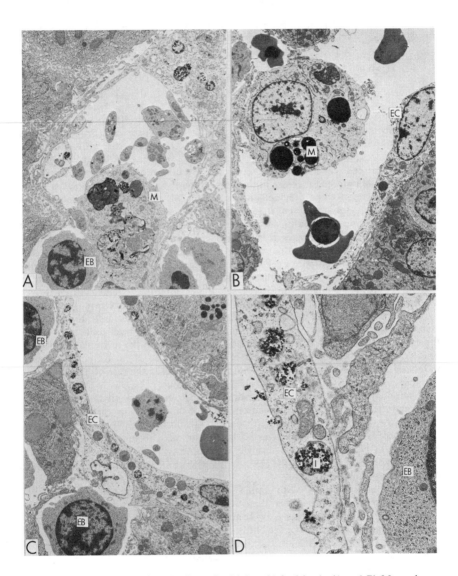

FIGURE 2. Phagocytic cells in the liver of a 24-day-old fetal lamb. (A and B) Macrophages in the liver sinuses. The cell in (A) contains ingested particles of india ink. The cell in (B) contains nuclear fragments of red cells. (C and D) Endothelial cells lining the liver sinuses containing india ink particles. M—macrophage, EB—erythroblast, EC—endothelial cell, I—india ink. (Original magnifications: (A) ×3000, (B) ×5000, (C) ×5000, (D) ×22,000; each has been reduced to 64% of original size.) Courtesy of Mr. M. Al Salami.

several months of gestation; by birth they have disappeared. In adult life these cells are confined to the peripheral lymph and the tissue fluid. The fixed phagocytic reticuloendothelial cell population persists in the liver sinuses, lymph nodes, and spleen.

Lymphocytes

Lymphocytes first appear in the blood of fetuses around 40 days gestation and their numbers increase rapidly from this time onward. These cells originate in the thymus and carry no Ig on their surface membrane. Lymphocytes with Ig on their surface are present in the blood of fetuses at least as young as 56 days gestation.[5] At this time these cells constitute about 0.3% of the total lymphocyte population in the blood. There is a gradual increase in the proportion of Ig-positive lymphocytes in the blood up until term when they constitute some 2-4% of the total lymphocytes. Ig-positive lymphocytes are present in the lymph of fetuses at least as early as 82 days gestation. The immunoglobulin isotype on these cells is exclusively IgM.[4, 6]

The number of lymphocytes in the fetus increases rapidly during the last 60 days *in utero,* as reflected by the output of cells in the thoracic duct lymph of fetal lambs of different ages.[2] The output of cells in the thoracic duct lymph at 100 days gestation is around 10.0×10^6 cells per hour; in fetuses of 150 days gestation it has risen to 200×10^6 cells per hour. When the thoracic duct lymph of the fetus is drained over a period of weeks, the cell output falls rapidly during the first few days as the recirculating pool of cells is depleted. After this time it reaches a steady or slowly increasing level of output (FIGURE 3). This steady state has been used to calculate the rate of production of lymphocytes and their addition to the recirculating pool of cells drained by the thoracic duct. It is of the order of $20-30 \times 10^6$ cells per hour in fetuses of 140 days gestation. In thymectomized fetuses the rate of production of lymphocytes is reduced to around 10-20% of this value.

Lymphocytes in the fetus have an established pattern of recirculation between the blood and the lymph by 80 days gestation and probably somewhat earlier.[2] Migrating lymphocytes can be found in transit through the endothelium of blood capillaries in the cortex of lymph nodes as early as 80 days gestation. This metastatic aspect of the life history of lymphocytes is intrinsically determined. It is part of the genetic ethos of these cells and it develops in the absence of antigenic stimulation and in the absence of circulating immunoglobulins.

There is no evidence that migrant subpopulations of lymphocytes discriminate between tissues in the fetus other than that their migration is directed through the lymphoid organs.[7] Experiments have been reported which suggest that lymphocytes collected from certain tissues of the body have a predilection to return to these tissues during their migrations after birth and this finding has been interpreted in terms of an effect of antigen on the behavior of these cells.[8, 9]

THE IMMUNE RESPONSE IN SINGLE LYMPH NODES IN THE FETUS

The immune response to a putative primary or a secondary antigenic challenge can be studied in a single lymph node in adult sheep by following the events that occur in the efferent lymph coming from the node.[10] If an antigen is injected into the cannulated lymph node via an afferent lymphatic, the immune response is confined to the node provided the cellular and humoral products leaving the node in the lymph are drained from the animal. The immune response that ensues is comprised of a sequence of events that begins with the uptake and phagocytosis of the antigen; the reordering of the cellular traffic through the lymph node; the proliferation and differentiation of antigen-reactive cells into antibody-forming cells; the synthesis and secretion of antibody and the subsequent establishment of an immunological memory for the antigen. In the primary immune response in adult sheep each of these components of the response follows sequentially one after the other, giving rise finally to the appearance of specific antibody. It remains uncertain, however, as to which of

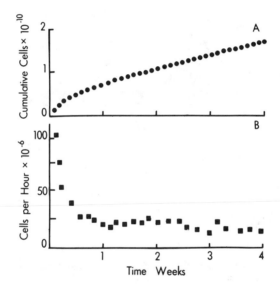

FIGURE 3. The output of cells in the thoracic duct lymph of a fetal lamb. The thoracic duct was cannulated at 115 days gestation and lymph collected continuously over the following 28 days. The fetus was born at 143 days gestation. (A) Cumulative cell output. (B) Hourly cell output.

these events are part of the authentic primary response to antigen and which result from previous conditioning of the immune system and the lymphoid apparatus by natural antigenic contacts. A study of immune responses in fetal lambs provides evidence that there are certain events which distinguish the authentic primary interaction between an antigen and the unmodified lymphoid apparatus from primary responses that occur in animals after birth.

It is possible to collect lymph from single lymph nodes in fetal lambs as early as 90 days gestation[11, 12] and to study immune responses by a modification of the experimental approach that is used in adult sheep. If both the prescapular nodes are cannulated at the same time one can be challenged with antigen and the contralateral node used as a control. This allows primary and secondary immune responses to be followed in the efferent lymph of the lamb *in utero* for periods of weeks without compromising its normal physiological status. Cannulated fetuses develop and are born normally, often with their cannulas intact and the lymph still flowing.[13]

Lymph nodes of fetuses 100 days and older are capable of giving primary responses to a variety of antigens. These responses have some features of the primary response in adult sheep and involve the recruitment of cells into the challenged node and the subsequent proliferation and differentiation of lymphocytes into blast cells and their appearance in the lymph (FIGURE 4). The lymph node enlarges and becomes filled with a population of blast cells and occasional plasma cells. However, in most of these

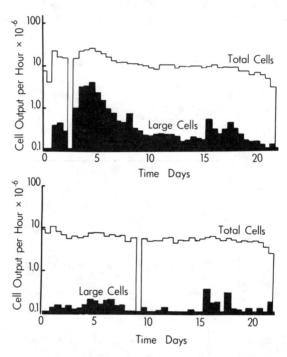

FIGURE 4. The output of cells from the prescapular lymph nodes of a fetal lamb. The right and left efferent prescapular lymph ducts were cannulated at 132 days gestation and lymph was collected continuously. The lamb was born alive with both fistulas intact and flowing at 154 days gestation, 22 days after cannulation. (Top) Right node challenged with killed *Brucella abortus* organisms injected subcutaneously at time of cannulation. (Bottom) Left node not challenged.

authentic primary responses there is little evidence of specific antibody formation or of the appearance of specific antibody-forming cells in the lymph.

Cell proliferation is the most characteristic aspect of these primary responses and in terms of the clonal selection theory, this proliferative response would be interpreted as the process whereby those antigen-sensitive cells carrying the specific cell surface determinants for the particular antigen have been stimulated to proliferate so as to establish the cellular basis for a secondary response in which specific antibody synthesis would be a dominating feature. In fact, many cells in the fetus, other than Ig-positive lymphocytes, are stimulated to proliferate and the primary response is not just confined to the expansion of specific clones of B cells.

Fetal lymph nodes challenged with antigen at around 65 days and removed at around 80 days contain large numbers of blast cells in which the endoplasmic reticulum is poorly developed (FIGURE 5A and B). However, a few cells can be found in the nodes which have the ultrastructural characteristics of plasma cells (FIGURE 5C). It is almost certain that, in response to the antigenic challenge, these cells are synthesizing and secreting some form of immunoglobulin molecule. This immunoglobulin has no specificity for the stimulating antigen in terms of the immunological assays used.

THE ACQUISITION OF IMMUNOLOGICAL COMPETENCE IN THE FETAL LAMB

Although antibody formation is not a distinguishing feature of most primary responses in fetal lymph nodes to many antigens, fetal lambs are able to produce specific humoral antibody responses quite early in development.[14-16] This capability can be demonstrated to be present at a time when the lymphoid apparatus is quite poorly developed and histologically immature.[17, 18] Polymeric and monomeric flagellin injected intramuscularly into the fetus at 70 days gestation gives rise to specific IgM antibody in the blood within 14 days[19] and fetuses infected with Akabane virus have specific neutralizing antibodies in their blood at around 80 days gestation.[20] Fetuses of 90 days gestation produce systemic titers of both specific mercaptoethanol (ME)-sensitive and ME-resistant antibodies to a variety of antigens.[16]

Fetal lambs younger than 60 days gestation do not produce specific antibody following antigenic challenge although antigens injected before 60 days can be shown to have effects on the immune system. In this regard fetuses of 55 days gestation given a primary challenge with polymerized flagellin produce no specific antibody, but when they are challenged a second time at around 70 days, they produce both IgM and IgG specific antibodies some 10 days earlier than fetuses of the same age given only a primary challenge.[19]

The probability of a fetal lamb producing specific antibody to antigens such as ferritin, chick red blood cells, polymerized flagellin, monomeric flagellin, chicken gamma globulin, and ovalbumin increases from 60 days gestation onward.[16] Most fetuses injected with these antigens in Freund's adjuvant between 66 and 75 days gestation produce specific antibody within 14 days of challenge. When antigens are given without adjuvant, antibody responses are significantly weaker and occur later. Some fetuses are able to give a weak antibody response around 75 days to the soluble antigen ovalbumin given in Freund's adjuvant although it is not until they reach 100 days gestation that specific antibody is produced regularly.

There are some antigens, such as the somatic antigens of salmonella organisms, that evoke no specific antibody production in fetal sheep of any age. These antigens do, however, cause a proliferative cellular response in fetal lymph nodes with the formation of plasma cells and nonspecific IgM immunoglobulins.

The capacity of fetuses to synthesize specific antibody increases throughout gestation and the humoral responses of older fetuses are qualitatively and quantitatively different from the first responses elicited in 65- to 70-day-old fetuses. The first specific antibody produced by fetuses around 65-70 days is IgM and not until later than 90 days gestation is the fetal lamb able to produce IgG_1 specific antibody in response to

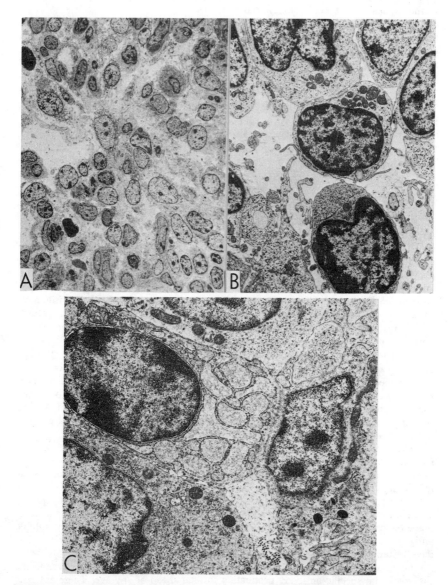

FIGURE 5. Sections through the popliteal lymph node of a fetal lamb of 85 days gestation challenged with 100 μg polymerized flagellin 15 days previously. (A and B) Blast cells in the cortex of the node. (C) A plasma cell with dilated ergastoplasm. (Original magnifications: (A) ×1000, (B) ×4500, (C) ×14,000; each has been reduced to 78% of original size.) Courtesy of Mr. M. Al Salami.

a primary challenge. IgG_2 and IgA antibodies are produced only in trace amounts, if at all, by the fetal lamb. The maximum titers of specific antibody reached and the total amount of antibody produced are much greater in older fetuses (TABLE 1).

There are thus several features of the immune response in the fetal lamb that can be dissociated within a time frame of development that allows their separate study. The capacity to recognize and phagocytose foreign materials develops as early as 24 days gestation, 40-50 days before the fetus is able to synthesize antibodies. This defense system is caducous and the free-floating macrophages have largely gone from the blood by the time the lamb is born. After birth these cells are relegated to the tissues and to the peripheral lymph where they function throughout life as a phylogenetic relic of the first primitive, defense mechanism.

The appearance of lymphocytes in the circulation at around 40 days gestation precedes the establishment of humoral and cell-mediated immune responses by some 30 days. The mature pattern of lymphocyte recirculation between the blood and lymph is not present at this time as it must await the development of the various lymphoid

TABLE 1. Passive Hemagglutinating Antibody Titers (Log_2) in Fetal Sheep of Different Ages[a]

Age of Fetus (days)	Days after Challenge													
	2		4		6		8		10		12		14	
	T	M	T	M	T	M	T	M	T	M	T	M	T	M
70	0	0	4.0	0	5.2	0	5.0	0	5.6	0	4.4	0	4.0	0
82	0	0	7.0	0	7.1	0	7.1	0	6.1	0	5.6	0	4.2	0
99	0	0	4.6	0	8.0	0	7.6	0	7.0	0	6.0	0	4.8	0
119	0	0	6.4	0	9.6	3.0	10.6	4.6	10.4	4.6	8.6	1.6	8.0	1.8

[a] The fetuses were injected with 100 μg of polymerized flagellin. T = Total antibody. M = 2-mercaptoethanol-resistant antibody. (See Reference 19.)

organs through which this cell traffic is directed. The lymph nodes, Peyer's patches, and spleen are not organized structurally for some weeks after lymphocytes first appear and the comprehensive migration of lymphocytes does not occur in the fetal lamb until the second half of gestation. The recirculation of lymphocytes is clearly not conditional on any interactions with antigen and is not crucial for the development of immunological competence.[2]

The response of an authentic primary encounter of the lymphoid system with antigen results much more obviously in the proliferation of cells than in the production of specific antibody. Many cells in the fetus that are stimulated primarily by antigen are T cells and it remains an open question as to whether or not these are responding in any specific way to the antigen.

The maturation of the immune response in the fetal lamb could reflect the role of an evolving population of regulatory T cells which act both in the inductive and reductive phases of the immune response. Just how these cells exert control over the proliferation and differentiation of antigen-specific B cells is not known but it seems certain that they must do so through the production of regulatory factors which would not be detected in conventional experimental systems and which play an unknown role in the development and regulation of the immune response. The fetal lamb provides a novel experimental model in which to study these phenomena.

ACKNOWLEDGMENTS

We thank Dr. K. J. Fahey, Dr. J. Reynolds, and Mr. M. Al Salami for allowing us to report some of their experimental results in this paper.

REFERENCES

1. COLE, G. J. & B. MORRIS. 1971. The growth and development of lambs thymectomized *in utero.* Aust. J. Exp. Biol. Med. Sci. **49:** 33.
2. PEARSON, L. D., M. W. SIMPSON-MORGAN & B. MORRIS. 1976. Lymphopoiesis and lymphocyte recirculation in the sheep fetus. J. Exp. Med. **143:** 167.
3. REYNOLDS, J. D. 1976. The Development and Physiology of the Gut-Associated Lymphoid System in Lambs. Ph.D. Thesis. Australian National University. Canberra, Australia.
4. GERBER, H. A., W. TREVELLA & B. MORRIS. 1985. The role of gut-associated lymphoid tissues in the generation of immunoglobulin-bearing lymphocytes in sheep. *In* Proceedings of a symposium held at Basel Institute of Immunology (Switzerland, November 1984). In press.
5. BINNS, R. M. & D. B. A. SYMONS. 1974. Ontogeny of immunoglobulin positive blood lymphocytes in foetal sheep. J. Int. Res. Commun. **2:** 1324.
6. GERBER, H. A. 1979. Functional Studies in Gut-Associated Lymphoid Tissues. Ph.D. Thesis. Australian National University. Canberra, Australia.
7. CAHILL, R. N. P., I. HERON, D. C. POSKITT & Z. TRNKA. 1980. *In* Blood Cells and Vessel Walls: Functional Interactions. Ciba Foundation Symposium 71, p. 145. Excerpta Medica. Amsterdam, the Netherlands.
8. SCOLLAY, R. G., J. HOPKINS & J. G. HALL. 1976. Possible role of surface Ig in non-random recirculation of small lymphocytes. Nature (London) **260:** 582.
9. CAHILL, R. N. P., D. C. POSKITT, H. FROST & Z. TRNKA. 1977. Two distinct pools of recirculating T lymphocytes: migratory characteristics of nodal and intestinal T lymphocytes. J. Exp. Med. **145:** 420.
10. HALL, J. G. & B. MORRIS. 1963. The lymph-borne cells of the immune response. Q. J. Exp. Physiol. Cogn. Med. Sci. **48:** 235.
11. SMEATON, T. C., G. J. COLE, M. W. SIMPSON-MORGAN & B. MORRIS. 1969. Techniques for the long-term collection of lymph from the unanaesthetized foetal lamb *in utero.* Aust. J. Exp. Biol. Med. Sci. **47:** 565.
12. CAHILL, R. N. P., D. C. POSKITT, I. HERON & Z. TRNKA. 1979. The collection of lymph from single lymph nodes and the intestines of fetal lambs *in utero.* Int. Arch. Allergy Appl. Immunol. **59:** 117.
13. SIMPSON-MORGAN, M. W., W. TREVELLA, A. R. HUGH, S. J. McCLURE & B. MORRIS. 1985. The long-term collection of lymph from single lymph nodes of foetal lambs *in utero.* Aust. J. Exp. Biol. Med. Sci. In press.
14. SILVERSTEIN, A. M. & R. J. LUKES. 1962. Fetal response to antigenic stimulus. I. Plasma cellular and lymphoid reactions in the human fetus to intrauterine infection. Lab. Invest. **11:** 918.
15. SILVERSTEIN, A. M., J. W. UHR, K. L. KRANER & R. J. LUKES. 1963. Foetal response to antigenic stimulus. II. Antibody production by the foetal lamb. J. Exp. Med. **117:** 799.

16. FAHEY, K. J. & B. MORRIS. 1978. Humoral immune responses in foetal sheep. Immunology **35:** 651.
17. SILVERSTEIN, A. M. & R. A. PRENDERGAST. 1970. Lymphogenesis, immunogenesis and the generation of immunological diversity. *In* Developmental Aspects of Antibody Formation and Structure. J. Sterzl & I. Riha, Eds.: 69. Academia. Prague, Czechoslovakia.
18. FAHEY, K. J. & B. MORRIS. 1974. Lymphopoiesis and immune reactivity in the foetal lamb. Ser. Haematol. **7:** 548.
19. FAHEY, K. J. 1976. Humoral Immune Responses in Foetal Sheep. Ph.D. Thesis. Australian National University. Canberra, Australia.
20. McCLURE, S. 1983. Personal communication.

Thymic Lymphopoiesis: Protected from, or Influenced by, External Stimulation?[a]

MAX W. HESS,[b] CHRISTOPH MUELLER,[b]
THOMAS SCHAFFNER,[b] HEINZ A. GERBER,[b]
PETER EGGLI,[c] AND HANS COTTIER[b]

[b]Institute of Pathology
[c]Institute of Anatomy
University of Bern
Bern, Switzerland

INTRODUCTION

Both generation and maturation of T lymphocytes in the thymus are generally considered to proceed in the absence of peripheral antigenic experience. Yet, production of differentiated T cells is apparently guided by peripheral demand. Mechanisms regulating thymic lymphopoiesis are still a matter of debate. Intracortical differentiation of thymocytes is thought to be controlled by locally produced humoral factors and/or by close contact with epithelial, possibly also phagocytic, cells and to be restricted by products of the major histocompatibility complex. Parenterally introduced antigens fail to induce histological changes in the thymus cortex that can be compared to the changes elicited in peripheral lymphoid organs.

The absence in the thymic cortex of an obvious and marked immune reaction to antigens—given most often by the intravenous route—has been attributed to both the immaturity of cortical thymocytes[1-3] and a barrier exclusion of antigenic material. The existence of an efficient, though not absolute, blood-thymus barrier at the level of cortical capillaries has been confirmed for a variety of macromolecules and small particulates: upon introduction by the intravenous route, minute amounts of these materials were observed to be confined to perivascular macrophages.[5] In view of the fact that other routes of entry of macromolecules and particles into the thymic cortex have rarely been considered, and taking into account the importance macrophage-

[a]Supported by Swiss National Science Foundation Grant 3.141.81.

processed materials may have on thymocyte proliferation and differentiation,[6] we addressed ourselves to the following problems:

(1) Light microscopic studies showed that the thymic cortex of mice was accessible to colloidal carbon injected into the peritoneal cavity which, among others, is drained by lymphatics leading to parathymic lymph nodes.[7] We, therefore, attempted to define the pathways of this translocation of particles from the abdominal cavity into the cortical parenchyma of the thymus by the use of transmission electron microscopy.

(2) While studying the kinetic responses of cortical thymocytes in aging mice to peripheral antigenic stimulation, we found a distinct peak in proliferative activity of thymic lymphocytes in the outermost cortex at 14 days after primary, but not after secondary, injection of tetanus toxoid in the hind leg footpads.[8] This apparent thymic response to peripheral stimulation prompted us to investigate whether or not this reaction might be different in cortical areas close to, and distant from, parathymic lymph nodes, a possible source of potentially stimulating material.

ACCESSIBILITY OF CORTICAL THYMOCYTES TO PARTICULATES INTRODUCED INTO THE PERITONEAL CAVITY

Balb/c mice, at the age of 2 months, were each given an intraperitoneal (i.p.) or intravenous (i.v.) injection of Percoll particles (Pharmacia); each particle consists of an electron-dense silica core with a polyvinylpyrrolidone (PVP) coat and measures from 20 to 30 nm in diameter. The thymus and perithymic tissue were removed in one block, fixed in cacodylate-buffered glutaraldehyde, and processed for electron microscopy (for details see Reference 9).

In less than 2 hr a small portion of the i.p.-injected particles reached the lymphatics surrounding the thymus and, floating free in interstitial fluid, traversed the thymic capsule (FIGURE 1A). In the outer parenchyma of the cortex considerable numbers of thymocytes were seen with endocytosed particles (FIGURE 1B), while larger clusters of Percoll were identified within cytoplasmic vesicles of macrophages located alongside cortical capillaries (FIGURE 1C).

Following injection of Percoll by the i.v. route, particles could only be found within perivascular macrophages, but were never present in intercellular spaces or in the cytoplasm of lymphocytes of the thymic cortex.

The rapid translocation via lymphatics of particulate matter from the peritoneal cavity to the mediastinum and to parathymic lymph nodes was reported years ago.[10] Transport along this route appears to be facilitated by the combined effect of respiration and a valvular function at the level of the diaphragm. The bulk of i.p.-injected particles reached the bloodstream as demonstrated by the very early appearance of Percoll within the lumen of thymic and extrathymic capillaries. The most important result of our study was the observation that small amounts of the injected material attained a network of lymphatics surrounding the thymic capsule and from there passed into the cortical parenchyma. The relative ease with which Percoll particles reached the intercellular spaces of the lymphoid thymic cortex may be taken as strong evidence in favor of an incomplete blocking function of the thymic capsule as compared to the much more efficient blood-thymus barrier.

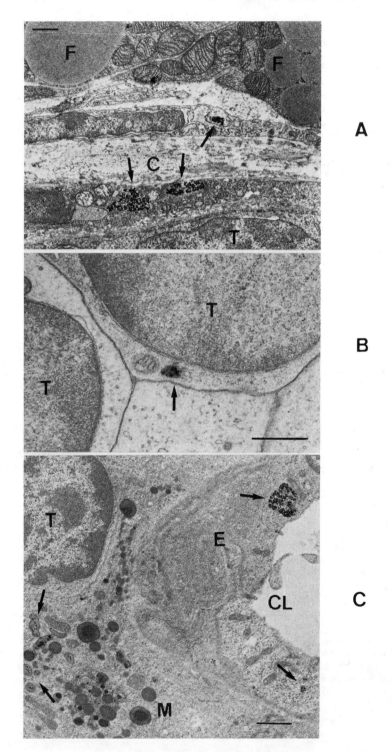

THE PROLIFERATIVE RESPONSE OF CORTICAL THYMOCYTES FOLLOWING PERIPHERAL STIMULATION IN RELATION TO NEIGHBORING PARATHYMIC LYMPH NODES

Swiss albino mice, 4 weeks old, were stimulated by an i.p. injection of aluminum phosphate-adsorbed tetanus toxoid; controls received an equivalent dose of aluminum phosphate only. The animals received an i.v. injection of 1.0 μCi/g body weight of [^{3}H]deoxycytidine (Amersham) 1 hr before being killed at from 6 hr to 21 days after stimulation. Thymus and parathymic lymph nodes were fixed in buffered 4% Formalin, embedded in methacrylate, and sectioned so that the anatomical relationship between the two types of tissues was maintained. Histological sections were processed for radioautography and evaluated as described earlier.[8]

The results clearly demonstrate a significantly increased proliferative activity of cortical thymocytes in the areas close to the draining parathymic lymph nodes as compared to those at opposite sides of the lobes. This difference was most pronounced in the outermost cortical zone at between 1 and 3 weeks after i.p. stimulation (FIGURE 2). A marked decrease in cellularity was noted within 24 hr after stimulation, again most marked in the subcapsular zone of the cortex, but evident both in the vicinity of and at a distance from parathymic lymph nodes (FIGURE 3), and manifesting itself in deeper cortical zones with a delay of 1 day.

It is noteworthy that control values obtained in lymph node-adjacent areas of animals injected with aluminum phosphate only were generally higher at the end of the observation period. This indicates that the observed changes are not, or not only, to be attributed to antigenic stimulation, but that penetrating particles as such might exert direct or indirect influence on thymocyte production.

CONCLUSIONS

A comparison of findings after i.p. and i.v. injection of Percoll demonstrates that the blood-thymus barrier is much more efficient than the "lymph-capsule" barrier of the thymus. This conclusion pertains also to capillaries in the subcapsular area of the thymic cortex which have been shown to possess fenestrated endothelia.[5] The question of whether or not some Percoll particles might have been carried to the thymic cortex by immigrating macrophages has not been addressed by the present studies.

The possible immunological implications of the finding of a "leaky" lymph-capsule barrier of the thymus are difficult to assess. The observed stimulatory effect of i.p.-injected particulates on the proliferative activity of cortical thymocytes in the vicinity of draining parathymic lymph nodes corroborates and partly explains the results of earlier studies, e.g., the induction of thymic cortical hyperplasia following the i.p.

FIGURE 1. Thymic cortex of mice following the injection of Percoll particles (transmission electron microscopy). (A) Percoll particles (arrows) within the thymic capsule, C, 2 hr after i.p. injection. F: perithymic fat cells; T: subcapsular thymocyte. (B) A subcapsular thymocyte, T, exhibits interiorized particles within a lysosome (arrow) at 4 hr after i.p. injection. (C) At 24 hr after i.p. injection of Percoll, particles (arrows) are almost exclusively found in the walls of cortical capillaries (CL: capillary lumen; E: endothelium) and in perivascular macrophages, M. This pattern of particle distribution is identical to the one observed after i.v. injection. (Scale bars = 1 μm.)

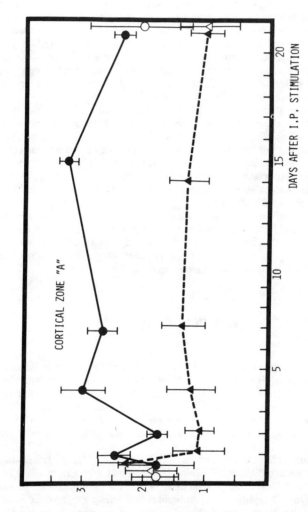

FIGURE 2. Absolute numbers of labeled thymocytes in the outermost cortical zone (zone "A") of thymic sections 1 hr after i.v. injection of [³H]deoxycytidine, and as a function of both time after i.p. stimulation with aluminum phosphate-adsorbed tetanus toxoid and location with regard to parathymic lymph nodes (for legend see FIGURE 3).

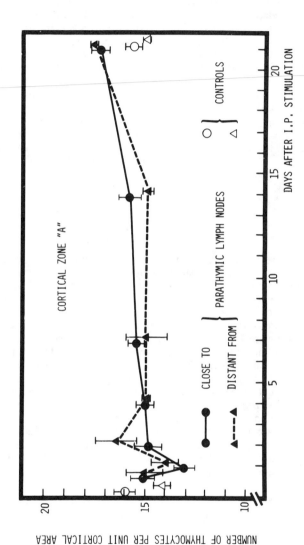

FIGURE 3. Cell density of the outermost thymic cortical zone (zone "A") as a function of both time after i.p. stimulation with aluminum phosphate-adsorbed tetanus toxoid and location with regard to parathymic lymph nodes.

injection of a *Viscum album* preparation,[11] a proliferative response of cortical thymocytes following stimulation with *Bacillus Calmette-Guérin* (BCG),[12] ovalbumin,[13] or oxazolone,[14] and the massive emigration of thymic lymphocytes 12 hr after phytohemagglutinin (PHA) given by the i.p. route.[15] Since the serosal surface of the peritoneal cavity represents one of the largest resorptive areas of the body, considerable amounts of blood plasma constituents, including agents with the potential to affect lymphocyte kinetics, continuously pass from the blood into this extravascular compartment and eventually reach the parathymic lymph nodes. Details of how and to what extent this constant exposure to minute quantities of materials from the peritoneal cavity, under physiological conditions, directly or indirectly influences proliferation, differentiation, and migration of cortical thymocytes are unknown. One might imagine that an indirect influence might be exerted by mediators (e.g., interleukins) produced in parathymic lymph nodes. Although the consequences of endocytosis of i.p.-injected particles by thymic lymphocytes in the outermost cortex remain unclear, this observation may be indicative of a more direct effect. In any event, the sum of available data appears to indicate that peripheral stimulation, especially via the peritoneal cavity, might play a role in the overall process of differentiation within the thymic cortex.

SUMMARY

The mechanisms regulating thymic lymphopoiesis are still a matter of debate. Intracortical proliferation and differentiation of thymocytes are thought to be controlled by locally produced humoral factors and close contact with epithelial, possibly also phagocytic, cells, and restricted by products of the major histocompatibility complex. The observation of a translocation of intraabdominally introduced PVP-coated silica particles (Percoll) via parathymic lymph vessels and through the thymic capsule into the cortical parenchyma demonstrates that the thymic cortex is accessible to materials carried with the transcapsular flux of interstitial fluid, and that this barrier is less effective than the blood-thymus barrier. The proliferative activity of cortical thymocytes following an intraabdominal injection of particulate tetanus toxoid was compared in sites adjacent to, and distant from, parathymic lymph nodes. Absolute numbers of DNA-synthesizing thymocytes were found to be much higher in cortical areas close to the lymph nodes, where lymphatic vessels are most numerous, than on the opposite sides of the thymic lobes. Taken together, these findings indicate that—in addition to intrinsic control mechanisms—cortical thymocyte production may be influenced by peripheral stimulation to some extent, and that materials from sites which are drained by parathymic lymph nodes may be important in this respect.

REFERENCES

1. RAFF, M. C. 1973. T and B lymphocytes and immune responses. Nature **242**: 19.
2. WAGNER, H., C. HARDT, R. BARTLETT, M. ROELLINGHOFF & K. PFIZENMAIER. 1980. Intrathymic differentiation of cytotoxic T lymphocyte (CTL) precursors. I. The CTL immunocompetence of peanut-agglutinin positive (cortical) and negative (medullary) Lyt 123 thymocytes. J. Immunol. **125**: 2532.
3. CEREDIG, R., H. R. MacDONALD & E. J. JENKINSON. 1983. Flow microfluorometric analysis of mouse thymus development in vivo and in vitro. Eur. J. Immunol. **13**: 185.

4. MARSHALL, A. H. E. & R. G. WHITE. 1961. The immunological reactivity of the thymus. Br. J. Exp. Pathol. **42:** 379.
5. RAVIOLA, E. & M. J. KARNOVSKY. 1972. Evidence for a blood-thymus barrier using electron-opaque tracers. J. Exp. Med. **136:** 466.
6. UNANUE, E. R. 1981. The regulatory role of macrophages in antigenic stimulation. Part Two: Symbiotic relationship between lymphocytes and macrophages. Adv. Immunol. **31:** 1.
7. LAENG, H., C. W. KIM, M. W. HESS & H. COTTIER. 1978. Hinweise auf eine Zugaenglichkeit der Thymusrinde fuer partikulaeres Material und deren moegliche Bedeutung. Schweiz. Med. Wochenschr. **108:** 467.
8. LUSCIETI, P., P. GRAFF, M. LEUTHI, H. COTTIER, M. W. HESS, R. KRAFT & R. D. STONER. 1983. Distinct kinetic responses in vivo of cortical thymocytes of ageing mice to primary as compared to secondary peripheral antigenic stimulation. Clin. Exp. Immunol. **52:** 455.
9. EGGLI, P., TH. SCHAFFNER, H. A. GERBER, M. W. HESS & H. COTTIER. 1983. Thymic cortical lymphocytes are accessible to particles injected into the peritoneal cavity. In preparation.
10. TILNEY, N. L. 1971. Patterns of lymphatic drainage in the adult laboratory rat. J. Anat. **109:** 369.
11. RENTEA, R., E. LYON & R. HUNTER. 1981. Biologic properties of Iscador: a *Viscum album* preparation. I. Hyperplasia of the thymic cortex and accelerated regeneration of hematopoietic cells following X-irradiation. Lab. Invest. **44:** 43.
12. KHALIL, A., H. RAPPAPORT, D. DANTCHEV, I. FLORENTIN & C. BOURUT. 1976. The effects of certain immunity system adjuvants, PHA, and human gammaglobulin on the thymic cortex of mice: a light and electron microscope study. Biomedicine **25:** 396.
13. DURKIN, H. G., J. M. CARBONI & B. H. WAKSMAN. 1978. Antigen-induced increase in migration of large cortical thymocytes (regulatory cells?) to the marginal zone and red pulp of the spleen. J. Immunol. **121:** 1075.
14. MYKING, A. O. 1979. Responses of the thymus and the paracortex of draining lymph nodes to repeated applications of oxazolone to mouse skin. Virchows Arch. B Cell. Pathol. **32:** 11.
15. BRYANT, B. J., M. W. HESS & H. COTTIER. 1975. Thymus lymphocytes. Efflux and restoration phases after peripheral exposure of mice to phytohaemagglutinin. Immunology **29:** 115.

Induction of Allogeneic Unresponsiveness in Adult Dogs by Irradiation and Bone Marrow Transplantation: Implication of Ia-Positive Bone Marrow Stem Cells[a]

FELIX T. RAPAPORT, RADOSLAV J. BACHVAROFF,
HIDEO ASARI, KOSHI SATO, ARJUN D. CHANANA,[b]
DARRELL D. JOEL,[b] AND EUGENE P. CRONKITE[b]

Transplantation Service
Department of Surgery
School of Medicine
Health Sciences Center
State University of New York at Stony Brook
Stony Brook, New York 11794

[b]Medical Department
Brookhaven National Laboratories
Upton, New York 11973

Alter and her associates,[1] Haot et al.,[2] and a number of other investigators have suggested in recent years that placement of hemopoietic cells into an irradiated host milieu may trigger such cells to undergo a transient cycle of replication and differentiation which recapitulates the events of immunological ontogeny—including fetal erythropoiesis, production of newborn γ-chains in adults, and generation of fetal and newborn-type lymphoid cells. In an extension of this hypothesis to transplantation, supralethally irradiated dogs were reconstituted with their own stored marrow, followed within 12 to 18 hr by the transplantation of a kidney allograft obtained from a DLA identical donor. This sequence resulted in long-term unresponsiveness to the transplanted kidneys in the recipients without further treatment.[3-5] The 60% incidence of success obtained with this procedure could be improved further if the host's own stored marrow was treated *in vitro* with methylprednisolone (MPd) prior to replacement of the marrow following irradiation.[6-8]

In an attempt to analyze the possible changes in the cellular composition of marrow that might have been associated with this result, a serial cytofluorographic analysis

[a]Supported by Grant AI 14453-07 from the National Institutes of Health, Bethesda, Md.

of marrow before and after treatment with MPd was performed. For this purpose, cell samples obtained before and after exposure of bone marrow to MPd were studied in an Ortho 50H Cell Sorter after staining with acridine orange by using green fluorescence for DNA and red fluorescence for RNA, or, alternatively, using 90° scatter for the X axis and a narrow forward scatter for the Y axis, without addition of any stain.[6-8]

The components of normal bone marrow obtained from untreated dogs were separated by flow cytometry into six main clusters, including three central clusters of predominantly myeloid cells at various stages of differentiation (including 85% of the sorted cells); a smaller cluster on the left, composed mainly of normoblasts and small lymphocytes and their precursors (10-12% of the sorted cells); and two clusters of more central cells, mainly located below and to the left of the myeloid cell mass (3-5% of the sorted cells), which were comprised largely of cells of the leukocyte series, corresponding in size and shape to monocytoid cells and/or their precursors. Exposure of marrow to MPd *in vitro* results in the elimination of the clusters of monocytoid-like cells.[6-8] In further study of this observation, whole bone marrow samples were purified by treatment with carbonyl iron and adenosine diphosphate (ADP), followed by Ficoll-Isopaque flotation. The resulting cell suspension was then analyzed by flow cytometry, yielding a predominantly monocytoid cell cluster (Population I) and a large cluster of myeloid cells at various stages of development (Population II). Exposure of this purified cell population to MPd *in vitro* again eliminated Population I cells, with no detectable effect upon Population II.

Further studies were then performed on the relative distribution of Population I and II cells in canine marrow, with particular regard to their location within the intraosseous marrow cavity of the host's long bones. For this purpose, four normal dogs were exsanguinated and the iliac arteries were cannulated bilaterally. The lower extremities were then perfused with normal saline solution until the venous effluent was cleared of erythrocytes. The animals were then sacrificed; each long bone was split longitudinally and the marrow cavities were exposed. At that time, the cavities were lined with a loosely adherent brownish-red pulp which was removed, minced, and filtered. The resulting suspension of marrow cells was then exposed, purified by the carbonyl iron-ADP-Ficoll-Hypaque flotation method, and the resulting suspension was once again analyzed by flow cytometry. The results indicated that the process of flushing out the marrow cavity of its loosely adherent (or unattached) cellular components left a cell population in the remaining adherent marrow interstitium that consisted predominantly (i.e., up to 70%) of *Population I* cells, while the concentration of *Population II* cells in this preparation was decreased to about 30% (from 85% in the whole marrow aspirates). Aliquots of Population I cells prepared in this fashion were then incubated in plastic tissue culture dishes containing fetal calf serum, and the nonadherent cells were washed off with balanced salt solution (BSS). The adherent cells were detached by adding lidocaine to each dish, and then analyzed once again in the cell sorter. It is of particular interest that this plastic-adherent cell population consisted almost exclusively (99%) of *Population II* cells, while the nonadherent or poorly adherent cells were almost exclusively Population I (i.e., monocytoid-like) cells.

The next series of studies was concerned with testing some of the cell surface properties of the cells isolated by these techniques. For this purpose, bone marrow aspirates were tested with a battery of murine monoclonal antibodies directed against distinctive human lymphocyte surface determinants. These reagents (Ortho Labs.) are currently in widespread use for the identification of various human lymphocyte and monocyte subpopulations. The monoclonal antibody OKIa-1, in particular, has been used recently in this laboratory[6-8] and by Iwaki *et al.*[9] for studies of canine monocytes, because of an apparent cross-reactivity between human and canine Ia core antigen(s).

Other antibodies used included OKT3 (for prepared T lymphocytes); OKT4 (for inducer/helper T lymphocytes); OKT6 (for thymocytes); OKT8 (for suppressor/cytotoxic T lymphocytes); and OKM1 (for some monocytes and null cells). These reagents were used with a standard fluorescein-labeled rabbit anti-mouse globulin as the indicator system.

Tests with the OKIa-1 reagent indicated that 19% of all canine whole marrow aspirate cells are Ia positive—a finding that is in agreement with similar observations by Iwaki et al.[9] The rabbit anti-mouse IgG alone only stained a minimal number of cells (<2%). Following study of complete bone marrow aspirates, the cell *Populations I and II* were separated, and each was tested with the anti-Ia antibody. While almost 50% of the cells in Population I were Ia positive, only 5.9% of the cells in Population II were Ia positive, with a control uptake of rabbit anti-mouse IgG of 3%, demonstrating that virtually all Ia-positive cells occurring in this marrow sample were in Population I.

In summary, the development of allogeneic unresponsiveness following total-body irradiation and reconstitution with autologous marrow appears to be associated with the elimination from the marrow of a cell population(s) which is Ia positive, non-phagocytic, and poorly adherent to plastic and glass surfaces. Such cells are closely associated with the reticular matrix of intraosseous bone marrow. They have been found to be negative to histochemical staining for neutral esterase, acid phosphatase, and peroxidase. The cells are susceptible to the action of corticosteroids, and are IgG and IgM negative. The cells also do not appear to bear any detectable surface characteristics of lymphocytes.

Taken together, these results suggest a striking resemblance between the properties of Population I monocytoid cells isolated in this study and those of cells of the dendritic series.[10-13] This raises the possibility that the bone marrow interstitial cells described in this report may include a highly enriched population of bone marrow precursors of the dendritic cell series at various stages of differentiation. Such a possibility is in keeping with the key role which has been ascribed to dendritic cells in the modulation of transplantation reactions. It is also in harmony with the demonstrated origin of dendritic cells from radiosensitive, as yet unidentified, bone marrow precursors.[14-16] The occurrence of high concentrations of this kind of Ia-positive cells in the intraosseous interstitial matrix of bone marrow may also be of interest in view of the special role which has been ascribed to the bone marrow microenvironment as a key determinant of the host's immunological reactivity after irradiation and reconstitution with allogeneic or autologous marrow.[12-21]

REFERENCES

1. ALTER, B. P., J. M. RAPPEPORT & T. H. J. HUISMAN. 1976. Blood **48**: 843-853.
2. HAOT, J., E. H. BETZ & L. J. SIMAR. 1974. Acta Haematol. (Basal) **51**: 170-178.
3. RAPAPORT, F. T., D. B. AMOS, R. J. BACHVAROFF, K. WATANABE, H. HIRASAWA, F. D. CANNON, N. MOLLEN, D. A. BLUMENSTOCK & J. W. FERREBEE. 1978. J. Clin. Invest. **61**: 790-800.
4. RAPAPORT, F. T., R. J. BACHVAROFF, K. DICKE & G. SANTOS. 1979. Transplant. Proc. **11**: 1028-1031.
5. RAPAPORT, F. T., R. J. BACHVAROFF, N. MOLLEN, H. HIRASAWA, T. ASANO & J. W. FERREBEE. 1979. Ann. Surg. **190**: 461-473.
6. RAPAPORT, F. T., R. J. BACHVAROFF, T. SATO, H. ASARI, A. D. CHANANA & E. P. CRONKITE. 1982. Immunological reconstitution of irradiated recipients with autologous

marrow. *In* Regulation of the Immune Response (Proceedings, 8th International Convocation on Immunology, Amherst, New York, 1982). P. L. Ogra & D. M. Jacobs, Eds.: 350-359. S. Karger. Basel, Switzerland.
7. RAPAPORT, F. T., R. J. BACHVAROFF, T. SATO, H. ASARI, A. D. CHANANA & E. P. CRONKITE. 1983. Transplant. Proc. **15:** 326-329.
8. ANAISE, D., H. ATKINS, H. ASARI, Z. OSTER, W. WALTZER, R. J. BACHVAROFF & F. T. RAPAPORT. 1983. Fed. Proc. **42:** 1088.
9. IWAKI, Y., P. I. TERASAKI, T. KINUKAWA, T. H. THAI, T. ROOT & R. BILLING. 1983. Transplantation **36:** 189-191.
10. STEINMAN, R. M. & Z. A. COHN. 1973. J. Exp. Med. **137:** 1142-1162.
11. STEINMAN, R. M., G. KAPLAN, M. D. WITMER & Z. A. COHN. 1979. J. Exp. Med. **149:** 1-16.
12. STEINMAN, R. M. & M. C. NUSSENZWEIG. 1980. Immunol. Rev. **53:** 127-147.
13. STEINMAN, R. M. 1981. Transplantation **31:** 151-155.
14. STEINMAN, R. M., D. S. LUSTIG & Z. A. COHN. 1974. J. Exp. Med. **139:** 1431-1445.
15. TAMAKI, K. & S. I. KATZ. 1980. J. Invest. Dermatol. **75:** 12-13.
16. HART, D. N. J. & J. W. FABRE. 1981. J. Exp. Med. **154:** 347-361.
17. LEVEY, R. H. 1972. Transplant. Proc. **4:** 395-399.
18. LEVEY, R. H. 1973. Transplant. Proc. **5:** 893-896.
19. RAPAPORT, F. T., R. J. BACHVAROFF, K. WATANABE, F. D. CANNON, J. H. AYVAZIAN, D. BLUMENSTOCK & J. W. FERREBEE. 1975. Transplant. Proc. **7:** 472-474.
20. BACHVAROFF, R., K. WATANABE & J. W. FERREBEE. 1975. Surg. Forum **26:** 329-330.
21. RAPAPORT, F. T. 1977. New approaches to the induction of allogeneic unresponsiveness. *In* Immune Effector Mechanisms in Disease—Irwin Strasburger Memorial Seminar on Immunology. G. W. Siskind, Ed.: 67-75. Grune & Stratton, Inc. New York, N.Y.

Regulation of Granulopoiesis by T Cells and T-Cell Subsets[a]

G. CHIKKAPPA[b] AND P. G. PHILLIPS

Medical and Research Services
Veterans Administration Medical Center
Albany, New York 12208

Albany Medical College
Albany, New York 12208

There is evidence suggesting that the thymus-dependent lymphocytes (T cells)[c] modulate granulopoiesis. However, there is controversy regarding the nature of this modulation (TABLE 1). Normal human blood (PB) T cells (sheep erythrocyte receptor-positive cells) have been shown to promote the growth of autologous and allogeneic bone marrow (BM) granulocytic-macrophagic progenitors (CFC) in *in vitro* cultures in some studies[1,2] and to inhibit[3,4] or to have no effect in others.[3-5] Such variability has also been observed when T cells derived from BM have been co-cultured with autologous or allogeneic BM cells.[2,4,7] Methodological variations such as the type of target cells, day of culture analysis, and source of colony stimulating activity (CSA) may have been responsible for the observed differences.

We performed these studies to clarify the influence of the normal human PB T cells on the growth of the autologous BM CFC. Additional studies were done to determine the influence of the PB T cells and T-cell subsets on the growth of the PB CFC. Results indicated that the T cells consistently promoted the growth of the PB CFC, inhibited the d_7 BM CFC (cultures assayed on day 7) in most studies, and neither stimulated nor inhibited the d_{14} CFC (cultures assayed on day 14). The T suppressor cell, which inhibits immune functions in the classical immune system, was found to be responsible for the PB CFC growth promotion. From results of this study and of others in the literature, we speculate that the CFC are heterogeneous cells. The d_7 BM CFC are more mature and ontogenically closer to the myeloblast than

[a] Supported by the Veterans Administration.

[b] Address correspondence to: G. Chikkappa, M.D., Hematology Division, Medical Service, Veterans Administration Medical Center, Albany, N.Y. 12208.

[c] **Abbreviations:** BM = bone marrow; CFC = granulocytic-macrophagic aggregate forming cells in culture; CSA = CFC growth stimulating activity; d_7 CFC = CFC counted on culture day 7; d_{14} CFC = CFC counted on culture day 14; ECM = endothelial cell conditioned medium; GCM = giant cell conditioned medium; HPCM = human placental conditioned medium; LDBM = T-cell- and Mo-depleted light-density BM cells; Leuk-feeder = underlayer containing normal human blood leukocytes; Mo = monocyte; MoCM = Mo conditioned medium; PB = peripheral blood; PHSC = pluripotent hemopoietic stem cell; T cell = T lymphocyte; T_4 cell = T cell capable of binding with OKT$_4$ monoclonal antibody; T_8 cell = T cell capable of binding with OKT$_8$ monoclonal antibody.

TABLE 1. Review of the Reported Studies on the Influence of Lymphocytes from the Blood (PB) and Marrow (BM) on the Growth of Bone Marrow CFC[a]

Reference	Type of BM Target Cells	Day of Culture Reading	CSA Source	PB MNC	PB T	BM T	BM T_4	BM T_8
Abdou et al.[5] (1978)	Whole ?	Not given	None	↕	↕	—	—	—
Bacigalupo et al.[6] (1980)	Whole ?	10	Leuk-feeders	—	—	↕	—	—
Ascensao et al.[3] (1981)	LDBM(−T, −Mo)	8-10	ECM, leuk-feeders	—	↕	↕	—	—
Bagby[7] (1981)	LDBM(−T)	7	HPCM	—	↓	—	—	—
Spitzer & Verma[2] (1982)	LDBM(−T, −Mo)	8-14	HPCM	—	↓	↑↓	—	—
This study (1983)	LDBM(−T, −Mo)	7	HPCM, GCM, MoCM	—	↕	—	↕	↕

[a] MNC = Ficoll-Hypaque-separated light-density cells; T = sheep erythrocyte rosettable cells; T_4 = OKT_4 antibody binding cells; T_8 = OKT_8 antibody binding cells. Type of target BM cells: whole = all nucleated cells, ? = not clear, LDBM = light-density BM cells, −T = T depleted, −Mo = monocyte depleted. Leuk-feeders = normal blood leukocytes in the underlayers; HPCM = human placental conditioned medium; ECM = endothelial cell CM; GCM = giant cell CM. ↕ = neither stimulation nor inhibition; ↑ = growth promotion; ↓ = growth inhibition; — = not tested.

the d_{14} BM CFC. The PB CFC are the most immature CFC and are ontogenically closer to the pluripotent hemopoietic stem cell (PHSC). We believe that a small fraction of the BM CFC are maturationally equivalent to the PB CFC. The nature of the T-cell influence on the CFC growth seems to be determined by the maturity of the CFC. It is one of stimulation on the most immature CFC and inhibition or indifference on the more mature cell. Those delicately balanced and controlled effects of the T cells on the CFC seem to contribute to the maintenance of normal granulopoietic homeostasis.

METHODS

The blood and bone marrow samples were obtained from normal healthy subjects after obtaining informed written consent as required by the Institutional Studies Committee. Preservative-free heparin was used as an anticoagulant.

Cell Separation

The procedure was as described previously[8,9] and is summarized in FIGURE 1. Briefly, the blood and marrow samples were mixed with one and three times their volumes, respectively, with McCoy's 5A medium, layered over Lymphoprep (sp gr 1.077), and centrifuged at $400 \times g$ for 35 min. The interphase mononuclear cells (MNC) from the blood and light-density cells from the marrow samples were collected, washed twice with and suspended in McCoy's medium containing 10% (v/v) heat-treated (55°C for 30 min) fetal bovine serum. The cells were then incubated in a petri dish at 37°C for 1 hr to deplete monocytes (Mo). The free-floating cells were decanted and mixed with 2-aminoethylisothiouronium bromide (AET)-treated sheep erythrocytes (SRBC) to rosette the T cells. In some studies, the T cells were rosetted using non-AET-treated as well as AET-treated SRBC to study the comparative influences of the T cells of these two sources on BM CFC. These cells were layered over Isolymph and centrifuged at $400 \times g$ for 35 min. The interphase populations containing B cells and null cells (BNull cells) from the blood and the T-cell- and Mo-depleted light-density cells (LDBM) from the marrow samples were collected and used as CFC-enriched fractions. The pelleted T rosettes of the PB samples were collected separately. The SRBC from the T rosettes were lysed with tris-buffered ammonium chloride and the free T cells were collected. In some studies, the SRBC from the T rosettes were lysed by two separate methods, with distilled water as well as ammonium chloride, and the influences of these T cells were compared on BM CFC.

Separation of T-Cell Subsets

OKT_4 and OKT_8 monoclonal antibodies were obtained from Ortho Pharmaceutical Corporation. The OKT_4 reactive helper cells (T_4) and OKT_8 reactive suppressor

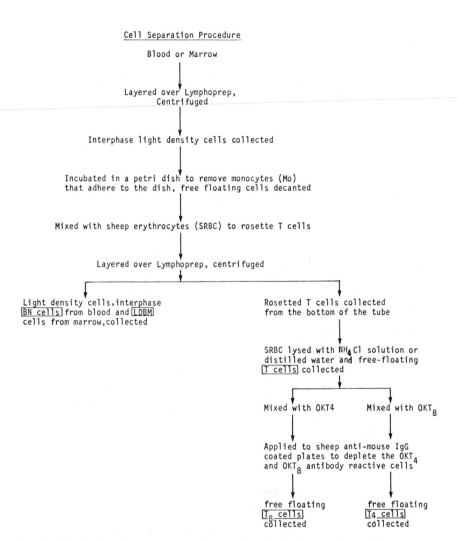

FIGURE 1. Outline of procedures used in separation of cells from peripheral blood and bone marrow. Squares indicate the cells used in culture studies. See footnote *c* for abbreviations. (Reprinted, by permission, from Reference 8.)

populations (T_8) were separated by a negative-enrichment immunoadherence "panning" method.[8,10,11]

Purity of the Cells

The purity of the various fractions was evaluated on Wright-Giemsa stained smears by counting 500 cells as well as by more specific methods. The T cells were verified by the SRBC rosetting method, Mo by their diffuse cytoplasmic staining for α-naphthylacetate esterase, and B cells by the presence of surface immunoglobulin.[12,13] The T_4 and T_8 populations were recognized by their capacity to react with OKT_4 and OKT_8 monoclonal antibodies, using an immunofluorescent technique.[8]

CFC Assay

The CFC culture procedure was as described previously.[9] The cells to be cultured and co-cultured were mixed in 0.3% agar gel in a nutrient medium. The agar medium-cell suspension was pipetted in volumes of 1 ml into 30 × 10-mm petri dishes containing GCM (giant cell conditioned medium, GIBCO), human placental conditioned medium (HPCM), or Mo conditioned medium (MoCM) as a source of colony stimulating activity. For a given study, however, a constant volume of a source of CSA was used for all culture dishes. The dishes were incubated at 37°C with 5% CO_2 flow in a maximally humidified atmosphere. Unless stated otherwise the PB cultures were analyzed at day 14 and the BM cultures at day 7-8.

At the time of harvesting, the agar gel disks were mounted on microscope slides and stained by hematoxylin for overall CFC growth evaluation or with the triple-stain technique for simultaneous analysis of neutrophilic, eosinophilic, and macrophagic growth.[14] With the triple-stain technique, chloracetate esterase-positive cells were recognized as neutrophils, α-naphthylacetate esterase-positive cells as macrophages, and luxol-fast blue-positive cells as eosinophils. Aggregates with less than eight cells were not counted.

Source of Colony Stimulating Factor Activity

The HPCM and MoCM were prepared as described elsewhere.[9]

RESULTS

The purity of the cells used in cultures is shown in TABLE 2. The BNull, T, T_4, and T_8 cells were minimally contaminated with neutrophilic and eosinophilic cells.

TABLE 2. Purity of the Cells Used in Cultures[a]

	% Cells, on Wright-Giemsa Smears				% Cells, by Special Studies				
	Lymph	M_{1-4}	M_{5-7}	EOS	$SRBCR^+(T)$	$sIg^+(B)$	$ANAE^+(Mo)$	$OKT_4^+(T_4)$	$OKT_8^+(T_8)$
BNull(PB)	69.0 ± 20.0	0	0.7 ± 0.9	1.2 ± 2.0	6.0 ± 2.0	24.0 ± 3.0	25.0 ± 8.0	NT	NT
T(PB)	94.5 ± 5.7	0	0.1 ± 0.0	1.8 ± 2.4	93.0 ± 5.0	1.4 ± 1.4	6.9 ± 8.0	NT	NT
T_4(PB)	87 ± 7.0	0	0.2 ± 0.0	0.3 ± 0.2	NT	NT	6.7 ± 7.5	88.0 ± 4.2	15.0 ± 1.4
T_8(PB)	75.3 ± 11.0	0	0.7 ± 0.5	0.2 ± 0.2	NT	NT	6.6 ± 8.0	4.9 ± 1.6	99.5 ± 0.7
LDBM	5.5 ± 3.0	54.5 ± 13.5	13.0 ± 7.0	1.0 ± 1.0	NT	4.0 ± 1.4	13.5 ± 7.0	NT	NT

[a] Lymph=lymphocyte; M=myeloblast; M_2=promyelocyte; M_3 and M_4=large and small myelocytes; M_5=metamyelocyte; M_6=band form; M_7=segmented form; EOS=eosinophil; $SRBCR^+(T)$=sheep erythrocyte receptor-positive T cell; $sIg^+(B)$=surface immunoglobulin-positive B cell; $ANAE^+(Mo)=\alpha$-naphthylacetate esterase-positive monocyte; $OKT_4^+(T_4)=OKT_4$ monoclonal antibody reactive T helper cell; $OKT_8^+(T_8)=OKT_8$ monoclonal antibody reactive T suppressor cell; NT=not tested. See text for other abbreviations.

Mo contamination of the BNull cells was about 25% and that of the T, T_4, or T_8 cells 7%. Approximately 88% of the T_4 cells reacted with OKT_4 antibody and 99% of the T_8 cells reacted with OKT_8 antibody. Neutrophils of all stages constituted 70%, Mo 14%, and lymphocytes 6% of the LDBM (T-cell- and Mo-depleted) cells.

The numbers of CFC (only colonies) that proliferated from separate cultures of LDBM and co-culture of LDBM with PB T cells are shown in TABLE 3. In separate cultures, 0.5×10^5 LDBM per dish were incorporated. In co-cultures, 0.5×10^5 LDBM per dish were incorporated with varying numbers of T cells, as shown in the table. All dishes contained a constant volume of a source of CSA. The numbers of CFC that proliferated from the LDBM alone varied with different donors. None or very few (<2 per dish) CFC proliferated from the separate cultures of T cells (results not shown). In co-cultures with T cells, the number of CFC proliferated from LDBM decreased in three studies and was unchanged in two. The pattern of CFC that proliferated from the LDBM was the same whether or not the AET-treated sheep erythrocytes were used in T-cell rosetting and also whether the tris-buffered ammonium

TABLE 3. Number ($\bar{x} \pm SD$) of CFC (Only Colonies with $>$ 32 Cells per Aggregate) Proliferated from T-Cell- and Monocyte-Depleted Light-Density Marrow Cells (LDBM) with and without Autologous Blood T Cells[a]

Study	LDBM	LDBM + T (Ratio)		
		1:1	1:4	1:8
1	261 ± 35	179 ± 63	218 ± 68	175 ± 26
2	236 ± 4	152 ± 52	178 ± 11	—
3	803 ± 61	683 ± 49	526 ± 9	—
4	59 ± 39	51 ± 3.5	70 ± 2	—
5	50 ± 5	18 ± 4	21 ± 7	19 ± 3

[a] LDBM cultures contained 0.5×10^5 per dish. In co-cultures, 0.5×10^5 LDBM per dish and variable numbers, as shown, of T cells were added. All cultures were added with a source of CSA, and two to four plates were prepared for each point. Cultures evaluated at day 7-8.

chloride solution or distilled water was used for lysing SRBC to free T cells (results not shown).

FIGURE 2 depicts results of a study of PB T-cell influence on the BM CFC evaluated both on cultures d_7 and d_{14}. The d_7 CFC decreased significantly (p <0.05), almost to the same extent in three different ratios of LDBM co-cultures with T cells. Although a reduction in the total d_{14} CFC was noted in co-cultures, the differences were not significant (p $>$ 0.05). These results indicate that the T cells suppress the d_7 CFC but not the d_{14} CFC. Similar results were noted in another study.

The numbers of CFC (only colonies) that proliferated from separate cultures of PB BNull cells and co-cultures of BNull with T cells in varying ratios are shown in TABLE 4. In the separate cultures the number of cells incorporated was 10^5 per dish and in co-cultures the same number of BNull cells and variable numbers of T cells, as shown in the table, were incorporated. The culture dishes were prepared without and with a constant volume of a source of CSA. Variable numbers of CFC proliferated from BNull cells of different donors. None or very few (<2 per dish) CFC proliferated

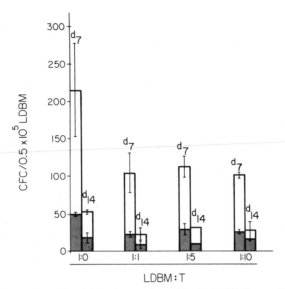

FIGURE 2. The numbers ($\bar{x}$ and SD of two to four dishes) of CFC that proliferated from the T-cell- and monocyte-depleted light-density bone marrow cells in co-cultures (at various ratios) with autologous blood T cells are shown. The cultures were evaluated at days 7 (d_7) and 14 (d_{14}), as noted at the top of each bar. The open bars represent clusters (8 to 32 cells per aggregate) and hatched bars represent colonies (> 32 cells per aggregate).

from the cultures of T cells alone (results not shown). The CFC that proliferated from the BNull cells in co-cultures increased significantly ($p < 0.05$; $r^2 = 0.9$) in a T-cell dose-dependent manner. The proliferation of CFC from cultures of BNull cells alone or in co-cultures of BNull cells with T cells was observed only in dishes with CSA and it was poor or nonexistent in dishes without CSA.

TABLE 4. Number ($\bar{x} \pm$ SD) of CFC (Only Colonies with > 32 Cells per Aggregate) Proliferated from T-Cell- and Monocyte-Depleted Light-Density Blood Mononuclear Cells (BNull Cells) with and without Autologous Blood T Cells[a]

Study	BNull	BNull + T (Ratio)		
		1:1	1:4	1:8
1	9.0 ± 7.0	14.0 ± 0	21.0 ± 1.4	20.0 ± 6
2	40.0 ± 9.0	60.8 ± 10.0	110.0 ± 12.0	—
3	9.0 ± 3.0	—	24.0 ± 7.0	29.0 ± 3.0
4	1.0 ± 0.7	—	64.0 ± 9.0	67.0 ± 12.0
5	23.0 ± 5.0	—	123.0 ± 24.0	115.0 ± 12.0

[a] BNull cell cultures contained 10^5 per dish. The same number of BNull cells was incorporated into co-cultures and the numbers of T cells added varied as shown. All cultures were added with a source of CSA and two to four plates were prepared for each point.

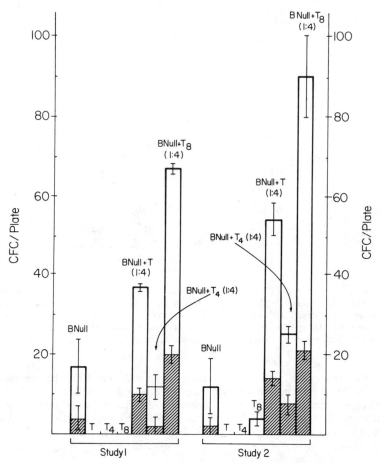

FIGURE 3. The numbers ($\bar{x}$ and SD of two to four dishes) of CFC that proliferated from cultures of autologous blood BNull, T, T_4, and T_8 cells and from co-cultures of BNull cells with T, T_4, or T_8 cells at a 1:4 ratio are shown. The number of cells plated was 10^5 per dish in cultures of individual populations. The same number of BNull cells and four times as many T cells and T-cell subsets were added for co-cultures.

The numbers of CFC that proliferated from separate cultures of BNull, T, T_4, and T_8 cells and co-cultures of BNull with T, T_4, and T_8 cells are shown in FIGURE 3. In the separate cultures 10^5 cells per dish were incorporated and the same number of BNull cells was added into the co-cultures. The number of co-cultured T, T_4, and T_8 cells added was four times the number of BNull cells. Each dish also contained 0.1 ml HPCM. None or very few CFC proliferated from the T, T_4, and T_8 populations. The number of CFC proliferated increased significantly ($p < 0.001$) in co-cultures of BNull cells with T and T_8 cells. T_8 cells promoted the CFC growth better ($p < 0.01$) than did the unseparated T cells.

The numbers of neutrophil, macrophage, eosinophil, and mixed cellular aggregates proliferated from cultures of BNull cells alone and cultures of BNull cells with T, T_4, and T_8 cells at 1:4 ratio were evaluated by the triple-stain method.[14] The results indicated that although the various cell types of aggregates formed from the BNull cells varied among the groups, the differences were not significant ($p > 0.05$).

The CFC (clusters plus colonies) proliferated from co-cultures of a constant, 10^5 per dish, number of BNull cells with increasing numbers of T, T_4, and T_8 cells are shown in FIGURE 4. Each dish also contained 0.1 ml of HPCM. The results are expressed as percentages of total aggregates formed from BNull cells alone. Data of three separate studies are pooled. The results indicate that both the unseparated T and T_8 cells promoted the CFC growth from the BNull cells in a dose-dependent manner. This effect was greater ($p < 0.01$) with T_8 cells than with unseparated T cells. Minimal CFC promotion was noted by the T_4 cells only at the BNull-to-T_4 cell ratio of 1:8.

Addition of OKT_4 and OKT_8 antibodies to BNull cell cultures did not modulate the CFC growth, indicating that the CFC promoting effect of the T_8 cells is not due to residual OKT_4 antibody.

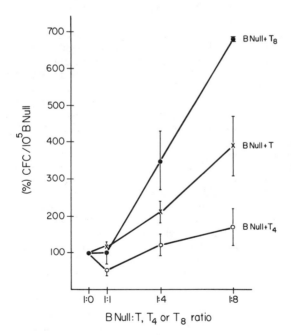

FIGURE 4. Dose-response effects of CFC proliferation from co-cultures of autologous blood BNull cells with T, T_4, or T_8 cells in various ratios are shown. CFC proliferation from co-cultures is expressed as a percentage of that from BNull cells alone.

DISCUSSION

We and others have demonstrated that the CFC are present in the light-density population of the marrow and BNull fraction of the blood and not in the T population or its subpopulations.[2,3,7,8] The T cells are heterogeneous, consisting of many distinct subpopulations which can be recognized by their unique surface membrane markers delineated by monoclonal antibodies.[15-17] Not only do these subsets have distinct functions in the classical immune system, they also exert growth regulatory influences on the hemopoietic stem cells. Unseparated T cells promote proliferation-differentiation of the pluripotent hemopoietic stem cell (CFU-S) of the mouse.[18-22] The most immature erythroid committed stem cell, the burst forming unit (BFU-E), which constitutes almost all of normal human blood erythroid precursors, requires T cells for its growth.[23-25] Further studies indicated that the BFU-E growth promoting effect resides in the T helper (T_4) population.[26,27]

The growth of the d_7 BM CFC was inhibited in most of our studies under the T-cell influence but no such inhibition was observed on the d_{14} BM CFC. The exact mechanism by which this interaction between the T cells and BM CFC occurs and the T-cell subset or subsets responsible for such effects are not known. The growth of the PB CFC is consistently promoted by the unseparated T cells and is due to the presence of a T_8 population contained within the T cells. As demonstrated in this study, the T cells exert the CFC growth promoting effect only in the presence of another source of CSA. This may be very important physiologically since there are other cells which are, directly or indirectly, known to influence the CFC growth. They include the monocyte-macrophage system, endothelial cells, "marrow stromal cells," etc.[28,29]

The CFC are heterogeneous[30,31] with cells varying in maturation from one extreme, the most immature that are closer in ontogeny to the PHSC, to the other, the most mature that are closer to the myeloblast. The PB CFC appears to be the former population and the d_7 BM CFC to be the latter, while the d_{14} BM CFC seem to fall in between these extremes. The basis for such classification is shown in TABLE 5 which depicts the distinct properties of these three CFC populations demonstrated by various investigators.[9,30-33] There is an analogy between these three stages of CFC and those of the erythroid committed precursors.[25] The stages of the PB CFC are similar to those of the PB BFU-E and those of the d_{14} and d_7 BM CFC to those of the BM BFU-E and CFU-E, respectively. The PB BFU-E progeny have been shown to synthesize significant amounts of fetal hemoglobin, while the progeny of the BM cells synthesize primarily the adult type. The cells that proliferate to produce progeny that are capable of synthesizing fetal hemoglobin are considered to be the most immature erythroid precursors.[34] Although the existence has not been clearly documented, we hypothesize that the BM has some CFC that are identical to the PB CFC. As shown in FIGURE 5, these CFC exchange randomly between the two compartments. The reason for such a hypothesis is the finding of a transient elevation in the number of PB CFC following administration of a dose of endotoxin to normal humans.[35] The transient elevation was thought to be due to a flux of the CFC from the marrow into the blood.

The T-cell subsets along with monocytes-macrophages and "marrow stromal cells" form components of the "hemopoietic inductive microenvironment" of the marrow. The concentration of the T_8 cells is 8 to 16 times higher than that of the T_4 cells in the marrow.[36] It is reasonable to assume that the proliferation and differentiation of the hemopoietic stem cells are influenced at the local level by the T cells since they are anatomically located in close proximity to each other.

TABLE 5. Differences between the Blood- and Bone Marrow-Derived CFC in *in Vitro* Cultures

	Bone Marrow		Blood	
	d_7	d_{14}	$d_{14}(?)$	References
Peak day in culture	7-8	Not done	> 14(21)	9, 30, 32, 33
No. of aggregates per 10^5 LDBM($-$Mo, $-$T) or BNull cells	1400	700	125	9
Growth response to CSA	+ + + +	+ +	+	9, 30
Growth in absence of CSA	+ +	+	±	9, 30
CSA requirement for growth	+	+ +	+ + + +	9
Thymidine suicide (%)	30-40	11-39 (?)	0-19	4, 31
T-cell influence on growth	Indifference or inhibition	Indifference	Promotion	7, this study
Sedimentation velocity (mm/hr)	8-9 —	6-7 5-6	— 4	30 31

As stated earlier, the proliferation promoting effect of the T cells is seen on the more immature CFC. Through this effect, coupled with the inhibitory or indifferent effect at the more mature CFC level, the T cell may contribute to the maintenance of granulopoiesis at a steady state. There are many unanswered questions with regard to T-cell-CFC interactions which consequently do not permit for construction of a clear and complete model of T-cell regulation of granulopoiesis. Some of the unanswered questions include: (a) Will the nature of the T-cell effect on the CFC change appropriately with altered requirements for granulocytes as in a bacterial infection? (b) Does it happen by change in concentrations of T-cell subsets? (c) How do T cells sense the need for granulocytes? What is the mechanism of action of T cells on the

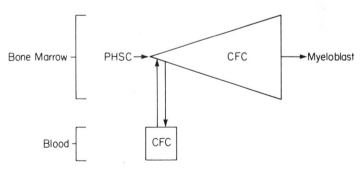

FIGURE 5. A model of the kinetics of CFC between the bone marrow and peripheral blood compartments is shown. The most immature CFC are closer to the PHSC and the most mature closer to the myeloblast. The bidirectional arrows indicate the postulated exchange of the most immature CFC between the two compartments. PHSC = Pluripotent hemopoietic stem cell. CFC = Granulocytic-macrophagic committed stem cell.

CFC, via cell-cell interaction or a humoral mechanism? In addition to these, under-standing of the T-cell interaction with other hemopoietic cells will be essential for full understanding of the role of T cells in granulopoiesis.

ACKNOWLEDGMENTS

We thank Mrs. Elena Turley for her patience and expertise in preparing the manuscript and Mrs. Marti McSharry for her excellent technical assistance.

REFERENCES

1. SINGER, J. W., K. C. DONEY & E. D. THOMAS. 1979. Blood **54**(1): 180-185.
2. SPITZER, G. & D. S. VERMA. 1982. Blood **60**(3): 758-766.
3. ASCENSAO, J. L., N. E. KAY, M. BANISADRE & E. D. ZANJANI. 1981. Exp. Hematol.: 473-478.
4. CHIKKAPPA, G. & P. G. PHILLIPS. Unpublished.
5. ABDOU, N. I., C. NAPOMBEJARA, L. BALENTINE & N. L. ABDOU. 1978. J. Clin. Invest. **61**: 739-743.
6. BACIGALUPO, A., M. PODESTA, M. C. MINGARI, L. MORETTA, M. T. VAN LINT & A. MARMONT. 1980. J. Immunol. **125**(4): 1449-1453.
7. BAGBY, G. C. 1981. J. Clin. Invest. **68**: 1597-1600.
8. CHIKKAPPA, G. & P. G. PHILLIPS. 1984. Blood **63**(2): 356-361.
9. CHIKKAPPA, G., P. G. PHILLIPS & P. BRINSON. 1982. Exp. Hematol. **10**(10): 852-858.
10. PAYNE, S. M., S. O. SHARROW, G. M. SHEARER & W. E. BIDDISON. 1981. Int. J. Immunopharmacol. **3**(3): 227-232.
11. WISNIEWSKI, D., C. PLATSOUCAS, A. STRIKE, C. LAMBEK & B. CLARKSON. 1982. Exp. Hematol. **10**(10): 817-829.
12. KNOWLES, D. M., T. HOFFMAN, M. FERRARINI & H. G. KUNKEL. 1978. Cell. Immunol. **35**: 112-123.
13. RABELLINO, E., S. COLON, H. M. GREY & E. R. UNANE. 1971. J. Exp. Med. **133**: 156-167.
14. PHILLIPS, P. G., G. CHIKKAPPA & P. BRINSON. 1983. Exp. Hematol. **11**: 10-12.
15. REINHERZ, E. L. & S. F. SCHLOSSMAN. 1980. N. Engl. J. Med. **303**: 370-373.
16. REINHERZ, E. L., P. C. KUNG, G. GOLDSTEIN & S. F. SCHLOSSMAN. 1979. J. Immunol. **123**: 2894-2896.
17. REINHERZ, E. L., P. C. KUNG, G. GOLDSTEIN & S. F. SCHLOSSMAN. 1980. J. Immunol. **124**: 1301-1307.
18. LORD, B. I. & R. SCHOFIELD. 1973. Blood **42**: 395-404.
19. SHARKIS, S. J., J. L. SPIVAK, A. AHMED, J. MISITI, R. K. STUART, W. WIKTOR-JEDRZEJCZAK, K. SELL & L. L. SENSENBRENNER. 1980. Blood **55**: 524-527.
20. ZIPORI, D. & N. TRAININ. 1975. Exp. Hematol. **3**: 1-11.
21. ZIPORI, D. & N. TRAININ. 1975. Exp. Hematol. **3**: 389-398.
22. ZIPORI, D. & N. TRAININ. 1973. Blood **42**: 671-678.
23. NATHAN, D. G., L. CHESS, D. G. HILLMAN, B. CLARKE, J. BREARD, E. MERLER & D. E. HOUSMAN. 1978. J. Exp. Med. **147**: 324-339.
24. MANGAN, K. F. & J. F. DESFORGES. 1980. Exp. Hematol. **8**: 717-727.
25. NATHAN, D. G. 1981. Int. J. Immunopharmacol. **3**(3): 223-247.
26. TOROK-STORB, B., P. J. MARTIN & J. A. HANSEN. 1981. Blood **58**: 171-174.
27. MANGAN, K. F., G. CHIKKAPPA, L. Z. BEILER, W. B. SCHARFMAN & D. R. PARKINSON. 1982. Blood **59**: 990-995.

28. KURLAND, J. 1977. *In* Experimental Hematology Today. S. J. Baum & G. D. Ledney, Eds.: 47-60. Springer-Verlag. New York, N.Y.
29. VERMA, D. S. & G. SPITZER. 1979. Blood **54**(6): 1376-1383.
30. JOHNSON, G. R., C. DRESCH & D. METCALF. 1977. Blood **50**(5): 823-831.
31. TEBBI, K., S. RUBIN, D. H. COWAN & E. A. MCCULLOCH. 1975. Blood **48**(2): 235-243.
32. CHERVENICK, P. A. & D. R. BOGGS. 1971. Blood **37**(2): 131-135.
33. KURNICK, J. E. & W. A. ROBINSON. 1971. Blood **37**(2): 136-141.
34. CLARKE, B. J. & D. E. HOUSMAN. 1977. Proc. Natl. Acad. Sci. **74**: 1105-1109.
35. CLINE, J. J. & D. W. GOLDE. 1977. Exp. Hematol. **5**: 186-190.
36. JANOSSY, G., N. TIDMAN, W. S. SELBY, J. A. THOMAS, S. GRANGER, P. C. KUNG & G. GOLDSTEIN. 1981. Int. J. Immunopharmacol. **3**(3): 209-225.

The Status of Pulmonary Host Defense in the Neonatal Sheep: Cellular and Humoral Aspects[a]

R. A. WEISS

Department of Pathology
Health Sciences Center
State University of New York
Stony Brook, New York 11794

A. D. CHANANA AND D. D. JOEL[b]

Medical Research Center
Brookhaven National Laboratory
Upton, New York 11973

INTRODUCTION

During the period following birth the neonate is challenged with multiple forms of antigenic stimuli present in its environment. The defense mechanisms employed by adults of a species to deal with these entities are not fully developed in the newborn. An observed incompetency can reflect deficiencies in quantity, function, and/or regulation of one or several components of host defense. Due to the lack of appropriate animal models for study, many aspects of human neonatal host defense have been examined directly. Noninvasive sampling of cord blood can provide sufficient cellular and humoral material for analysis. Although the observations are not free of contradictions, such studies have suggested that the neonate (premature and term) is deficient in multiple components of host defense.[1] It has been inferred that such deficiencies may contribute to the heightened susceptibility to respiratory infections prevalent in this age group. Among the cellular and humoral aspects examined and found to be

[a] Research supported by the U.S. Department of Energy under Contract DE-AC02-76CH00016. Accordingly, the U.S. Government retains a nonexclusive, royalty-free license to publish or reproduce the published form of this contribution, or allow others to do so, for U.S. Government purposes. The research described in this report involved animals maintained in animal care facilities fully accredited by the American Association for Accreditation of Laboratory Animal Care. Portions of this work will be submitted by R. A. Weiss in partial fulfillment of the requirements for the Doctor of Philosophy degree at SUNY at Stony Brook, School of Medicine, Basic Sciences Department.

[b] Author to whom reprint requests should be sent.

40

insufficient relative to maternal or normal adult controls, are: neutrophil (PMN) chemotaxis *in vitro*[2–13]; microbicidal activities of blood granulocytes and mononuclear cells[14–17]; complement protein levels[18–22]; and the ability to generate chemotactic complement fragments.[3,6,23–27] The interdependent nature of these functions suggests that both cellular and humoral factors must attain a certain level of competence for successful host defense. These studies are limited in that the information provided is only relevant to the function of neonatal circulating leukocytes. Although it is generally accepted that bone marrow-derived blood monocytes are a source of alveolar macrophages (AMs), it is presumptive to extrapolate from studies of blood leukocytes to functional capabilities of AMs.

Consideration of the respiratory tract as a site of environmental antigenic exposure requires a more conventional approach, i.e., the use of an appropriate animal model. Bronchoalveolar lavage (BAL) permits sampling of the lung free cell (LFC) population, as well as proteins, peptides, and lipids present in bronchial secretions.[28,29] In the normal adult lung, cells obtained by lavage are predominantly mononuclear; of these, the primary cell is the AM. The role of the AM in the maintenance of the integrity of the alveolar spaces has long been established. Critical functions of AMs include: binding and ingestion of animate and inanimate particles; killing of bacteria; and elaboration of factors chemotactic for circulating leukocytes, specifically PMNs. Whereas the first two functions involve direct AM interactions, the last provides a means of blood cell recruitment to augment pulmonary host defense.

Since newborns can be thought of as compromised hosts, it is not unreasonable to suspect that they might constitute a population with an increased susceptibility to the harmful effects of inhaled pollutants. With this in mind we have initiated a study whose objective is to critically define the development of pulmonary host defense in an acceptable animal model.

THE LUNG FREE CELL POPULATION

During the first week of life the LFC population in the lamb is dynamic. Both relative and absolute changes in subpopulations were observed. Lavage samples obtained at birth or shortly thereafter were rather acellular, but did contain epithelial-like cells. At 1 day of age, PMNs constituted 74% of all cells, whereas AMs represented only 19%. This cell distribution pattern changed rapidly; a sharp decrease in PMNs was accompanied by an even sharper increase in AMs. PMNs declined rapidly until day 8, when they accounted for 8% of all cells, and then gradually until day 90. At this age, LFC distributions were comparable to those observed in adults. AMs represented 91% of all cells at day 8; this decreased to 88% at day 21 and 83% at day 90. Lymphocytes, which were negligible during the early neonatal period (< 1% of the LFC population at day 8), increased gradually and at day 90 constituted 14% of all cells (FIGURE 1). The composition of LFCs at specific neonatal time points may be reflected in age-related functional performance to be described later. Factors contributing to observed differences in performance may include the relative proportion of certain cell classes and cellular functional maturity.

Few comparable studies have been reported for other species. Rothlein *et al.*[30] examined the development of AMs in specific pathogen-free (SPF) and germfree miniature swine. Their findings were similar to ours in that: (1) only epithelial-like cells were observed in lavage fluids obtained 3 days prior to term or immediately following birth; (2) in 12-hr-old SPF piglets, PMNs accounted for 74% of all cells and AMs for 11%; (3) by day 4, the proportions were 48 and 50%, respectively; and (4) at 1 week of age, AMs constituted 83% of all cells, and PMNs, 15%. However, in the SPF piglet, adult LFC distributions were attained by 2 weeks of age, far earlier than in the lamb. Zeligs *et al.*[31] reported that, in the rabbit, AMs were obtained by lavage as early as 1 day prior to term. In addition, the LFC population was described as predominantly mononuclear; no mention was made of granulocytes being observed in perinatal and neonatal lavage samples.

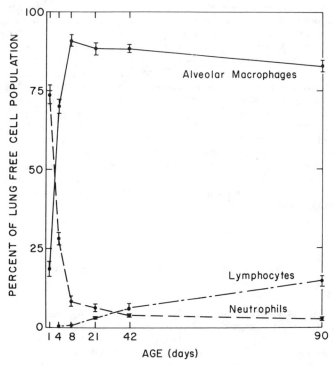

FIGURE 1. Changes in LFC subpopulations during the first 90 days of life. LFCs were obtained from anesthetized (halothane) lambs by lavaging with 150 ml of 0.9% pyrogen-free saline (pH 7.4) at room temperature. A pediatric fiberoptic bronchoscope was introduced via an endotracheal tube. Cell counts were made using a Coulter Counter, Model ZBI. Cytocentrifuge preparations were stained with Wright-Giemsa stain. A minimum of 500 cells/lamb were identified for differential counts.

The changes in cell subpopulation proportions and numbers described above are for conventionally reared lambs, i.e., lambs housed with their dams in a relatively antigenic environment and allowed to suckle freely, thus receiving passive immunization via colostrum. A question arises as to whether the initial PMN extrusion into the air spaces is attributable to an endogenous or exogenous factor(s). Observations made in colostrum-deprived lambs maintained in isolators either under germfree conditions or exposed to ambient air suggest that environmental exposure modulates both the magnitude and time course of the PMN response. In one germfree lamb sampled at day 1, PMNs accounted for only 23% and AMs for 70% of all cells. PMNs were negligible as early as day 4, representing only 1.3% of the LFCs in two germfree lambs. At days 8 and 10, 98.2% of cells obtained by lavage from four germfree lambs were identifiable as AMs, while <1% were PMNs. Cell proportions in two isolator-maintained but non-germfree lambs of this same age were intermediate between those in conventionally reared lambs and those in germfree lambs, i.e., 95% of the cells were AMs and 3.4% were PMNs. Rothlein *et al.*[30] reported that, although the number of AMs in germfree piglets sampled at 3 to 4 days and 2 weeks of age was comparatively low, cell distributions paralleled those noted in SPF piglets. Our findings differ in that: (1) the total number of LFCs obtained from germfree lambs at days 8 and 10 was 90% of the corresponding value in conventional lambs; and (2) at all ages sampled, the percentage of PMNs was greatly reduced.

Mononuclear LFCs had characteristic morphological features. At day 1, the cytoplasm was relatively scant and foamy in appearance. This vacuolization was very apparent at day 4 (FIGURE 2) and was still partially evident until day 42, when the cytoplasm became more homogeneous. Sudan Black B staining indicated that the vacuolar material was, in part, phospholipids and neutral lipids. This observation is in agreement with that reported[31,32] for neonatal rabbit AMs and lends support to a proposed surfactant scavenging function for these cells in the period immediately following birth. At day 4 an additional distinctive morphological characteristic became apparent, i.e., mononuclear cells were very heterogeneous with respect to size. Size heterogeneity was not as predominant at day 8.

Metaphase figures were frequently seen in LFCs obtained on day 8 (FIGURE 3). This, too, is in accord with the observations of Zeligs *et al.*[31] DNA-labeling studies suggested that, in lambs, a relatively large portion of lavageable mononuclear cells are capable of *in situ* regeneration during the first postnatal week. Fourteen to 24% of all AMs sampled on days 1, 4, and 8 incorporated [^{3}H]thymidine, indicating that from 0.7-4.8 $\times$ 10^4 AMs/ml were in the S phase of the cell cycle (TABLE 1). At subsequent ages, i.e., day 21 onward, both the percentage and number of AMs incorporating [^{3}H]thymidine decreased, limiting the phenomenon to the early neonatal period.

While there is agreement that histiocytic lineages are primarily derived from monocyte precursors in the bone marrow, the degree to which histiocytes can proliferate *in situ* is disputed. Lung macrophages are located both in the interstitium and the air spaces. The *in vitro* DNA-labeling studies provide no information on the proliferative capacity of interstitial macrophages; however, they do indicate that the mononuclear cells present in the lung air spaces during the early neonatal period are capable of considerable self-renewal. While this observation is itself of interest, it may have further implications for cell function.

INTERACTION WITH BACTERIA

Host defense against inhaled bacteria can be viewed as a composite of sequential cellular events requiring humoral mediators for optimal performance. Recognition is the initial step, followed by binding, ingestion, and killing. Our studies were designed to examine these functional capacities in neonatal LFCs and circulating PMNs.

The binding of *Staphylococcus aureus* (ATCC 25923) by sheep LFCs (AMs and PMNs) is a ligand-mediated process. Interaction between effector and target cells was

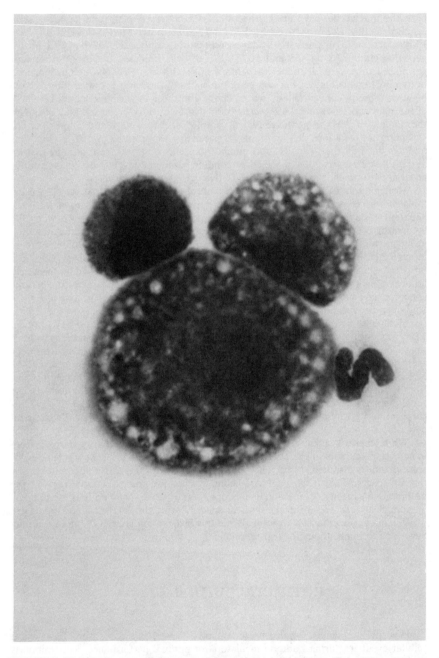

FIGURE 2. Wright-Giemsa-stained cytocentrifuge preparation of LFCs obtained from a lamb at day 4. Characteristic features include cytoplasmic vacuolization and size heterogeneity of mononuclear cells. PMN presence is still marked at this age. (Magnification, ×1000.) Photomicrography by W. Marin.

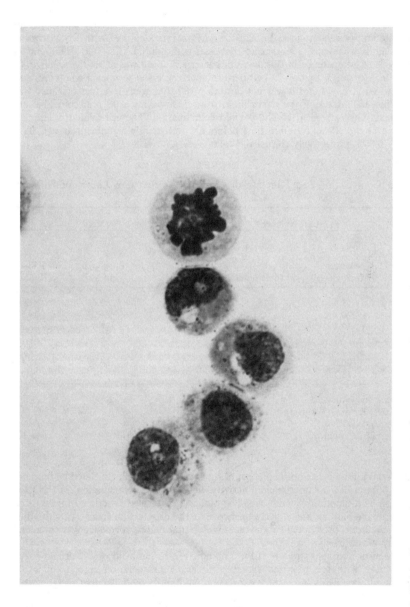

FIGURE 3. Wright-Giemsa-stained cytocentrifuge preparation of LFCs obtained from a lamb at day 8. Mitotic figures such as this were frequently observed. (Original magnification, ×1000; reduced to 90% of original size.) Photomicrography by W. Marin.

negligible ($\overline{Y}$ = 2.6 at 90 min coincubation; three experiments) in the absence of serum components. FIGURE 4 describes the average binding kinetics observed during a 90 min coincubation of LFCs with preopsonized *S. aureus* at a target:effector ratio of 2:1. The phagocytic index, an expression of the percentage interaction, increased with incubation time. A gradual enhancement of functional capacity was apparent during the first postnatal week. In fact, the performance obtained with LFCs from 8-day-old lambs was nearly identical to that seen with adult LFCs. The attainment of adult levels of competence in this assay of bacteria binding was short-lived, however. As seen in FIGURE 5, by day 21 cell performance regressed to a level comparable to that observed at day 4 and it was not until day 180 that adult-level performance was again achieved. Although the curve in FIGURE 5 describes a 90 min coincubation, similar results were seen at 15 and 30 min coincubation. The age-related differences in binding at the 30- and 90-min time points are statistically significant at $p < 0.05$ and $p < 0.005$, respectively (Kruskal-Wallis Test).

TABLE 1. Composition and Function of Lung Free Cells from Lambs of Different Ages

	Cell Number ($\times$ 10⁴)/ml			Cell Function	
Age (days)	Alveolar Macrophage	Neutrophil	Alveolar Macrophage in S Phase	Phagocytic Index[a, b]	Killing Index[c]
1	3.8	15.3	0.7	62.6	ND[d]
4	20.1	7.0	4.8	81.2	29.9
8	30.8	2.4	4.4	94.4	45.7
21	23.5	1.4	1.5	85.8	31.7
42	23.5	0.9	1.2	82.8	32.5
90	20.8	0.6	0.8	84.2	35.4
180	23.7	1.9	0.7	92.1	ND

[a] 90 min coincubation.
[b] p <0.005, Kruskal-Wallis Test.
[c] 30 min coincubation.
[d] ND = not determined.

Bacterial killing is the optimal effect of the sequence of events initiated by binding. FIGURE 6 describes the microbicidal activity, at 30 min of coincubation, of the LFC population as a function of lamb age. The biphasic pattern of functional maturation, observed in the binding assay, was repeated, i.e., the progression from day 4 to adult was a gradual one, broken only at day 8, at which time cell performance was enhanced relative to all other ages examined.

The question arises as to why LFCs, obtained from lambs at day 8, are so adept at interaction with preopsonized target particles. An association among cell cycle stage, magnitude of Fcγ2a receptor expression, and antibody-dependent phagocytosis in P388D1 cells was recently reported by Gandour and Walker.[33] Cells in the G2 and M phases of the cell cycle expressed twice the number of Fcγ2a receptors. Receptor avidity was, however, unaffected by cell cycle phase. In the lamb at day 8, approximately 91% of the lung free cells were identifiable as AMs on the basis of light microscopic morphology. Of these cells, 14% incorporated [³H]thymidine. Should the

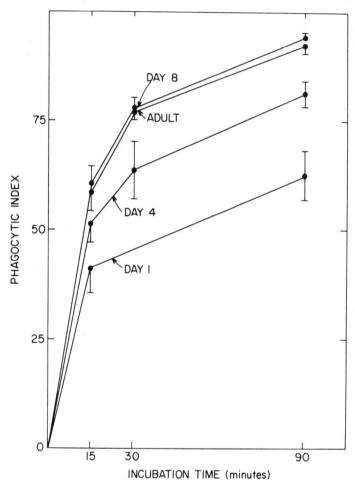

FIGURE 4. Interaction between LFC and *S. aureus*: kinetics of days 1, 4, 8, and adult. An 18-hr trypticase soy broth culture of *S. aureus* (ATCC 25923) was incubated with pooled adult normal sheep serum (PANSS) (37-39°C; 60 min), washed extensively, and resuspended in 0.1% gelatin Hanks' balanced salt solutions (gHBSS) at a concentration of 2×10^7/ml. Bacterial concentrations were estimated with a Klett-Summerson colorimeter and ascertained by colony counts following an 18 hr incubation (34-36°C). LFCs were centrifuged twice (650 $\times$ g; 4°C) and adjusted to a concentration of 10^7 LFC/ml gHBSS. LFCs and bacteria were coincubated at a target:effector ratio of 2:1 for time periods ranging from 0 to 90 min (39°C; 8 rpm). Bacteria were also incubated in the absence of LFCs to control for growth under assay conditions. All samples were processed in duplicate. At selected intervals, aliquots were removed, quenched by dilution, and differentially centrifuged, and the supernatant was diluted and plated on blood agar plates. At 18 hr incubation, the number of colony forming units (CFU) was determined. The phagocytic index describes the percentage of LFC-associated bacteria, corrected for bacterial growth.

observations of Gandour and Walker be applicable, enhanced performance may simply reflect increased Fcγ receptor expression associated with increased mitotic activity. This suggests that the functional competence observed *in vitro* may not be an appropriate indicator of cell function *in vivo*. Neonatal lung washings contained very low levels of IgG1 and IgA at this time. The availability of endogenous opsonins *in vivo* may be the limiting factor in pulmonary host defense.

Consideration must also be given to the dynamic character of the neonatal LFC population. As shown in TABLE 1, the calculated numbers of AMs in S phase were very similar at days 4 and 8, yet bacterial binding and killing activity were considerably different. This observed difference in performance may be the result of the changing proportion of PMNs in the lavage cell suspensions. PMNs have been reported to differ from mononuclear phagocytes in both the magnitude and avidity of Fcγ receptor expression.[34,35] In a series of three experiments, the binding capacity of circulating PMNs obtained from a single adult sheep was examined. At 15, 30, and 90 min of coincubation, the average phagocytic indices were 2.4, 17.0, and 39.2, respectively, as compared to 58.2, 77.5, and 99.2 for adult AMs. It appears that circulating PMNs do not perform as well as LFCs in this assay. While PMNs constituted 26% of the phagocytic cell population sampled at day 4, by day 8 they accounted for only 7%. The PMN presence may also physically impede interactions between mononuclear cells and bacteria. Two aspects require further thought: (1) Is the performance of circulating PMNs representative of PMNs obtained by lavage? (2) What is the magnitude of animal to animal variability in ovine PMN binding capacity? Several investigators have examined the functional heterogeneity of circulating human PMNs[36,37] and have concluded that only a portion of the circulating PMN population is functionally similar to exudative cells. If the LFC PMN is an exudative cell, then circulating PMNs may not be appropriate cells to study. The second concern is prompted by reports of intra- and inter-animal variability in bovine mammary gland PMN phago-

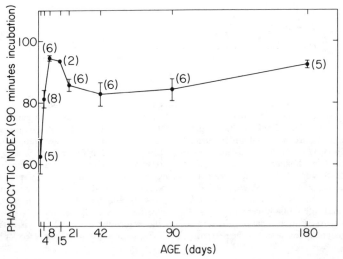

FIGURE 5. Interaction between LFC and *S. aureus*: Days 1 to 180 at 90 min coincubation. For experimental details, see the caption for FIGURE 4.

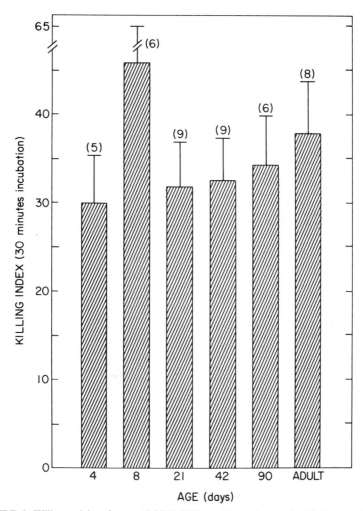

FIGURE 6. Killing activity of neonatal LFC. LFCs and bacteria were handled as described in the caption for FIGURE 4, with the following exceptions: (1) the final coincubation medium contained 10% PANSS; (2) sampling time points were 0, 30, and 60 min; and (3) when removed, aliquots were diluted 1:10 in sterile distilled water and subjected to three freeze-thaw cycles. The lysate was diluted and plated, and the CFUs were enumerated at 18 hr of incubation. The killing index describes the percentage of bacteria killed, corrected for bacterial growth.

cytic capacity.[38,39] Additional studies addressing both issues are necessary before conclusions can be drawn.

To ensure that the functional performance observed in LFCs of sequentially lavaged lambs was not affected by repeated sampling, individual lambs were lavaged only once at day 8, 21, or 42. The binding performance of LFCs was comparable and statistical analyses confirmed that no differences existed.

IMMUNOGLOBULINS IN BAL

Samples of lung washings obtained from lambs aged 1 to 180 days were analyzed for immunoglobulin and albumin content. At all ages, both IgM and IgG2 were undetectable, suggesting that the levels of these immunoglobulins were less than 9 μg/ml and 150 ng/ml, respectively. As shown in TABLE 2, IgG1 and albumin were present in lung washings as early as day 1, whereas IgA was not detected until day 21. At all subsequent ages, the IgA concentration was four- to fivefold greater than that of IgG1. Two samples obtained from germfree colostrum-deprived lambs aged 1 and 8 days contained albumin but lacked detectable immunoglobulins. Due to the structure of the ungulate placenta, transfer of maternal immunoglobulins does not occur *in utero,* but is delayed until just after birth, at which time the neonatal gut is highly permeable to immunoglobulins present in colostrum.

The biphasic change in albumin concentrations, i.e., a peak at day 21, a trough at day 90, and subsequent increases, is in agreement with findings from saliva samples

TABLE 2. Average Concentrations[a] (μg/ml) of Albumin, IgG1, and IgA in Lavage

Age (days):	1	4	8	21	42	90	180
Albumin:	11.0	27.1	34.8	55.5	36.8	26.9	44.9
	(1.1)[b]	(3.7)	(7.2)	(13.4)	(8.4)	(4.9)	(12.2)
IgG1:	7.8	11.5	16.2	10.3	28.8	87.0	162.5
	(2.4)	(2.1)	(3.3)	(2.7)	(7.0)	(16.2)	(39.7)
IgA:	ND[c]	ND	ND	8.6	128.5	373.0	857.5
				(1.4)	(37.0)	(85.2)	(193.3)
Number of Samples:	6	4	6	6	6	6	4

[a] Concentrations of albumin, IgG1, and IgA were determined by radioimmunoassay performed by A. J. Husband and A. Cripps.
[b] Data are presented as the mean ± (1 SEM).
[c] ND = not detectable.

obtained from human neonates. It is thought that this pattern may reflect serum transudation secondary to increased mucosal permeability. (A. J. Husband, personal communication). The critical observation to be made is that the levels of endogenous IgG1 prior to day 21 are quite low, suggesting that *in vivo* opsonic capacity may limit pulmonary host defense effectiveness.

CHEMOTACTIC FACTORS: RECOGNITION AND SYNTHESIS

Due to the brief *in vivo* doubling time of pathogenic bacteria, efficient mobilization of phagocytes is undoubtedly critical for successful defense. A bacterial inoculum of modest size requires only a short period of unmonitored growth in which to become an overwhelming challenge. Experimental evidence suggests that the neonate is deficient in its response to inflammatory stimuli. *In vivo* studies on the neonatal rat indicated that the inflammatory response to Group B streptococci was both delayed and of lesser magnitude than that of adult rats.[40] *In vitro* studies have shown that human neonatal cord blood PMNs are relatively deficient in response to known chemotactic factors, suggesting defects at the level of membrane receptor expression[5] and membrane deformability.[41] Whether or not this defect in PMN chemotaxis contributes to increased susceptibility to respiratory infection is unknown. The number and types of cells present in the lungs of newborn infants have not been adequately studied because of the obvious restrictions on sampling.

The presence of PMNs in lavage cell suspensions obtained from newborn sheep and pigs indicated that, in these species, emigration from the vasculature into the lung air spaces occurred readily. Increased permeability of pulmonary capillaries may have facilitated the process, for endothelial junctions in neonatal mice have been shown to be more permeable than those in adult mice.[42] To further characterize our *in vivo* observations, the ability of neonatal PMNs to respond to chemotactic stimuli was examined. In three newborn lambs, PMNs isolated from both the blood (93.0% PMNs) and the lung air spaces (66.7% PMNs) were simultaneously tested in a standard chemotaxis assay. Comparisons were always made to the performance of blood PMNs obtained from a single adult sheep. The depth of migration of the leading front of cells was the endpoint assessed. Statistical treatment included one-way analysis of variance and pairwise *t* tests employing Bonferroni probabilities. When the data were examined in this manner, it became apparent that: (1) random migration of day 2 blood PMNs was equivalent to or greater than that of adult cells ($p < 0.01$); (2) migration in response to sodium caseinate, a chemoattractant, by both day 1 and 2 blood PMNs was equivalent to or greater than that of adult cells ($p < 0.01$); (3) neonatal blood PMN migration, random and stimulated, was equivalent to or exceeded that of autologous LFC PMNs ($p < 0.05$); and (4) adult blood PMN migration, random and stimulated, exceeded that of day 2 LFC population PMNs ($p < 0.001$). The presence of fewer PMNs in the LFC population may explain observations (3) and (4). A standard approach to the analysis of chemotaxis data is the comparison of chemotactic indices. Differences between blood and LFC PMN performances were masked when chemotactic indices were compared. Regardless of the method of analysis, sheep neonatal PMNs clearly demonstrated both random and directed migration comparable to that of adult PMNs. In a separate experiment, migration of day 4 and adult blood PMNs was tested in response to a LFC culture supernatant, sodium caseinate, and medium. All cells performed comparably. In addition, the depths of migration recorded in response to sodium caseinate and the LFC culture supernatant were equivalent, suggesting the presence of a putative chemotactic activity in the LFC culture supernatant and, most important, the ability of day 4 blood PMNs to recognize and respond to it appropriately.

AMs of several species have been shown to synthesize chemoattractants *in vitro*[43–47] and the major AM-derived chemotactic factor is thought to be an hydroxyeicosatetraenoic acid.[48,49] Observed differences in the ability of AMs and PMNs to handle bacterial challenges[50,51] suggest that recruitment of circulating blood neutrophils by AMs may be an important facet of pulmonary host defense. In the context of our study, LFCs obtained from lambs aged 8 days and older were examined for their ability to elaborate chemotactic factors *in vitro*. LFC populations obtained at days 1 and 4 were not included due to the large number of PMNs present in the cell suspensions. Following an 18 hr incubation with opsonized zymosan, LFC culture supernatants were tested for chemotactic activity. Chemotactic indices, i.e., the ratio of the depth of migration of the leading front of cells in response to a chemoattractant to that in response to medium lacking chemotactic activity, were used for comparisons between experiments. LFCs obtained from lambs at day 8 did not elaborate chemotactic factors recognized by adult blood PMNs, as indicated by the difference in chemotactic indices in FIGURE 7 ($p < 0.03$; Wilcoxon's Signed-Ranks Test). However, at day 21 and thereafter (days 42, 90, and adult), similar chemotactic responses to LFC culture supernatants and sodium caseinate were observed, suggesting the presence of a putative chemotactic factor. Supernatants obtained from cultures containing only opsonized zymosan lacked chemotactic activity (average chemotactic index $\pm$ 1 SD $= 1.08 \pm 0.010$; 17 experiments). Preliminary checkerboard analysis indicated that the activity present was chemotactic and not just chemokinetic. Whether this AM-derived chemotactic activity is similar to those described in other species remains to be examined.

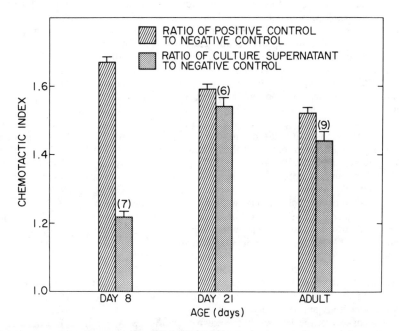

FIGURE 7. Comparison of chemotactic indices generated in response to sodium caseinate and LFC culture supernatants. A PMN-enriched cell suspension ($> 88\%$ PMNs) was prepared by the method of Boyum[52] from venous blood obtained from a single donor sheep. Chemotaxis studies were done in duplicate in blind well chambers using 3-μm nitrocellulose filters to separate the cells from: (1) sodium caseinate (5 mg/ml saline); (2) Gey's balanced salt solution containing 2% bovine serum albumin, 100 U penicillin/ml, and 100 μg streptomycin/ml (GBSS); and (3) LFC culture supernatants obtained from 18-hr cultures of LFCs and opsonized zymosan. PMNs were exposed to test substances for 30 min (5% CO_2; 39°C). Filters were removed and processed. The depth of migration of the leading front of cells was determined for five randomly selected high-power fields. Chemotactic indices represent the depth of migration in response to a chemoattractant relative to that in response to GBSS.

SUMMARY

In consideration of the sheep neonate as a compromised host, we have examined the status of cellular and humoral pulmonary host defense components at selected developmental time points. The dynamic character of the early neonatal LFC population, reflected in changes in subpopulations and proliferative capacity, most probably contributed to the observed changes in *in vitro* cell function. While certain cell responses, e.g., blood and LFC PMN chemotaxis, appeared intact by day 1, others developed subsequently. The ability of AMs to elaborate a chemotactic factor(s) was first noted at day 21. Bacteria binding and killing presented a biphasic maturation pattern, with full competence not present until day 180. Although the *in vitro* binding and killing activity of day 8 LFCs was comparable to that of the adult, it may be a poor indicator of *in vivo* host defense capacity, given the relative paucity of endogenous opsonins at that age. In fact, the interdependence of mediators suggests that the sheep neonate may remain a compromised host during the first 3 months of life. Thereafter, cellular and humoral parameters begin to approximate those of adult sheep and by 180 days of life pulmonary defense, as assessed in this study, is fully developed.

ACKNOWLEDGMENTS

We thank Drs. A. J. Husband and A. Cripps of the University of Newcastle, New South Wales, Australia for quantitating immunoglobulins and albumin in lung washings. In addition, we note the excellent technical assistance of Mrs. K. Conkling, Mrs. A. Alberico, Mr. T. Weldon, Mr. J. Pedersen, and Mr. F. O. Lawson and the expert secretarial skills of Ms. L. Wasson and Mrs. M. Susa.

REFERENCES

1. LOKE, Y. W. 1978. Immunology and Immunopathology of the Human Foetal-Maternal Interaction. Pp. 51-70. Elsevier/North-Holland Biomedical Press. Amsterdam, the Netherlands.
2. KLEIN, R. B., T. J. FISCHER, S. E. GARD, M. BIBERSTEIN, K. C. RICH & E. R. STEIHM. 1977. Pediatrics 60: 467-472.
3. MILLER, M. E. 1971. Pediatr. Res. 5: 487-492.
4. MILLER, M. E. 1979. Pediatrics 64(Suppl.): 709-712.
5. MILLER, M. E. 1980. *In* Immunologic Disorders in Infants and Children. E. R. Steihm & V. A. Fulginiti, Eds.: 165-180. Saunders. Philadelphia, Pa.
6. MEASE, A. D., G. D. FISCHER, K. W. HUNTER & F. B. RUYMANN. 1980. Pediatr. Res. 14: 142-146.
7. PAHWA, S. G., R. PAHWA, E. GRIMES & E. SMITHWICK. 1977. Pediatr. Res. 11: 677-680.
8. REPO, H., A. M. M. JOKIPII, M. LEIRSALO & T. U. KOSUNEN. 1980. Clin. Exp. Immunol. 40: 620-626.
9. BONER, A., B. J. ZELIGS & J. A. BELLANTI. 1982. Infect. Immun. 35: 921-928.
10. ANDERSON, D. C., B. J. HUGHES & C. W. SMITH. 1981. J. Clin. Invest. 68: 863-874.
11. ANDERSON, D. C., B. R. BRINKLEY, G. PERRY & C. W. SMITH. 1982. Pediatr. Res. 16: 219A.

12. RAGHUNATHAN, R., M. E. MILLER, S. EVERETT & R. D. LEAKE. 1982. J. Clin. Immunol. 2: 242-245.
13. KIMURA, G. M., M. E. MILLER, R. D. LEAKE, R. RAGHUNATHAN & A. T. W. CHEUNG. 1981. Pediatr. Res. 15: 1271-1273.
14. QUIE, P. G. & E. L. MILLS. 1979. Pediatrics 64(Suppl.): 719-721.
15. SHIGEOKA, A. O., R. P. CHARETTE, M. L. WYMAN & H. R. HILL. 1981. J. Pediatr. 98: 392-398.
16. BECKER, I. D., O. M. ROBINSON, T. S. BAZAN, M. LOPEZ-OSUNA & R. R. KRETSCHMER. 1981. Infect. Immun. 34: 535-539.
17. KRETSCHMER, R. R., P. B. STEWARDSON, C. K. PAPIERNIAK & S. P. GOTOFF. 1976. J. Immunol. 117: 1303-1307.
18. JOHNSTON, R. B., JR., K. M. ALTENBURGER, A. W. ATKINSON, JR. & R. H. CURRY. 1979. Pediatrics 64(Suppl.): 781-785.
19. STOSSEL, T. P., C. A. ALPER & F. S. ROSEN. 1973. Pediatrics 52: 134-137.
20. COLTEN, H. R. 1977. In Development of Host Defenses. M. D. Cooper & D. H. Dayton, Eds.: 165-174. Raven Press. New York, N.Y.
21. DAVIS, C. A., E. H. VALLOTA & J. FORRISTAL. 1979. Pediatr. Res. 13: 1043-1046.
22. ADINOLFI, M. 1971. Ontogeny of Acquired Immunity. Pp. 65-85. Elsevier Excerpta Medica/North-Holland. Amsterdam, the Netherlands.
23. DOSSETT, J. H., R. C. WILLIAMS, JR. & P. G. QUIE. 1969. Pediatrics 44: 49-57.
24. MCCRACKEN, G. H., JR. & H. F. EICHENWALD. 1971. Am. J. Dis. Child. 121: 120-126.
25. WINKELSTEIN, J. A., L. E. KURLANDSKY & A. J. SWIFT. 1979. Pediatr. Res. 13: 1093-1096.
26. MILLS, E. L., B. BJORKSTEIN & P. G. QUIE. 1979. Pediatr. Res. 13: 1341-1344.
27. ANDERSON, D. C., B. J. HUGHES, M. S. EDWARDS, G. J. BUFFONE & C. J. BAKER. 1983. Pediatr. Res. 17: 496-502.
28. REYNOLDS, H. Y. & R. E. THOMPSON. 1973. J. Immunol. 111: 358-368.
29. ROLA-PLESZCZYSNKI, M., P. SIROIS & R. BEGIN. 1981. Lung 159: 91-99.
30. ROTHLEIN, R., R. GALLILY & Y. B. KIM. 1981. J. Reticuloendothel. Soc. 30: 483-495.
31. ZELIGS, B. J., L. S. NERURKAR & J. A. BELLANTI. 1977. Pediatr. Res. 11: 197-208.
32. SHERMAN, M., E. GOLDSTEIN, W. LIPPERT & R. WENNBERG. 1977. Am. Rev. Respir. Dis. 116: 433-440.
33. GANDOUR, D. M. & W. S. WALKER. 1983. J. Immunol. 130: 1108-1112.
34. PHILLIPS-QUAGLIATA, J. M., B. B. LEVINE, F. QUAGLIATA & J. W. UHR. 1970. J. Exp. Med. 133: 589-601.
35. FLEIT, H. B., S. D. WRIGHT & J. C. UNKELESS. 1982. Proc. Natl. Acad. Sci. USA 79: 3275-3279.
36. HARVATH, L. & E. J. LEONARD. 1982. Infect. Immun. 36: 443-449.
37. KLEMPNER, M. S. & J. I. GALLIN. 1978. Blood 51: 659-669.
38. PAAPE, M. J., R. E. PEARSON & W. D. SCHULTZE. 1978. Am. J. Vet. Res. 39: 1907-1910.
39. WILLIAMS, M. R. & K. J. BUNCH. 1981. Res. Vet. Sci. 30: 298-302.
40. SCHUIT, K. E. & R. DE BIASIO. 1980. Infect. Immun. 28: 319-324.
41. MILLER, M. E. & K. A. MYERS. 1977. In Development of Host Defenses. M. D. Cooper & D. H. Dayton, Eds.: 175-185. Raven Press. New York, N.Y.
42. MEYRICK, B. & L. H. REID. 1977. In Development of the Lung. W. A. Hodson, Ed.: 145. Marcel Dekker. New York, N.Y.
43. KAZMIEROWSKI, J. A., J. I. GALLIN & H. Y. REYNOLDS. 1977. J. Clin. Invest. 59: 273-281.
44. HUNNINGHAKE, G. W., J. I. GALLIN & A. S. FAUCI. 1978. Am. Rev. Respir. Dis. 117: 15-23.
45. HUNNINGHAKE, G. W., J. E. GADEK, H. M. FALES & R. G. CRYSTAL. 1980. J. Clin. Invest. 66: 473-483.
46. MERRILL, W. W., G. P. NAEGEL, R. A. MATTHAY & H. Y. REYNOLDS. 1980. J. Clin. Invest. 65: 268-276.
47. GADEK, J. E., G. W. HUNNINGHAKE, R. L. ZIMMERMAN & R. G. CRYSTAL. 1980. Am. Rev. Respir. Dis. 121: 723-733.
48. VALONE, F. H., M. FRANKLIN, F. F. SUN & E. J. GOETZL. 1980. Cell. Immunol. 54: 390-401.

49. FELS, A. O. S., N. A. PAWLOWSKI, E. B. CRAMER, T. K. C. KING, Z. A. COHN & W. A. SCOTT. 1982. Proc. Natl. Acad. Sci. USA **79:** 7866-7870.
50. HOF, D. G., J. E. REPINE, P. K. PETERSON & J. R. HOIDAL. 1980. Am. Rev. Respir. Dis. **121:** 65-71.
51. PIERCE, A. K., R. C. REYNOLDS & G. D. HARRIS. 1977. Am. Rev. Respir. Dis. **116:** 679-684.
52. BOYUM, A. 1974. Tissue Antigens **4:** 269-274.

Comparison of Pulmonary and Intestinal Lymphocyte Migrational Patterns in Sheep[a]

D. D. JOEL AND A. D. CHANANA

Medical Department
Brookhaven National Laboratory
Upton, New York 11973

INTRODUCTION

Following the intrabronchial instillation of antigen, specific immune effector cells can be consistently demonstrated in lung lavage cell suspensions and lung parenchyma.[1-10] The source of these cells remains, however, to be fully clarified. There are two fundamentally different mechanisms by which the lung may become populated with antigen-sensitive lymphocytes following intrabronchial immunization. One is the local production of these cells from precursors present in subepithelial lymphoid tissues scattered throughout the respiratory tract. The second mechanism involves the production of effector lymphocytes in regional and/or systemic lymphoid tissues and entrance of these cells into the circulation with subsequent extravasation or recruitment into the lung.

In sheep a major portion of the lung is drained by the caudal mediastinal lymph node (CMLN).[11] Cannulation of the efferent duct of the CMLN permits continuous access to lymphocytes emerging from a regional pulmonary lymph node. We have shown that intrabronchial immunization results in the appearance of large numbers of specific antibody-forming cells and lymphoblasts in efferent pulmonary lymph.[12] The fate of these cells following their entry into the blood is, however, unknown.

It is well documented in experimental animals, including sheep, that lymphoblasts from the thoracic duct, intestinal lymph or mesenteric lymph nodes preferentially localize in the lamina propria of the intestine.[13-21] The lung, like the intestine, has a mucosal cell lining which is constantly exposed to environmental materials, including antigens. Lymphoblasts isolated from bronchial lymph nodes have a propensity to relocate in the lungs rather than the intestine,[22-26] suggesting that with respect to these two "mucosal" organs immunoblast distribution is nonrandom and dependent upon cell origin. Cells isolated from minced lymph nodes may not, however, be representative of those cells which normally enter the circulation via efferent lymph.[27]

[a] Work supported by U.S. Department of Energy under Contract DE-AC02-76CH00016 and by U.S. Public Health Service Grant HL 30865-01. Accordingly, the U.S. Government retains a nonexclusive, royalty-free license to publish or reproduce the published form of this contribution, or allow others to do so, for U.S. Government purposes.

This problem can be circumvented in sheep by cannulation of the efferent lymph duct of the CMLN. The purpose of the present study was to use such preparations to compare the migrational patterns and tissue distribution of lymphoblasts from efferent pulmonary lymph to those of lymphoblasts from thoracic duct lymph, which is principally efferent intestinal lymph.

MATERIALS AND METHODS

Animals and Cannulation Techniques

Dorset-cross young adult sheep weighing 25 to 40 kg were used. A week prior to surgery sheep were conditioned to limited restraint in chutes which allowed each animal to stand or lie down as desired with free access to water, pelleted chow, and alfalfa hay.

Cannulation of the efferent lymph duct of the CMLN was done under general anesthesia (halothane) using a modification[28] of the two-stage procedure described by Staub et al.[11] During the same surgical procedure, the thoracic duct was cannulated just posterior to the entry of the CMLN lymph duct. Cannulation of the efferent lymph duct of the prescapular lymph node was done as a separate surgical procedure a few days later.

Cannulas were composed of a Silastic rubber T-tube with a Teflon tip. Within 2 cm of the tip, heparin was infused at the rate of 130 units/hr to prevent clotting. An indwelling Silastic catheter was placed in the external jugular vein and lymph circulation was maintained in a closed system by a special pumping mechanism.

Lymph Collection and in Vitro Cell Labeling

Lymph was collected in sterile, siliconized glass bottles kept at 4°C. Lymphocytes (1 to 5 $\times$ 10^9) were concentrated to about 10^8 cells/ml in phosphate-buffered saline containing either 0.5 μCi [^{125}I]iododeoxyuridine (^{125}I-UdR, New England Nuclear, sp act > 2000 Ci/mM) alone, or ^{125}I-UdR plus 10 μCi Na$_2$^{51}CrO$_4$ (New England Nuclear, sp act 305-400 mCi/mg) per ml cell suspension and incubated for 45 min at 37°C. Cells were washed once and resuspended in 200 ml of cell-free autologous lymph. After aliquots were removed for cell counting and measurement of radioactivity, the labeled cell suspensions were slowly reinfused intravenously.

Sampling and Measurement of Radioactivity

Lymph samples (10-30 ml) were collected at 5 hr, 9 hr, and 1, 2, 3, and 6 days after infusion and cell counts determined using a Coulter Model ZBI. Cells were pelleted by centrifugation and washed twice in phosphate-buffered saline. Radioactivity was determined using a 2-channel well-type gamma scintillation counter. Counts were corrected for decay and channel spillover and expressed as cpm/10^6 or 10^7 lymphocytes.

In some experiments, free lung cells were obtained by bronchoalveolar lavage as previously described.[28] One subsegment each of the right and left diaphragmatic lobes was lavaged with 6 $\times$ 30 ml aliquots of room-temperature saline. Total and differential cell counts were made and radioactivity was determined as above.

Organ/Tissue Distribution of Radioactivity

Twenty to 24 hr after the infusion of labeled lymphocytes, sheep were anesthetized and exsanguinated, and the vascular system was "flushed" with 8 liters of saline via carotid artery and jugular vein cannulas. Organs were weighed and several representative samples taken for analysis. Each sample was weighed; radioactivity was determined and expressed as cpm/mg tissue or converted to the percentage of injected activity recovered in various organs.

To circumvent the possibility of passive intra-pulmonary trapping, labeled cell suspensions were infused intraarterially in two sheep.

Antigenic Stimulation

To increase the concentration of lymph-borne immunoblasts, the CMLN was antigenically stimulated by the intrabronchial instillation of 10^{11} horse red cells into the lower right diaphragmatic lobe. This resulted in a marked increase in proliferating lymphoblasts 4 to 6 days later.

RESULTS

Recirculation of Lymphoblasts Labeled with ^{125}I-UdR

Six separate studies were done in which either CMLN or thoracic duct (TD) lymph-borne lymphoblasts were labeled *in vitro* with ^{125}I-UdR and reinfused intravenously. Results of representative experiments are shown in FIGURES 1 and 2. When TD (intestinal) lymphoblasts were labeled, cell-associated radioactivity in TD lymph rose rapidly, reaching a peak 9 hr after infusion (FIGURE 1). At this time the specific activity in TD lymph was three times that found in lung lymph. By 2 days postinfusion, radioactivity was barely detectable. In contrast, when pulmonary lymphoblasts were labeled, the specific activity in efferent CMLN lymph was consistently higher than that in TD lymph (FIGURE 2). Cell-associated radioactivity peaked somewhat later, i.e., day 1, and was readily detectable in both pulmonary and intestinal lymph for 3 and even 6 days after infusion.

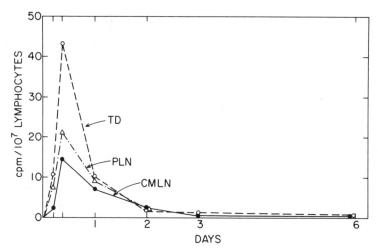

FIGURE 1. Specific activity in thoracic duct lymph (TD) and efferent lymph of the caudal mediastinal lymph node (CMLN) and prescapular lymph node (PLN) after the intravenous infusion of 3.3 × 10⁹ thoracic duct lymphocytes labeled with 1.0 × 10⁶ cpm ¹²⁵I-UdR.

In two experiments the efferent duct of the prescapular lymph node was cannulated in addition to the TD and the efferent duct of the CMLN. As shown in FIGURE 1, when labeled TD lymphoblasts were reinfused the specific activity in TD lymph was clearly greater than that in either the prescapular or pulmonary lymph. On the other hand, when pulmonary lymphoblasts were reinfused the specific activity in prescapular lymph was significantly higher than that in TD lymph, but still somewhat below that

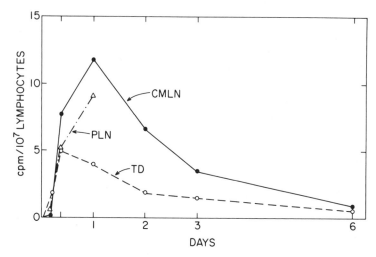

FIGURE 2. Specific activity in thoracic duct lymph (TD) and efferent lymph of the caudal mediastinal lymph node (CMLN) and prescapular lymph node (PLN) after the intravenous infusion of 5.5 × 10⁹ lymphocytes from efferent CMLN lymph labeled with 5.5 × 10⁵ cpm ¹²⁵I-UdR.

seen in pulmonary lymph (FIGURE 2). Unfortunately, in this study the prescapular node cannula was accidentally dislodged between days 1 and 2. A second study confirmed that pulmonary immunoblasts reappear in pulmonary lymph with a higher specific activity than in prescapular lymph.

Recirculation of Lymphocytes Labeled with ^{51}Cr

The recirculation patterns of lymphocytes labeled *in vitro* with Na$_2$ ^{51}CrO$_4$ and reinfused intravenously are shown in FIGURES 3 and 4. As shown in FIGURE 3, essentially no difference was observed in the specific activities of pulmonary and TD lymph following the infusion of ^{51}Cr-labeled TD lymphocytes. When pulmonary lymphocytes were labeled and reinfused, a slight but consistently (all four studies) higher specific activity was found in efferent CMLN lymph as compared to TD lymph (FIGURE 4).

Radioactivity Associated with Cells Recovered by Bronchoalveolar Lavage

In three studies with labeled pulmonary lymphocytes and one study with labeled intestinal lymphocytes, lung lavage cell suspensions were obtained 2 or 3 days after infusion. Cell-associated radioactivity was consistently detected; however, the amounts were very low. Estimates, based on the proportion of lung lavaged, suggest that on the average less than 0.1% of the ^{125}I activity and less than 0.02% of the ^{51}Cr activity

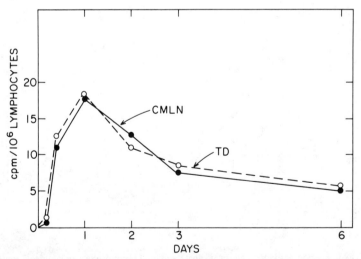

FIGURE 3. Specific activity in thoracic duct lymph (TD) and efferent lymph of the caudal mediastinal lymph node (CMLN) after the intravenous infusion of 3.3 × 10^9 thoracic duct lymphocytes labeled with 3.1 × 10^6 cpm ^{51}Cr.

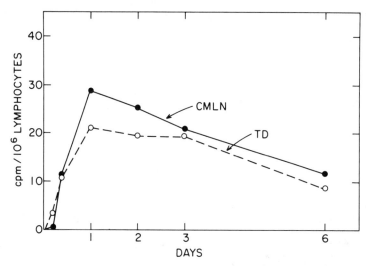

FIGURE 4. Specific activity in thoracic duct lymph (TD) and efferent lymph of the caudal mediastinal lymph node (CMLN) after the intravenous infusion of 5.5×10^9 CMLN lymphocytes labeled with 5.1×10^6 cpm ^{51}Cr.

injected as labeled pulmonary lymphocytes were present in the lavageable cell population at the time of sampling. In the single study with ^{125}I-labeled TD lymphoblasts, the estimated recovery was less than 0.02% of the injected radioiodine.

Organ / Tissue Distribution of Radioactivity

The percentages of injected radioactivity present in organs 20 to 24 hr after intravenous or intraarterial infusion of labeled lymphocytes are shown in TABLES 1 and 2. Clearly, ^{125}I-labeled TD lymphoblasts have a marked propensity to localize in the intestinal tract. Of the radioactivity recovered, 87% was in the intestinal tract and only 5% was lung associated (TABLE 3). In contrast, when ^{125}I-labeled pulmonary immunoblasts were infused, the largest fraction of radioactivity was present in the lung; however, significant amounts of radioiodine were also recovered from the intestinal tract and spleen.

The distribution of ^{51}Cr activity was also dependent upon the source of labeled cells. ^{51}Cr-labeled TD lymphocytes were nearly equally divided between intestine and lung (TABLE 2). On the other hand, when ^{51}Cr-labeled pulmonary lymphocytes were infused, very little radioactivity was found in the intestine. The highest fraction was recovered in the lung followed by the spleen and liver (TABLE 2).

The specific activities (cpm / mg tissue) of various lymph nodes are listed in TABLE 4. It is apparent that differences in lymph node activity were dependent upon the source of labeled lymphocytes. Labeled TD lymphocytes resulted in higher specific activities in the mesenteric lymph node while labeled pulmonary lymphocytes resulted in higher specific activities in the caudal mediastinal lymph node. The differences in ^{125}I activity were more apparent than the differences in ^{51}Cr activity.

TABLE 1. Percentages of Injected Radioactivity Present in Various Organs of Sheep 20-24 hr after the Injection of Autologous, Lymph-Borne Lymphoblasts Labeled *in Vitro* with ^{125}I-UdR[a]

		Lymphoblasts from Thoracic Duct Lymph			Lymphoblasts from Efferent Lymph of the CMLN		
Sheep No.:	511[b]	526[c]	530[b]	Mean	517[b]	539[c]	Mean
Small intestine	32.6	19.8	28.3	26.9	3.4	9.8	6.6
Large intestine	3.2	4.7	2.4	3.8	0.5	3.6	2.1
Lung	1.24	2.0	1.5	1.6	7.6	12.2	9.9
Spleen	0.6	1.5	0.8	1.0	4.6	3.9	4.3
Liver	0.4	0.8	0.9	0.7	1.9	2.1	2.0
MLN	1.0	1.4	1.0	1.1	0.2	0.9	0.5
CMLN	0.2	0.1	—	0.2	0.3	1.0	0.6
Combined recovery	39.2	30.3	35.9	35.3	18.5	33.5	26.0

[a] Abbreviations: MLN, mesenteric lymph node; CMLN, caudal mediastinal lymph node.
[b] Labeled cells infused intravenously.
[c] Labeled cells infused intraarterially.

DISCUSSION

The aims of this study were: (1) to ascertain whether or not lymphoblasts issuing from the caudal mediastinal lymph node preferentially localize in the lung, and (2) to compare the migrational patterns of lymph-borne pulmonary lymphocytes to the patterns of lymph-borne lymphocytes from another "mucosal" organ, namely, the intestine.

TABLE 2. Percentages of Injected Radioactivity Present in Various Organs of Sheep 20-24 hr after the Injection of Autologous, Lymph-Borne Lymphocytes Labeled with $Na_2^{51}CrO_4$ *in Vitro*[a]

		Lymphocytes from Thoracic Duct Lymph			Lymphocytes from Efferent Lymph of the CMLN		
Sheep No.:	511[b]	526[c]	530[b]	Mean	517[b]	539[c]	Mean
Small intestine	7.1	2.1	6.7	5.3	0.7	1.8	1.3
Large intestine	1.8	0.4	0.9	1.0	0.3	0.5	0.4
Lung	13.2	5.0	6.5	8.2	22.4	15.9	19.2
Spleen	4.1	4.7	4.1	4.3	14.1	9.7	11.9
Liver	2.6	1.8	2.8	2.4	7.1	7.5	7.3
MLN	8.0	3.4	4.0	5.1	0.9	5.3	3.1
CMLN	2.5	0.5	—	1.5	0.6	3.7	3.1
Combined recovery	39.3	17.9	25.0	27.8	46.1	44.4	45.4

[a] Abbreviations: MLN, mesenteric lymph node; CMLN, caudal mediastinal lymph node.
[b] Labeled cells infused intravenously.
[c] Labeled cells infused intraarterially.

TABLE 3. The Mean Percentage of Recovered Radioactivity Associated with Various Tissues 20-24 hr after Infusion of Labeled Lymphocytes[a]

	Lymphoblasts Labeled with ^{125}I-UdR		Lymphocytes Labeled with $Na_2^{51}CrO_4$	
	TD	CMLN	TD	CMLN
Intestinal tract	87	31	22	3
Lung	5	39	29	42
Spleen	3	18	18	26
Liver	2	8	9	16
MLN	3	2	18	7
CMLN	1	2	4	5

[a] Abbreviations: TD, thoracic duct lymphocytes labeled and reinfused; CMLN, lymphocytes in efferent lymph of the caudal mediastinal lymph node labeled and reinfused; MLN, mesenteric lymph node.

It is assumed in this study that the vast majority of lymphocytes in the TD originate from the intestine and associated lymph nodes and enter the TD via efferent intestinal lymphatics.[29] When lymphoblasts were labeled *in vitro* with ^{125}I-UdR and reinfused intravenously, recirculation patterns were clearly nonrandom and dependent upon the tissue of origin. Intestinal lymphoblasts preferentially reappeared in TD lymph. However, they remained in circulation for only a short period of time. ^{125}I activity of efferent lymph-borne cells was detectable but very low by 48 hr after the infusion of labeled TD lymphoblasts. In contrast, radiolabeled pulmonary blasts reappeared in efferent CMLN lymph with a significantly higher specific activity than in intestinal lymph. Pulmonary lymphoblasts also remained in circulation longer as indicated by significant cell-associated ^{125}I activity in efferent lymph, particularly pulmonary lymph, 3 days after infusion and even detectable amounts 6 days after infusion. This observation suggests that the time required for organ localization or "homing" may depend upon the initial source of lymphoblasts. If this is true, the analysis of organs 20-24 hr after infusion, as is frequently done, may not reflect the ultimate distribution of lymphoblasts, with the possible exception of intestinal lymphoblasts.

TABLE 4. The Specific Activity[a] of Lymph Nodes 20-24 hr after the Infusion of Labeled Lymphocytes[b]

Lymph Node	TD Lymphocytes Labeled		CMLN Lymphocytes Labeled	
	^{125}I	^{51}Cr	^{125}I	^{51}Cr
Mesenteric lymph node	551	9750	70	7650
Caudal mediastinal lymph node	176	6430	161	9350
Prescapular/prefemoral lymph nodes	177	4830	93	7930

[a] Specific activity is expressed as the mean cpm/mg lymph node.
[b] Abbreviations: TD, thoracic duct; CMLN, caudal mediastinal lymph node.

It should be emphasized that in the present studies, all lymph, with the exception of samples collected for analysis, was continuously returned to the blood via an indwelling jugular cannula. This may in part explain the more prolonged recirculation of ^{125}I-labeled lymphocytes than has been previously observed.[19] Also, it is not unreasonable to consider that the continuous return of lymph to the blood would allow a larger fraction of lymphoblasts to mature *in vivo* and enter the long-lived, recirculating pool of "small" lymphocytes.

It was somewhat surprising, in view of work published by Chin and Hay,[30] that clear differences in the migration of ^{51}Cr-labeled lymphocytes from blood to various lymph compartments were not observed in our studies. ^{51}Cr-labeled TD lymphocytes reappeared in pulmonary and thoracic duct lymph with almost identical specific activities. When pulmonary lymphocytes were labeled and reinfused, a small, but consistently higher, specific activity was found in pulmonary lymph as compared to TD lymph. It should be pointed out that Chin and Hay[30] were comparing lymphocyte migration through intestinal lymph nodes, subcutaneous lymph nodes, and inflammatory sites. Perhaps the migratory patterns through intestinal and pulmonary lymph nodes are more similar.

It is evident from the organ distribution experiments that lymph-borne immunoblasts emerging from the caudal mediastinal lymph node in response to intrabronchial immunization tend to relocate in the lung, although significant ^{125}I activity was also present in the intestine and to a lesser extent in the spleen. Specific organ localization or "homing" with pulmonary lymphoblasts was, however, not as dramatic as that seen with TD lymphoblasts which accumulated rapidly and almost exclusively in the intestinal tract. Part of the apparent difference may be a consequence of the 24-hr time interval between cell injection and analysis as discussed above. Studies varying this time interval, and in particular extending it beyond 24 hr, would help resolve this question.

Although substantial ^{125}I activity could be demonstrated in lung tissue following the infusion of labeled pulmonary lymphoblasts, only small amounts of radioactivity were present in cell samples obtained by bronchoalveolar lavage. Estimates based on the portion of lung lavaged would indicate that less than 0.1% of the injected radioactivity was in the lung air spaces at the time of sampling. Demonstration of immune effector lymphocytes in lavage cell suspension is often used as an assessment of pulmonary immune responsiveness. If the organ distribution data in the present study are meaningful, it is clear that the number of immune effector lymphoid cells obtained by lavage is only a minor fraction of those present in lung parenchyma. Nevertheless, the observation that a significantly larger fraction of ^{125}I activity, as compared to ^{51}Cr activity, was recovered would suggest that lymphocyte extrusion into lung air spaces is nonrandom.

Of interest was the finding that the largest fraction of radiochromium was recovered from the lung irrespective of the source of labeled cells. Assuming that $Na_2{}^{51}CrO_4$ labels all classes of lymphocytes, these data suggest that the lung contains a large pool of lymphocytes, particularly recirculating lymphocytes.

ACKNOWLEDGMENTS

The authors wish to thank A. Alberico, K. Conkling, F. Lawson, J. Pederson, C. Van Tuyle, and T. Weldon for their excellent technical assistance.

REFERENCES

1. WALDMAN, R. H. & C. S. HENNEY. 1971. Cell mediated immunity and antibody responses in the respiratory tract following local and systemic immunization. J. Exp. Med. **134:** 482-494.
2. NASH, D. R. 1973. Direct and indirect plaque forming cells in extrapulmonary lymphoid tissue following local vs. systemic injection of soluble antigen. Cell. Immunol. **9:** 234-241.
3. NASH, D. R. & B. HOLLE. 1973. Local and systemic cellular immune responses in guinea-pigs given antigen parenterally or directly into the lower respiratory tract. Clin. Exp. Immunol. **13:** 573-583.
4. KALTREIDER, H. B. & F. N. TURNER. 1976. Appearance of antibody-forming cells in lymphocytes of the lower respiratory tract of the dog after intrapulmonary or intravenous administration with sheep erythrocytes. Am. Rev. Respir. Dis. **113:** 613-617.
5. MCLEOD, E., J. L. CALDWELL & H. B. KALTREIDER. 1978. Pulmonary immune responses of inbred mice. Appearance of antibody-forming cells in C57BL/6 mice after intrapulmonary or systemic immunization with sheep erythrocytes. Am. Rev. Respir. Dis. **118:** 561-571.
6. HILL, J. O. & R. BURRELL. 1979. Cell-mediated immunity to soluble and particulate inhaled antigens. Clin. Exp. Immunol. **38:** 332-341.
7. CALDWELL, J. L. & H. B. KALTREIDER. 1980. Cytolytic activity of pulmonary and systemic lymphoid cells from C57B1/6 mice following intrapulmonary or intraperitoneal immunization with allopeneic tumor cells. Exp. Lung Res. **1:** 99-110.
8. BICE, D. E. & C. T. SCHNIZLEIN. 1980. Cellular immunity induced by lung immunization of Fischer 344 rats. Int. Arch. Allergy Appl. Immunol. **63:** 438-447.
9. BICE, D. E., D. L. HARRIS, J. O. HILL, B. A. MUGGENBURG & R. K. WOLFF. 1980. Immune responses after localized lung immunization in the dog. Am. Rev. Respir. Dis. **5:** 755-760.
10. LIPSCOMB, M. F., C. R. LYONS, R. M. O'HARA & J. STEIN-STREILEIN. 1982. The antigen-induced selective recruitment of specific T lymphocytes to the lung. J. Immunol. **128:** 111-115.
11. STAUB, N. C., R. D. BLAND, K. L. BRIGHAM, R. DEMLING, A. J. ERDMANN III & W. C. WOOLVERTON. 1975. Preparation of chronic lung fistulas in sheep. J. Surg. Res. **19:** 315-320.
12. JOEL, D. D., A. D. CHANANA & P. CHANDRA. 1980. Immune responses in pulmonary lymph of sheep after intrabronchial administration of heterologous erythrocytes. Am. Rev. Respir. Dis. **122:** 925-932.
13. GOWANS, J. L. & E. J. KNIGHT. 1964. The route of recirculation of lymphocytes in the rat. Proc. R. Soc. London Ser. B **159:** 257-282.
14. HALL, J. G., O. M. PARRY & M. E. SMITH. 1972. The distribution and differentiation of lympho-borne immunoblasts after intravenous injection into syngeneic recipients. Cell Tissue Kinet. **5:** 269-281.
15. GUY-GRAND, D., C. GRISCELLI & P. VASSALI. 1974. The gut-associated lymphoid system: nature and properties of the large dividing cells. Eur. J. Immunol. **4:** 435-443.
16. PARROTT, D. M. V. & A. FERGUSON. 1974. Selective migration of lymphocytes within the mouse small intestine. Immunology **26:** 571.
17. PIERCE, N. F. & J. L. GOWANS. 1975. Cellular kinetics of the intestinal immune response to cholera toxoid in rats. J. Exp. Med. **142:** 1550-1563.
18. MCWILLIAMS, M., J. M. PHILLIPS-QUAGLIATA & M. F. LAMM. 1975. Characteristics of mesenteric lymph node cells homing to gut-associated lymphoid tissue in syngeneic mice. J. Immunol. **115:** 54.
19. HALL, J. G., J. HOPKINS & E. ORLANS. 1977. Studies on the lymphocytes of sheep. III. Destination of lymph-borne immunoblasts in relation to their tissue of origin. Eur. J. Immunol. **7:** 30-37.
20. HUSBAND, A. J. & J. L. GOWANS. 1978. The origin and antigen-dependent distribution of IgA-containing cells in the intestine. J. Exp. Med. **148:** 1146-1160.
21. HUSBAND, A. J. 1982. Kinetics of extravasation and redistribution of IgA-specific antibody containing cells in the intestine. J. Immunol. **128:** 1355-1359.

22. BIENENSTOCK, J., R. L. CLANCY & D. Y. E. PEREY. 1976. Bronchus associated lymphoid tissue (BALT): its relationship to mucosal immunity. *In* Immunologic and Infectious Reactions in the Lung. C. H. Kirkpatrick & H. Y. Reynolds, Eds.: 29-58. Marcel Dekker, Inc. New York, N.Y.

23. BIENENSTOCK, J. 1980. Bronchus-associated lymphoid tissue and the source of immuno-globulin-containing cells in the mucosa. Environ. Health Perspect. **35:** 39-42.

24. RUDZIK, O., R. L. CLANCY, D. Y. E. PEREY, R. P. DAY & J. BIENENSTOCK. 1975. Repopulation with IgA-containing cells of bronchial and intestinal lamina propria after the transfer of homologous Peyer's patch and bronchial lymphocytes. J. Immunol. **114:** 1599-1604.

25. MCDERMOTT, M. R. & J. BIENENSTOCK. 1979. Evidence for a common mucosal immu-nologic system. I. Migration of B immunoblasts into intestinal, respiratory and genital tissues. J. Immunol. **122:** 1892-1898.

26. SPENCER, J., L. A. GYURE & J. G. HALL. 1983. IgA antibodies in the bile of rats. III. The role of intrathoracic lymph nodes and the migration pattern of their blast cells. Immunology **48:** 687-693.

27. REYNOLDS, J., I. HERON, L. DUDLER & Z. TRNKA. 1982. T-cell recirculation in the sheep: migratory properties of cells from lymph nodes. Immunology **47:** 415-421.

28. CHANANA, A. D., P. CHANDRA & D. D. JOEL. 1981. Pulmonary mononuclear cells: studies of pulmonary lymph and bronchoalveolar cells of the sheep. J. Reticuloendo. Soc. **29:** 127-135.

29. MANN, J. D. & G. M. HIGGINS. 1950. Lymphocytes in thoracic duct, intestinal and hepatic lymph. Blood **5:** 177-190.

30. CHIN, W. & J. B. HAY. 1980. A comparison of lymphocyte migration through intestinal lymph nodes, subcutaneous lymph nodes and chronic inflammatory sites of sheep. Gas-troenterology **79:** 1231-1242.

Cell Replication in an Immunologically(?) Stimulated Cell Population in Human Bone Marrow[a]

MICHAEL L. GREENBERG[b] AND
FREDERICK P. SIEGAL[c]

[b]Polly Annenberg Levee Division of Hematology
[c]Division of Clinical Immunology
Mount Sinai School of Medicine
City University of New York
New York, New York 10029

INTRODUCTION

The acquired immune deficiency syndrome (AIDS)[1] is known to be associated with an alteration in T-lymphocyte subset ratios (defined by surface antigens) with T-suppressor cells outnumbering T-helper cells and a decreased T-cell proliferation response to mitogens.[2, 3] Humoral immunity may also be affected, resulting in an increase in serum immunoglobulins,[3] a decreased response to B-cell mitogens, and a diminished response to immunization with keyhole-limpet hemocyanin.[4] In this report we focus on the proliferation of the immunoglobulin-producing cells in the bone marrow of five patients with AIDS.

Others have found that 4-6% of normal marrow lymphocytes and plasma cells are in DNA synthesis, i.e., labeled with [³H]thymidine ([³H]TdR).[5] In antigen-stimulated mice, lymph node plasmablasts and proplasmacytes were actively replicating cells which produced the more mature plasma cells.[6] In patients with multiple myeloma both lymphocytic and plasmacytic marrow cells produced the idiotypic immunoglobulin.[7] Killmann et al. noted that both large and small myeloma cells incorporated [³H]TdR.[8] These various studies generally lacked objective criteria for the definition of cell types, however, so we felt that such a system was required.

[a]Supported in part by the Irma T. Hirschl Charitable Trust, the Chemotherapy Foundation, and National Institutes of Health Grant CA/AI 34980.

MATERIALS AND METHODS

Five hospitalized patients with AIDS were studied. Four were male homosexuals, and one was a female drug addict. Blood T-helper lymphocyte:T-suppressor lymphocyte ratios (Leu 3:Leu 2) were 0.17-0.87. The patients had decreased mitogen responses to phytohemagglutinin, concanavalin A, and pokeweed mitogen. They had polyclonal hyperglobulinemia with IgG 2.3-12.8 g/dl, IgA 180-735 mg/dl, and IgM 220-525 mg/dl. All were febrile at the time of study. Four had opportunistic infections. Two had Kaposi's sarcoma. Their marrows had 15-28% plasma cells.

Each patient had bone marrow aspirated into 1% EDTA in saline. The marrows were then incubated for 1 hr with [³H]TdR, sp act 1.9 Ci/mmole, 1 μCi/ml. Slides were then made and fixed in methanol. Autoradiographs were made with NTB-2 Nuclear Tract Emulsion as previously described.[9]

On each slide a minimum of 1000 plasmacytic and lymphocytic cells was counted. Nuclear and cell diameters were measured in two perpendicular diameters (usually maximum and minimum diameters). Diameters were averaged for the nucleus and for the cell and used to calculate nucleus:cell ratios. Plasmablasts were defined as plasmacytic cells with eccentric nuclei, fine chromatin, and one or more nucleoli. The more mature plasma cells and cells morphologically transitional between lymphocytes and plasma cells were arbitrarily divided into plasma cells, lymphocytic plasma cells, and plasmacytic lymphocytes. These three cell types all had eccentric, slightly oval nuclei with the long axis of the nucleus generally perpendicular to the long axis of the cell. Arbitrary, but objective, definitions for the latter three cell types were made on the basis of the nucleus:cell ratios. For plasma cells nucleus:cell ratios were 0.70 or less, for lymphocytic plasma cells 0.71-0.83, and for plasmacytic lymphocytes 0.84 or more. Lymphocytes did not have eccentric nuclei, and the maximal diameters of nuclei and cell were not perpendicular to each other.

The labeling index (LI), i.e., the fraction of cells labeled with [³H]TdR, was determined for each cell type. For part of the analysis within a given cell type, the mean cell diameters were used to define the largest one-third of the population as *large*, the smallest one-third as *small*, and the rest as *medium*.

The analyses were done for the lymphocyte and plasma cell populations present in these marrows. Other cell types were excluded.

RESULTS

TABLE 1 shows the fraction of each morphologic cell type within the total population of lymphocytes and plasma cells. Lymphocytes, plasmablasts, and plasmacytic lymphocytes together constituted less than 10% of the total population. Lymphocytic plasma cells averaged 33% and plasma cells 57% of these cells.

TABLE 2 shows the fraction of each morphologic cell type found labeled with [³H]TdR in DNA synthesis. No lymphocytes were labeled and very few plasma cells. Small fractions of plasmablasts were in DNA synthesis, and plasmacytic lymphocytes had by far the largest population of cells in DNA synthesis in four of the five patients.

TABLE 3 shows the distribution of the cells that were in DNA synthesis. In all cases at least three out of four cells in DNA synthesis were lymphocytic plasma cells, more than twice the proportion of the total population with that morphology. Similarly,

TABLE 1. Fraction of Total Lymphocytes and Plasma Cells (%)

Patient No.	Lymphocytes	Plasmablasts	Plasmacytic Lympho- cytes	Lymphocytic Plasma Cells	Plasma Cells
1	3.2	0.7	5.3	41.4	49.4
2	5.6	3.5	4.4	47.7	38.9
3	5.7	2.3	0.9	23.8	67.3
4	5.0	1.3	1.0	28.1	64.6
5	7.7	0.6	1.2	24.7	65.7
Mean ± SD:	5.4 ± 1.6	1.7 ± 1.2	2.6 ± 2.1	33.1 ± 10.8	57.2 ± 12.5

plasmablasts and plasmacytic lymphocytes had disproportionately high fractions of the DNA synthesizing cells, and plasma cells had a markedly decreased proportion.

TABLES 4 and 5 show the LIs of plasma cells and lymphocytic plasma cells, respectively, by the sizes of the cells, i.e., large, medium, and small. In both cases the large cells had the largest fraction of DNA synthesizing cells. There were too few cells for each of the other cell types to obtain similar, reasonably reliable data.

DISCUSSION

Although much of the attention in AIDS has been directed at the T lymphocytes, it has been obvious that B lymphocytes are also affected.[2-4] The high serum levels of polyclonal immunoglobulins seen in many of these patients may reflect previous antigenic stimulus to a set of immunologically competent cells since the decreased responsiveness to B-cell mitogens *in vitro* or to keyhole-limpet hemocyanin *in vivo*[4] demonstrates that the disease depresses B-lymphocyte function for new stimuli, perhaps partly due to the decrease in T-helper lymphocytes. Our patients are typical in these respects. The plasmacytosis in their marrows may have been induced by previous immunologic stimuli. We did not test the possibility that, as demonstrated in normal human lymphocytes *in vitro*,[10] Epstein-Barr virus may have induced both immuno-globulin synthesis and B-cell replication in these patients. Their high serum levels of

TABLE 2. Fraction of Cells in DNA Synthesis (%)

Patient No.	Lymphocytes	Plasmablasts	Plasmacytic Lympho- cytes	Lymphocytic Plasma Cells	Plasma Cells
1	0	0	20.0	13.3	1.1
2	0	19.2	18.2	19.2	2.7
3	0	13.0	66.7	16.4	0.4
4	0	16.7	33.3	20.2	0.7
5	0	16.7	33.3	12.8	0.3
Mean ± SD:	0	13.1 ± 7.7	34.3 ± 19.5	16.4 ± 3.3	1.0 ± 1.0

TABLE 3. Fraction of All of the DNA Synthesizing Cells in Each Category (%)

Patient No.	Lymphocytes	Plasmablasts	Plasmacytic Lympho- cytes	Lymphocytic Plasma Cells	Plasma Cells
1	0	0	14.9	77.4	7.6
2	0	5.8	6.9	78.4	9.0
3	0	5.9	11.8	76.5	5.3
4	0	3.2	5.0	85.0	6.8
5	0	2.6	10.3	81.8	5.3
Mean ± SD:	0	3.5 ± 2.5	9.8 ± 3.9	79.8 ± 3.5	6.8 ± 1.6

immunoglobulins show that there is continued production of the globulins, and the DNA synthesis seen demonstrates that there is continuing turnover of those B lymphocytes and plasma cells. McMillan et al.[11] measured IgG production in marrow, spleen, blood, lymph node, and human thymic lymphocytes *in vitro* and suggested that as much as 97% of IgG may be synthesized in the marrow. This observation is consistent with the idea that marrow lymphocytes and plasma cells may be the most pertinent B cells to study in man.

The morphologic scheme used is admittedly arbitrary, but it is objective and reproducible. Therefore, the scheme could be used for comparison with activated B cells in other disease states with increased numbers of B cells and with malignant B cells, especially in multiple myeloma. Since plasma cells are derived from B lymphocytes, their mature morphology must necessarily have intermediate states such as the plasmacytic lymphocytes and lymphocytic plasma cells. The position of plasmablasts within this scheme is unclear, especially in view of the small fraction of cells in DNA synthesis in comparison with the plasmacytic lymphocytes. By contrast, large fractions of rodent lymph node plasmablasts synthesized DNA.[5] The low fraction of plasma cells in DNA synthesis does suggest that the nucleus:cell ratio was appropriately chosen to define an almost completely terminally differentiated compartment. We cannot directly compare the plasma cells as herein defined with plasma cells in other studies because a similar classification scheme has not been used in such studies.

Rodent studies have also shown that the marrow is a major site of B-cell formation and that the majority are turning over.[12, 13] In rodents, the small lymphocyte was not in DNA synthesis, as was also true in our studies. Whether any of our cells correspond to the large B-lymphocyte cells with cytoplasmic μ-chains which are in the cell cycle in rodents is not known since our cells were not studied in that way. At least the

TABLE 4. Plasma Cells—LI, by Size of Cell

Patient No.	Large	Medium	Small
1	2.1	0.6	0
2	4.3	1.0	4.2
3	0.4	0	0.9
4	1.9	0	0
5	0.5	0	0
Mean ± SD:	1.8 ± 1.6	0.3 ± 0.5	1.0 ± 1.8

morphologic observations are consistent with studies of normal humans[5] wherein the vast majority of marrow lymphocytes were B cells. Since continuing cell production in an apparent steady state implies cell death or migration out of the marrow both in rodents and in these patients and since it is not known which cells either die or migrate, it is not presently possible to determine the rates of transition from one morphologic compartment to another. Although both B-cell replication and B-cell maturation factors are produced by T cells,[12, 13] we did not test whether the B cells from these patients were T dependent or not.

When one considers only cells in DNA synthesis, plasmablasts, plasmacytic lymphocytes, and plasma cells each contribute only small numbers of newly produced cells if one assumes that DNA synthesis times are similar and that death within a compartment and migration into or out of the marrow are not greatly different among the various cell types. Furthermore, with these assumptions the fractional distribution would represent the contribution of each compartment to total cell production. The lymphocytic plasma cells were nearly 80% of the replicating cells. If there is equal division of cellular material among daughter cells, it is likely that those daughter cells would have the appearance of plasmacytic lymphocytes. The difference in numbers of DNA synthetic cells in those two compartments implies that most such cells would have to accumulate significantly more cytoplasm before they would redivide, if indeed

TABLE 5. Lymphocytic Plasma Cells—LI, by Size of Cell

Patient No.	Large	Medium	Small
1	24.0	11.5	5.4
2	37.3	11.6	10.7
3	22.9	13.5	4.4
4	49.4	12.3	2.1
5	18.5	15.3	2.5
Mean ± SD:	30.4 ± 12.7	18.8 ± 1.6	5.0 ± 3.5

they are capable of subsequent division. Perhaps the large immunoglobulin content in the plasma cells inhibits further DNA synthesis, thus explaining the few DNA synthetic cells in that category.

The differences in DNA synthesis in large, medium, and small cells within the lymphocytic plasma cell and plasma cell classes are consistent with data from leukemic blast cells,[9] where the larger cells were also more likely to be in DNA synthesis. In both cases, the average number of divisions and turnover times within the marrow cannot be determined from the available data.

SUMMARY AND CONCLUSIONS

1. In AIDS, although there is a lack of humoral responsiveness *in vitro* and *in vivo,* many patients persistently have an increased number of B cells which continue to produce increased amounts of immunoglobulin.

2. An objective, reproducible morphologic classification scheme for B cells was devised. Comparison of cell kinetic parameters in various disease states will require such a classification.

3. Although not immunologically responsive to new stimuli, the marrow B cells in the AIDS patients were shown to be replicating and turning over. The latter may be due to either death *in situ* or to migration.

4. Plasmacytic lymphocytes and lymphocytic plasma cells, morphologic transitions between lymphocytes and mature plasma cells, had the largest fractions in DNA synthesis. Because of their relative cell numbers, the lymphocytic plasma cells contained most of the cells in DNA synthesis.

5. The position of plasmablasts in the sequential compartments is unclear. Only small numbers are dividing.

6. Within a given morphologic category, large cells were more likely to be in DNA synthesis than smaller cells.

7. These studies can serve as a basis for comparison with marrow B-cell proliferation in other disease states.

REFERENCES

1. CENTERS FOR DISEASE CONTROL. 1982. Update on acquired immune deficiency syndrome (AIDS)—United States, 1982. Morbidity and Mortality Weekly Report **31:** 507-508, 513-514.
2. SIEGAL, F. P., C. LOPEZ, G. S. HAMMER, A. E. BROWN, S. J. KORNFELD, J. GOLD, J. HASSETT, S. Z. HIRSCHMAN, C. CUNNINGHAM-RUNDLES, B. R. ADELSBERG, D. M. PARHAM, M. SIEGAL, S. CUNNINGHAM-RUNDLES & D. ARMSTRONG. 1981. Severe acquired immunodeficiency in male homosexuals, manifested by chronic perianal ulcerative herpes simplex lesions. N. Engl. J. Med. **305:** 1439-1444.
3. GOTTLIEB, M. S., J. E. GROOPMAN, W. M. WEINSTEIN, J. L. FAHEY & R. DETELS. 1983. UCLA Conference: The acquired immunodeficiency syndrome. Ann. Intern. Med. **99:** 208-220.
4. LANE, H. C., H. MASUR, L. C. EDGAR, G. WHALEN, A. H. ROOK & A. S. FAUCI. 1983. Abnormalities of B-cell activation and immunoregulation in patients with the acquired immunodeficiency syndrome. N. Engl. J. Med. **309:** 453-458.
5. MELLSTEDT, H., D. KILLANDER & D. PETTERSON. 1977. Bone marrow kinetic studies on three patients with myelomatosis. Acta Med. Scand. **202:** 413-417.
6. SCHOOLEY, J. C. 1961. Autoradiographic observations of plasma cell formation. J. Immunol. **86:** 331-337.
7. SALMON, S. E. & B. A. SMITH. 1970. Immunoglobulin synthesis and total body tumor cell number in IgG multiple myeloma. J. Clin. Invest. **49:** 1114-1121.
8. KILLMANN, S. A., E. P. CRONKITE, T. M. FLIEDNER & V. P. BOND. 1962. Cell proliferation in multiple myeloma studied with tritiated thymidine in vivo. Lab. Invest. **11:** 845-853.
9. GREENBERG, M. L., A. D. CHANANA, E. P. CRONKITE, G. GIACOMELLI, K. R. RAI, L. M. SCHIFFER, P. A. STRYCKMANS & P. C. VINCENT. 1972. The generation time of human leukemic myeloblasts. Lab. Invest. **26:** 245-252.
10. BIRD, A. G., S. BRITTON, I. ERNBERG & K. NILSSON. 1981. Characteristics of Epstein-Barr virus activation of human B lymphocytes. J. Exp. Med. **154:** 832-839.
11. MCMILLAN, R., R. L. LONGMIRE, R. YELENOSKY, J. E. LANG, V. HEATH & C. G. CRADDOCK. 1972. Immunoglobulin synthesis by human lymphoid tissues: normal bone marrow as a major site of IgG production. J. Immunol. **109:** 1386-1394.
12. KINCADE, P. W. 1981. Formation of B lymphocytes in fetal and adult life. Adv. Immunol. **31:** 177-245.
13. MELCHERS, F., J. ANDERSSON, C. CORBEL, M. LEPTIN, W. LERNHARDT, W. GERHARD & J. ZEUTHEN. 1982. Regulation of B lymphocyte replication and maturation. J. Cell. Biochem. **19:** 315-332.

Bone Marrow Structure and Its Possible Significance for Hematopoietic Cell Renewal[a]

T. M. FLIEDNER, W. CALVO, V. KLINNERT,
W. NOTHDURFT, O. PRÜMMER, AND
A. RAGHAVACHAR

Department of Clinical Physiology and Occupational Medicine
University of Ulm
D-7900 Ulm / Donau, Federal Republic of Germany

INTRODUCTION

It is now nearly a quarter of a century since preparations were begun in several laboratories for a symposium on "The Kinetics of Cellular Proliferation"[1] to be held in Salt Lake City, Utah in January 1959 under the chairmanship of our unforgotten friend and colleague, the late Dr. Fred Stohlman. It turned out to be a milestone in the history of hematology since it marked the advent of a new approach to the study of hematopoietic cell renewal. The years between 1956 and 1959 were characterized by the introduction of cellular labeling by radioactive nuclides, such as tritiated thymidine, diisopropylfluorophosphate (DF^{32}P), and other compounds.[2–6] And it was at the Brookhaven National Laboratory (BNL) under the leadership and intellectual guidance of Dr. Eugene P. Cronkite, that a new conceptual thinking was introduced into the clinical, as well as experimental, approaches to the study of normal and abnormal blood cell formation. The first autoradiographs of human bone marrow smears to study the kinetics of hemopoietic cell renewal were prepared at the BNL in 1957. Dr. Cronkite opened the Salt Lake City Conference by giving a lecture on the Anatomic Hypothesis and Facts of Hemopoiesis and it was there that Dr. Victor P. Bond summarized our cell kinetic data on man.[7, 8]

A quarter of a century has passed since those most exciting days. We are happy to realize that most of us are still around to witness the scientific progress. We are here to celebrate the 70th birthday of our friend and teacher Gene Cronkite and we would like to contribute to the occasion by asking a very simple question: What have we learned about hematopoietic cellular proliferation since the Salt Lake City Conference? We would like to approach this question from the viewpoint of the bone marrow structure and function, recognizing fully that we will witness in the next few years the understanding of the functional relationship between hemopoietic replication

[a] Research supported by the Commission of the European Communities, Contract BIO-C 345-80-D Radiation Protection Programme, Contribution No. 2005, and by the Deutsche Forschungsgemeinschaft (SFB 112).

and differentiation and the microenvironment within which this unlimited self-renewal occurs.

First, we want to summarize what is known of the bone marrow structure and to suggest that the marrow composition is the result of a seeding of a cellular stroma, or matrix, by migrating hematopoietic stem cells. At the present time the first attempts are being made to characterize those factors that are produced by the microenvironmental cells to stimulate replication and differentiation. Second, we should like to summarize results of our experiments in which we use stem cell transplantation methods to establish models for the study of the *in vivo* regulation of stem cell replication and differentiation. These studies will show that it appears feasible to isolate from hemopoietic tissues those cells endowed with stem cell potentialities and to investigate the microecological conditions that may be important for the induction of replication and differentiation.

STRUCTURE AND DEVELOPMENT OF THE MARROW

There are two concepts about the genesis of the bone marrow as a hematopoietic organ. The first postulates that hemopoietic cell renewal originates from *reticular* and from *endothelial* cells and that these cell systems retain their hemopoietic potential throughout adult life, if called upon. Pioneered through the experimental work of Moore in Melbourne, Australia, and laid down best in the monograph of Metcalf and Moore[9] entitled "Haemopoietic Cells," the second concept indicates that the bone marrow matrix originates from mesenchymal cells of the embryo, particularly from the tissue around the embryonic skeletal parts, and that this matrix becomes populated by stem cells migrating from the blood into the vascularized, innervated stroma. The original source of stem cells is the extraembryonic tissues, i.e., the yolk sac and the body stalk. We have been able to provide morphological evidence for a "stem cell migration or seeding stream" from the yolk sac via fetal liver (as a transient site of stem cell amplification and restricted differentiation) to the marrow and other sites of hemopoiesis (Kelemen *et al.*[10]). Indeed, one is able to demonstrate in the fetal bone marrow a "pre-hemopoietic phase" that lasts for about 14 days in all bone studied and reminds one of a truly "aplastic marrow," consisting only of "stromal cells."[11] It is after that time that "stem cells" appear and settle in the microenvironment which is now ready to support hemopoietic cell replication and differentiation into all cell lineages while the fetal liver is restricted in its differentiation potential mostly to erythropoiesis.

The concept of the bone marrow as an organ composed of two major cellular components, the *stromal* elements and the *parenchymal* cells (erythropoietic, granulopoietic, and megakaryopoietic), was portrayed morphologically long ago, as evidenced by Maximow's textbook of 1927.[12] However, it took many years to characterize the stem cells *in vivo* and *in vitro*. The concept, however, that one is dealing with a small mononuclear cell with the properties of a stem cell, was suggested as early as 1909 in a paper by Maximow.[13] The bone marrow matrix receives a great deal of attention today, since it appears to be endowed with the functional potentiality to induce, maintain, and control replication, differentiation, maturation, and release of blood cells and their precursors. Members of the stroma cell family are presently identified morphologically as "endothelial cells," "endosteal cells," and "reticular cells."

Examples of these cells are given in the following figures, photographed from our material. In FIGURE 1 we see an endothelial cell lining a sinusoid of a rat marrow as well as a reticular cell. In FIGURE 2 the central sinus is reinforced by reticular cells and reticulin fibers which may sustain its otherwise very fragile structure. Also of interest and importance are the endosteal cells, since it is well known that hemopoietic regeneration in an aplastic bone marrow is associated regularly with early cell production along the endosteum. It is of more than passing importance to realize that the marrow shows a high degree of innervation. Calvo[14] counted almost 4000 unmyelinated nerve fibers in a cross section of the tibial marrow nerve of a 5-month-old human fetus. The nerve fibers reach all parts of the marrow and must play an

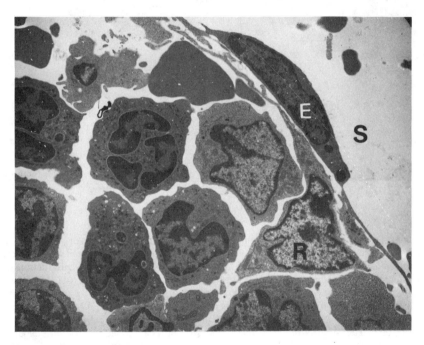

FIGURE 1. Marrow of a normal mouse showing a reticulum cell (R) with long cytoplasmic process reinforcing the endothelial cell (E) of a sinus (S). EM. (Magnification, ×3000.)

important, but still unexplored, role in hemopoietic cell renewal, a worthwhile field for future exploration.

THE ROLE OF THE MARROW STROMA IN HEMATOPOIESIS

The recent advances in the study of hemopoietic cell renewal are geared to the question of what role the stromal elements of the marrow may play. It would be too much to try to summarize all the work done in this field in order to characterize

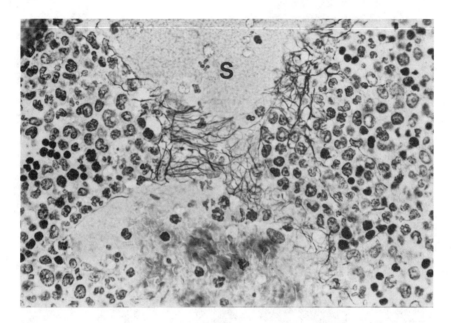

FIGURE 2. Bone marrow of a normal rat. A network of reticulum fibers reinforces the wall of the central sinus (S). Gömöri. (Original magnification, ×560; reduced to 94% of original size.)

what Trentin described as the hemopoietic inductive microenvironment. However, a few comments may be pertinent. It is now an established fact that a cell feeder layer, produced from "stroma cells" of the marrow, allows the continuous production of hemopoietic stem cells as shown by Dexter.[15] This basic experimental tool stimulated the search for the mechanisms that are operative in that system. What are the factors involved? Is a cell-to-cell interaction necessary? Which are the cells *in vivo* that are responsible *in vitro* for the induction and maintenance of stem cell replication? The work of Friedenstein *et al.*[16, 17] showed that stromal cells of the marrow are capable of maintaining hemopoietic cells cultured *in vitro* as "fibroblasts." FIGURE 3 shows a fibroblast culture prepared from stromal cells of the marrow in our group. Are the "adventitia-reticular cells" (AR cells) the important cells? If one studies these cells by means of electron microscopy, one finds that these cells have fine cytoplasmic processes extending between the hemopoietic cells and forming the important network within which cell renewal occurs. Chamberlain *et al.*[18] showed volume changes in these cells in cases of increased hemopoiesis. Around their processes there are, in particular, myelocytic cells and Trentin[19] postulated that these AR cells produce a granulocyte-macrophage colony stimulating factor (GM-CSF). On the other hand, Harigaya *et al.*[20] were able to culture stromal cells that carry the morphological and cytochemical properties of AR cells. These cells indeed seem to produce a colony stimulating factor (CSF) and prostaglandin E. They are also able to produce a labile factor that may inhibit granulopoiesis and one that may inhibit erythropoiesis. It appears quite conceivable that the stromal cells are cells that produce factors of different potentialities, depending on the local needs. The endothelial cells are part of this stroma cell concept. Several groups have investigated their potentialities to produce stimulatory and inhibitory substances. Knudtzon and Mortensen[21] showed that endothelial cells would produce a granulocyte-macrophage growth factor and also Quesenberry *et al.*[22] found colony stimulating activity in endothelial cells of the umbilical cord. Gartner and Kaplan[23] and Brennan *et al.*[24] found that endothelial cells in long-term cultures had a significant effect on hematopoiesis and that these cells produce chemically identifiable mediators of granulocytopoiesis. This, of course, leads to the question of how these capabilities of stimulatory and inhibitory activities are "turned on" or "turned off." In this context, attention should be placed on the fat cells of the marrow, which might well be "transformed" AR cells. Even these fat-containing AR cells seem to have an important function (Dexter *et al.*[25]). If serum of anemic mice is added to cultures, the "adipocytes" undergo lipolysis and lipids are released into the culture medium. This release is associated with granulopoietic and erythropoietic changes in the culture (Dexter[26]). These fat cells also play an important role in a number of other hemopoietic cell culture studies and seem to require particular attention. Gartner and Kaplan[23] showed that adipocytes are essential in the adherent cell layer for long-term culture of human bone marrow cells. If fetal calf serum (FCS) is present, these fat cells remain and are important in the maintenance of *in vitro* hemopoiesis. If horse serum is substituted for FCS, the adipocytes disappear and the adherent layer loses the capability to support hemopoiesis *in vitro* (Dexter *et al.*[26, 27]). However, too many fat cells inactivate CSF (Mendelow *et al.*[28] and Gordon *et al.*[29]).

We may summarize the "state of the arts" by saying that the search for microenvironmental mechanisms in the regulation and control of hemopoiesis and the availability of *in vitro* culture methods, as well as new approaches to characterizing regulatory factors, have opened up an entirely new field of research extending the

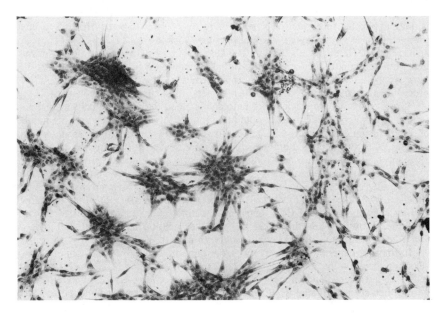

FIGURE 3. Colonies of fibroblasts cultured *in vitro*. The spindle-shaped cells form "stars" growing in all directions. May-Grünwald and Giemsa. (Original magnification, ×70; reduced to 94% of original size.)

"cell kinetic era" of hematology into the future "cell production regulation era." But, as before, the problem will be to relate *in vitro* observations to the understanding of regulation of hemopoietic cell production *in vivo*.

THE USE OF STEM CELL TRANSPLANTATION METHODS TO STUDY THE *IN VIVO* REGULATION OF STEM CELL REPLICATION AND DIFFERENTIATION

We are using dogs as our major experimental model since we think that the principles found in this species may well apply to the human situation. We collect stem cells from the dog and in the case of stem cells derived from the peripheral blood, we use leukocytapheresis after dextran sulfate mobilization.[30] A 4-hr leukapheresis is sufficient to obtain enough stem cells for hemopoietic reconstitution.[31] In the case of bone marrow stem cells, we aspirate marrow from different sites. To obtain fetal liver stem cells, we perform complete or partial hysterectomies on pregnant dogs. The cells collected are processed through a series of sedimentation procedures. In the case of blood-derived stem cells, the discontinuous albumin gradient as developed by Dicke and van Bekkum[32] has been found to be very useful. More recently, and in particular for humans, cell elutriation methods have been found to be quite adequate to isolate cells with stem cell capacity from other mononuclear cells with immunocompetence.[33, 34] Usually, we cryopreserve our cells (taken from blood, bone marrow, or fetal liver) in 10% dimethyl sulfoxide (DMSO) at $-196°C$. Our procedure, which is quite applicable to human cells, gives us recovery rates of better than 85 to 90%, if the content of granulocyte-macrophage colony forming units (GM-CFU) is used as an indicator.[35] The stem cells from these different sources are transfused (after thawing) into radiation-conditioned recipients. Initially, we used a total body dose of 12 Gy. Now we use a fractionated conditioning procedure of 3×6 Gy on alternate days, a procedure that gives very good results with fetal liver stem cell transfusions.

If one compares the efficiency of autologous blood-derived stem cells with that of stem cells from bone marrow, one obtains an interesting result, if one uses the number of colony forming units (GM-CFU) in culture present in the transfusate as an indicator of stem cell activity. If equal numbers of GM-CFU are in the transfusates, the animals receiving blood stem cells show a much faster early granulocyte recovery, compared to those receiving bone marrow.[36, 37] A histological evaluation supports this notion: 10 days after cell transfusion, the recipients of blood-derived stem cells show the best bone marrow cellularity (FIGURE 4). It is of interest to also note that the blood-derived cells showing GM-CFU potential are much more radiosensitive than those from the marrow. While the blood GM-CFU population has a D_0 of 26.1 rad, we find a bone marrow GM-CFU population with a D_0 of 60.0 rad.[38]

In another experiment we separated the bone marrow GM-CFU population by velocity sedimentation into small (II) (< 5.2 mm/hr) and large (III) (> 7.0 mm/hr) cells and injected equal numbers of autologous, cryopreserved GM-CFU from the unseparated suspension and from the separated suspension containing small and large mononuclear cells. The transfusion of small mononuclear cells gives the same results as unseparated cells (a speedy recovery), while the GM-CFU contained in the large fraction do not indicate the presence of repopulating stem cells (FIGURE 5). The same holds true with respect to lymphocyte and platelet regeneration.

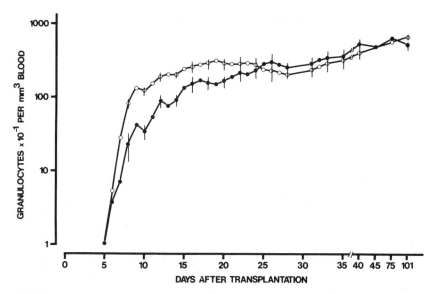

FIGURE 4. Pattern of reappearance of granulocytes in the peripheral blood of dogs after 3 ×
6 Gy of TBI and autotransfusion of equal numbers of GM-CFU from peripheral blood and bone
marrow. Source of autograft: ○, peripheral blood; ●, bone marrow.

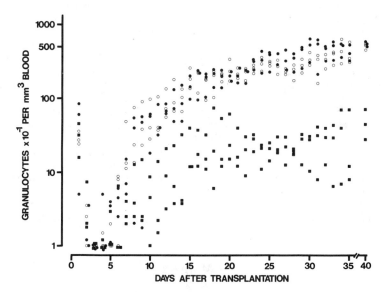

FIGURE 5. Pattern of reappearance of granulocytes in the peripheral blood of dogs after 3 ×
6 Gy of TBI and autotransfusion of equal numbers of GM-CFU from unseparated bone marrow
(○), small bone marrow MNC (●), and large bone marrow MNC (■).

From these results, we conclude that in the bone marrow there is a heterogenous population of GM-CFU with a wide range of velocity sedimentation rates indicating various cell sizes. And it is only the fraction of GM-CFU containing "small" mono-nuclear cells that also has the repopulating stem cells in it. It is of interest in this context that only a population of "small" GM-CFU is released into the peripheral blood. It is only after long-term leukapheresis that the velocity sedimentation profile of GM-CFU acquires the spectrum of normal bone marrow GM-CFU.

Thus we conclude that there are more pluripotent stem cells per GM-CFU in the blood than in the marrow and that this is the reason for the relatively slow regeneration of hemopoiesis if equal numbers of GM-CFU from blood and marrow are compared.

If one now compares hemopoietic reconstitution obtained from bone marrow and blood-derived stem cells with that obtained from fetal liver (FIGURE 6), one finds that fetal liver-derived cells give the best results, not so much in the early phase, but beyond 20 days. Very early, the bone marrow GM-CFU return to normal, while the blood GM-CFU population actually shows an overshoot, as compared to normal. These fetal liver stem cell transplantations were performed in dogs that were bred for this purpose. We made sure that dog leukocyte antigen (DLA)-identical dogs were paired. Two strategies were then used. The first strategy produced recipient dogs from the first pregnancy. During the second pregnancy, the fetal dogs were obtained on day 52 and their livers were removed and cryopreserved. In the second strategy, a partial hysterectomy was performed to obtain fetal liver for grafting, while the rest of the uterus was left in situ and normal delivery was obtained. None of these irradiated recipients of fetal liver cells required an immunosuppressive regimen and no severe graft-versus-host disease (GVHD) was observed.[39]

These results compare well with our earlier data on leukocyte transfusion. If one uses blood-derived stem cells, separated by the discontinuous albumin gradient (fraction 2 cells), then one finds a rapid hemopoietic regeneration without GVHD if allogeneic although DLA-identical cells are used. In contrast, the transfusion of cells from fractions 3 and 4 results in a severe GVHD. The granulocytic recovery correlates well with the number of GM-CFU present in the transfusate.[40]

We asked initially: What have we learned about hematopoietic cellular proliferation during the 25 years since the milestone set by the Salt Lake City Conference in 1959?

We are witnessing a new era of hemopoietic research, characterized by the opportunity to study mechanisms that control hemopoietic stem cell replication and differentiation.

We recognize now that this process of replication and differentiation requires an intricate interplay between a potent stem cell on the one hand and a microenvironment on the other, capable of modulating the stem cell response as required.

Although in vitro techniques are very important for studying these regulatory interplays between "adherent cells" and "stem cells," we think that refined cell transplantation techniques will allow us to answer the question of how this regulation occurs in vivo, allowing a cellular homeostasis from day to day. Also, one may well expect that progress in this field will allow us to understand the mechanism behind disturbed homeostasis as seen in leukemia and other hemopoietic disorders.

SUMMARY

The authors review the progress made during the last quarter of a century in the fields of hematopoietic cellular proliferation and differentiation in relation to the bone

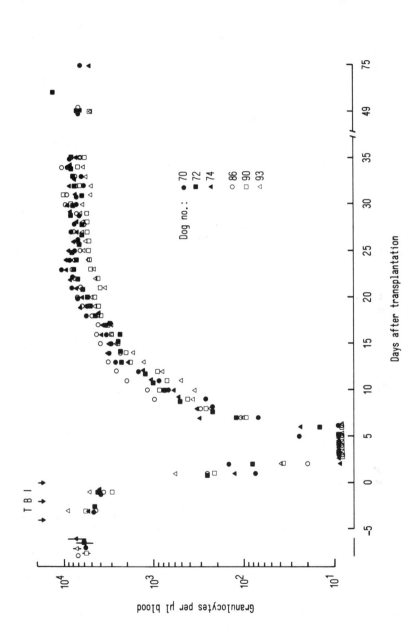

FIGURE 6. Regeneration of circulating granulocytes after 3 × 6 Gy TBI and transfusion of cryopreserved fetal liver cells from DLA-identical sibling dogs. GM-CFU content ranged from 0.9 × 10⁴ to 6.3 × 10⁴ GM-CFU per kg body weight.

marrow structure and the microenvironment provided by the marrow stroma in which unlimited self-renewal occurs.

The marrow is conceived of as an organ in which the stroma originates from local mesenchymal elements which form a vascularized and innervated matrix, seeded later by blood-borne stem cells.

Transplantation studies using total-body-irradiated dogs show that stem cells derived from the marrow, as well as those from the blood and from the fetal liver, are able to repopulate a marrow rendered aplastic by irradiation.

By grafting equal numbers of GM-CFU from peripheral blood and bone marrow, a faster hemopoietic reconstitution is provided by blood-derived stem cells. The most efficient stem cells in the long range are those derived from fetal liver.

Bone marrow and peripheral blood GM-CFU differ in some *in vitro* characteristics such as radiation sensitivity. These peripheral blood cells are more radiosensitive than those derived from the marrow.

Autografting of bone marrow mononuclear cell fractions obtained by velocity sedimentation techniques demonstrates that the fraction of small mononuclear cells holds a repopulating potential similar to that of circulating blood stem cells. The cells collected in fraction 2 of a discontinuous albumin gradient contain most of the blood stem cells and repopulate the marrow without causing GVHD, while cells collected in fractions 3 and 4 contain a minimal amount of stem cells and cause severe GVHD.

REFERENCES

1. STOHLMAN, F., JR. (Ed.). 1959. The Kinetics of Cellular Proliferation. Grune & Stratton. New York, N.Y.
2. MESSIER, B. 1959. Histological localization of newly-formed deoxyribonucleic acid by means of tritium-labelled thymidine. *In* Proceedings of the 3rd Canadian Cancer Research Conference. R. W. Begg, Ed. Academic Press. New York, N.Y.
3. HUGHES, W. L., V. P. BOND, G. BRECHER, E. P. CRONKITE, R. P. PAINTER, H. QUASTLER & F. G. SHERMAN. 1958. Cellular proliferation in the mouse as revealed by autoradiography with tritiated thymidine. Proc. Natl. Acad. Sci. USA **44:** 476-483.
4. CRONKITE, E. P., V. P. BOND, T. M. FLIEDNER & J. R. RUBINI. 1959. The use of tritiated thymidine in the study of DNA synthesis and cell turnover in hemopoietic tissues. Lab. Invest. **8:** 263-275.
5. CRONKITE, E. P., T. M. FLIEDNER, V. P. BOND, J. R. RUBINI, G. BRECHER & H. QUASTLER. 1959. Dynamics of hemopoietic proliferation in man and mice studied by H^3-thymidine incorporation into DNA. *In* Proceedings of the 2nd Geneva Conference on Peaceful Uses of Atomic Energy. Pp. 190-208. Pergamon Press. London, England.
6. ATHENS, J. W., A. M. MAURER, H. ASHENBRUCKER, G. E. CARTWRIGHT & M. M. WINTROBE. 1959. Leukokinetic studies: a method for labeling leukocytes with diisopropylfluorophosphate (DFP[32]). Blood **14:** 303-333.
7. CRONKITE, E. P., T. M. FLIEDNER, V. P. BOND & J. S. ROBERTSON. 1959. Anatomic and physiologic facts and hypotheses about hemopoietic proliferation systems. *In* The Kinetics of Cellular Proliferation. F. Stohlman, Ed.: 1-14. Grune & Stratton. New York, N.Y.
8. BOND, V. P., T. M. FLIEDNER, E. P. CRONKITE, J. R. RUBINI & J. S. ROBERTSON. 1959. Cell turnover in blood and in blood-forming tissues studied with tritiated thymidine. *In* The Kinetics of Cellular Proliferation. F. Stohlman, Ed.: 188-200. Grune & Stratton. New York, N.Y.
9. METCALF, D. & M. A. S. MOORE. 1971. Haemopoietic Cells. North-Holland. Amsterdam, the Netherlands.
10. KELEMEN, E., W. CALVO & T. M. FLIEDNER. 1979. Atlas of Human Hemopoietic Development. Springer-Verlag. Heidelberg, FRG.

11. FLIEDNER, T. M. & W. CALVO. 1978. Hematopoietic stem cell seeding of a cellular matrix: a principle of initiation and regeneration of hematopoiesis. *In* Differentiation of Normal and Neoplastic Hematopoietic Cells. B. Clarkson, P. A. Marks & J. E. Till, Eds.: 757-773. Cold Spring Harbor Laboratory. Cold Spring Harbor, N.Y.

12. MAXIMOW, A. 1927. Bindegewebe und blutbildende Organe. *In* Handbuch der mikroskopischen Anatomie des Menschen, Bd. 2/1. V. Möllendorf, Ed. Springer-Verlag. Berlin, Germany.

13. MAXIMOW, A. 1909. Der Lymphozyt als gemeinsame Stammzelle der verschiedenen Blutelemente in der embryonalen Entwicklung und im postfoetalen Leben der Säugetiere. Folia Haematol. (Leipzig) **8:** 125-134.

14. CALVO, W. 1981. Bone marrow hemopoiesis in the human fetus. *In* Advances in Physiological Sciences. Vol. 6. Genetics, Structure and Function of Blood Cells. S. R. Hollan, G. Gardos & B. Sarkadi, Eds.: 65-68. Akademiai Kiadó. Budapest, Hungary.

15. DEXTER, T. M. 1977. Regulation of hemopoietic stem cell proliferation in long-term bone marrow cultures. Biomedicine **27:** 344-349.

16. FREIDENSTEIN, A. J., R. K. CHAILAKHJAN & K. S. LALYKINA. 1970. The development of fibroblast colonies in monolayer cultures of guinea-pig bone marrow and spleen cells. Cell Tissue Kinet. **3:** 393-403.

17. FRIEDENSTEIN, A. J., R. K. CHAILAKHJAN, N. V. LATSINIK, A. F. PANASYNK & I. V. KEILISS-BOROK. 1974. Stromal cells responsible for transferring the microenvironment of hemopoietic tissues. Transplantation **17:** 331-340.

18. CHAMBERLAIN, J. K., P. F. LEBLOND & R. I. WEED. 1975. Reduction of adventitial cell cover: an early direct effect of erythropoietin on bone marrow ultrastructure. Blood Cells **1:** 655-674.

19. TRENTIN, J. J. 1978. Hemopoietic microenvironments. Transplant. Proc. **10:** 77-82.

20. HARIGAYA, K., E. P. CRONKITE, M. E. MILLER & R. K. SHADDUCK. 1981. Murine bone marrow cell line producing colony stimulating factor. Proc. Natl. Acad. Sci. USA **78:** 6963-6966.

21. KNUDTZON, S. & B. T. MORTENSEN. 1975. Growth stimulation of human bone marrow cells in agar culture by vascular cells. Blood **46:** 937-943.

22. QUESENBERRY, P. J., M. A. GIMBRONE, JR. & M. S. McDONALD. 1978. Endothelial derived colony stimulating activity. Exp. Hematol. 6(Suppl. 3): 4. (Abstract.)

23. GARTNER, S. & H. S. KAPLAN. 1980. Long-term culture of human bone marrow cells. Proc. Natl. Acad. Sci. USA 77(8): 4756-4759.

24. BRENNAN, J. K., M. A. LICHTMAN, J. F. DIPERSIO & C. N. ABBOUD. 1980. Chemical mediators of granulopoiesis. Exp. Hematol. **8:** 441-464.

25. DEXTER, T. M., T. D. ALLEN & L. G. LAJTHA. 1977. Conditions controlling the proliferation of hemopoietic stem cells in vitro. J. Cell. Physiol. **91:** 335-344.

26. DEXTER, T. M. 1982. Stromal cell associated hemopoiesis. J. Cell. Physiol. Suppl. **1:** 87-94.

27. DEXTER, T. M., E. SPOONCER, D. TOKSOZ & L. G. LAJTHA. 1980. The role of cells and their products in the regulation of in vitro stem cell proliferation and granulocyte development. J. Supramol. Struct. **13:** 513-524.

28. MENDELOW, B., D. GROBICKI, M. DE LA HUNT, J. KATZ & J. METZ. 1980. Characterization of bone marrow stromal cells in suspension and monolayer cultures. Br. J. Haematol. **46:** 15-22.

29. GORDON, M. Y., J. A. KING & E. C. GORDON-SMITH. 1980. Bone marrow fibroblasts, fat cells and colony stimulating activity. Br. J. Haematol. **46:** 151-152.

30. FLIEDNER, T. M., W. CALVO, M. KÖRBLING, H. KREUTZMANN, W. NOTHDURFT, W. ROSS & D. VASILEVA. 1978. Hematopoietic stem cells in blood: characteristics and potentials. *In* Hematopoietic Cell Differentiation. D. W. Golde, M. S. Cline, D. Metcalf & C. F. Fox, Eds.: 193-212. Academic Press. New York, N.Y.

31. FLIEDNER, T. M., W. CALVO, M. KÖRBLING, W. NOTHDURFT, H. PFLIEGER & W. ROSS. 1979. Collection, storage and transfusion of blood stem cells for the treatment of hemopoietic failure. Blood Cells **5:** 313-328.

32. DICKE, K. A. & D. W. VAN BEKKUM. 1970. Avoidance of acute secondary disease by purification of haematopoietic stem-cells with density gradient centrifugation. Exp. Hematol. **20:** 126-130.

33. WITTE, T. DE., E. SCHELTINGA-KOEKMAN, A. PLAS, G. GLANKENBORG, M. SALDEN, J. WESSELS & C. HAANEN. 1982. Enrichment of myeloid clonogenic cells by isopycnic density equilibrium centrifugation in percoll gradients and counterflow centrifugation. Stem Cells 2: 308-320.

34. MARTIN, H., M. NEUMANN, I. FACHE, T. M. FLIEDNER & H. PFLIEGER. 1985. Gradient separation of granulocytic progenitor cells (CFU-C) from human blood mononuclear leukocytes. Exp. Hematol. 13: 79-86.

35. KÖRBLING, M., T. M. FLIEDNER, E. RÜBER & H. PFLIEGER. 1980. Description of a closed plastic bag system for the collection and cryopreservation of leukapheresis-derived blood mononuclear leukocytes and CFU-C from human donors. Transfusion 20: 293-300.

36. RAGHAVACHAR, A., O. PRÜMMER, T. M. FLIEDNER & K. H. STEINBACH. 1983. Progenitor cell (CFU-C) reconstitution after autologous stem cell transfusion in lethally irradiated dogs: decreased CFU-C populations in blood and bone marrow correlate with the fraction mobilizable by dextran sulphate. Exp. Hematol. 11: 996-1004.

37. RAGHAVACHAR, A., O. PRÜMMER, T. M. FLIEDNER, W. CALVO & I. STEINBACH. 1983. Stem cells from peripheral blood and bone marrow: a comparative evaluation of the hemopoietic potential in the dog. Int. J. Cell Cloning 1: 191-205.

38. NOTHDURFT, W., K. H. STEINBACH & T. M. FLIEDNER. 1983. In vitro studies on the sensitivity of canine granulopoietic progenitor cells (GM-CFC) to ionizing radiation: differences between steady state GM-CFC from blood and bone marrow. Int. J. Radiat. Biol. 43: 133-140.

39. PRÜMMER, O., A. RAGHAVACHAR, W. CALVO, F. CARBONELL & T. M. FLIEDNER. 1983. Restoration of hemopoiesis by cryopreserved fetal liver cells in a canine model. In Recent Advances in Bone Marrow Transplantation. UCLA Symposia on Molecular and Cellular Biology. New Series, Vol. 7. R. P. Gale, Ed.: 857-863. Alan R. Liss, Inc. New York, N.Y.

40. KÖRBLING, M., T. M. FLIEDNER, W. CALVO, W. M. ROSS, W. NOTHDURFT, I. STEINBACH, I. FACHE & E. RÜBER. 1979. Albumin density gradient purification of canine hemopoietic blood stem cells (HBSC): long-term allogeneic engraftment without GVH-reaction. Exp. Hematol. 7: 277-288.

Lactoferrin: Its Role as a Regulator of Human Granulopoiesis?[a]

A. DELFORGE,[b,c] P. STRYCKMANS,[c] J. P. PRIEELS,[d]
C. BIEVA,[c] E. RONGÉ-COLLARD,[c] J. SCHLUSSELBERG,[d]
AND A. EFIRA[c]

[c]Service de Médecine Interne et
Laboratoire d'Investigation Clinique H. Tagnon
Institut J. Bordet
Brussels, Belgium

[d]Laboratoire de Chimie Générale
Université Libre de Bruxelles
Brussels, Belgium

INTRODUCTION

Previous reports have shown that granulocyte production is regulated by feedback mechanisms. Two groups of factors are implicated in this regulation *in vitro*. The first group, the colony stimulating activity (CSA), stimulates granulocyte and macrophage production *in vitro*. It is heterogenous and identified as glycoproteins produced by monocytes, stimulated lymphocytes, or placental cells.[1-4] The other group of factors, one of which is produced by mature polymorphonuclears,[5-7] inhibits granulocyte-monocyte progenitor (CFU-GM) growth. One of these factors has been identified as a glycoprotein inhibiting the CSA production by the monocytes/macrophages. It has been claimed that this glycoprotein is lactoferrin, an iron-binding glycoprotein first isolated from milk and also produced by mature polymorphonuclears.[8] Iron-saturated lactoferrin has been proposed by Broxmeyer to decrease both granulocyte and macrophage colony formation *in vitro* by inhibiting the monocyte CSA production. Human lactoferrin was shown in a murine system to inhibit granulopoiesis *in vivo* as well.[9] This view though has not been confirmed when using murine lactoferrin in a murine culture assay.[10] Recently Bagby *et al.* have shown that lactoferrin does not act directly on the CSA production by the monocytes but rather inhibits the production or release by monocytes of some factors which stimulate T-lymphocyte or fibroblast CSA production.[11,12]

We have tested the effect of lactoferrin from 10^{-18} to 10^{-8} M on the human marrow CFU-GM growth. No inhibitory activity of lactoferrin whether or not it was saturated with iron, was observed on the production of monocyte CSA.

[a]Supported by a fellowship from Pétrofina S.A., Belgium and by Euratom Grant 161-761-B10B.

[b]Address for correspondence: A. Delforge, Service d'Hématologie, Institut J. Bordet, 1, rue Héger-Bordet, Brussels, Belgium.

MATERIALS AND METHODS

Target Cell Separation

Bone marrows were obtained from normal subjects or from patients without hematological disease. Marrow cells were obtained by needle aspiration from the posterior iliac crest and anticoagulated with 10 units/ml preservative-free heparin (Upjohn Company, Kalamazoo, Mich.).

The mononucleated cell fraction was obtained by density cut gradient ($d = 1.077$ g/cm^3) on Ficoll-Hypaque (centrifugation, 20 min at $800 \times g$) or on bovine serum albumin (centrifugation, 10 min at $3000 \times g$). The mononucleated cells were removed and washed twice with Dulbecco's medium (GIBCO, Grand Island, N.Y.).

The non-adherent cell fraction containing the CFU-GM was separated from the monocytes producing the CSA by adherence to plastic. The mononucleated cells were submitted to adherence for 90 min on plastic dishes (Falcon 3033) in Dulbecco's medium containing 10% fetal calf serum (FCS).

CSA Production

CSA was produced either by feeder layers of normal peripheral blood mononucleated cells separated by density cut gradient as described above, or by endogenous marrow CSA-producing cells (spontaneous growth).

For exogenous stimulation, 0.5×10^6 mononucleated blood cells were plated in 1 ml Dulbecco's medium with 20% FCS and 0.6% agar and incubated for 2-3 days in 7.5% CO_2, 100% humidity at 37°C before assay. In some experiments, indomethacin (Merck Sharpe & Dohme, West Point, Pa.) at 10^{-6} M was added to the feeder layers to prevent the endogenous production of prostaglandin E_2 (PGE_2) by the monocytes.

Conditioned media were obtained after incubation of 1×10^6 mononucleated blood cells in Dulbecco's medium supplemented with 20% FCS. Conditioned medium was used as a 10% concentration to stimulate the CFU-GM growth. Iron-saturated human lactoferrin at concentrations ranging from 10^{-18} to 10^{-8} M was added to the feeder layers or to the conditioned medium.

CFU-GM Assay

For the exogenous stimulated CFU-GM growth, 1×10^5 nonadherent mononucleated cells were plated in 35-mm petri dishes (Sterrilin, Teddington, England) above a feeder layer of 0.5 or 1×10^6 normal peripheral mononucleated cells. For spontaneous growth, 3×10^5 mononucleated marrow cells were plated in 1 ml culture medium without exogenous CSA.

Before plating, marrow cells were placed in Dulbecco's medium containing 20% FCS and 0.3% agar. The plates were incubated 12 days for the spontaneous CFU-GM growth and 7 days for the exogenously stimulated CFU-GM assay in a 100% humidified incubator containing 7.5% CO_2 and at 37°C (Forma, Marietta, Ohio).

Colonies of more than 40 cells and clusters (3 to 39 cells) were scored using an inverted microscope at a 40-fold magnification (Olympus, Tokyo, Japan).

Leukemic Inhibitory Activity (LIA) Preparation

The peripheral blood leukemic blasts of three patients with acute nonlymphoblastic leukemia were used. LIA was obtained by incubation of 1×10^6 leukemic cells in Dulbecco's medium without FCS for 4 hr at 37°C, 7.5% CO_2, and 100% humidity. After incubation, the conditioned medium was centrifuged; the cells were discarded while the conditioned medium was stored at $-20°C$ until used. It was used in the culture assay at 10% to evaluate its inhibiting activity on normal CFU-GM growth.[13]

Purification of Human and Bovine Lactoferrin

Lactoferrin was obtained from two different sources. One lactoferrin was isolated from human milk by the method described by Querinjean *et al.*[14] The protein was homogeneous as judged by sodium dodecyl sulfate-polyacrylamide gel electrophoresis (SDS-PAGE), ion exchange chromatography on CM Sepharose 4B, and gel filtration with Sephadex G-100. The other human lactoferrin was provided by Dr. H. E. Broxmeyer (Memorial Sloan-Kettering Cancer Center, New York, N.Y.). Human lactoferrin was saturated with iron using the procedure described by Masson *et al.*[15] Bovine lactoferrin was purified as described by Castellino *et al.*[16]

Depletion of FCS from Endogenous Bovine Lactoferrin

Antiserum Preparation

Three rabbits were given three intramuscular injections of 1 mg of bovine lactoferrin with Freund's complete adjuvant at 2-week intervals. After 6 to 8 weeks, the rabbits were bled and the antibody was tested for specificity against normal calf serum and bovine lactoferrin by immunoelectrophoresis on 1% agar plates. A single precipitation line was observed with bovine lactoferrin, while no precipitation was observed with immunoadsorbed FCS.

Immunoadsorbent Preparation

Cyanogen bromide-activated (CNBr) Sepharose 4B was swollen and washed with 1 mM HCl. The anti-lactoferrin serum was coupled in large excess to the Sepharose at a ratio of 50 mg of protein to 5 ml of gel to ensure the removal of the entire lactoferrin content of the FCS. After washing with $NaHCO_3$ buffer, the immunoadsorbent was incubated with ethanolamine solution for 2 hr at room temperature and finally washed in a large amount of $NaHCO_3$ buffer, at pH 8.3, containing 0.5 M NaCl; 75 ml of FCS was passed through the column at a slow rate at room temperature. The column was then washed until no more protein was monitored at 280 nm by the Uvicord cell (LKB, Bromma, Sweden). Pure lactoferrin was eluted at acidic pH. The bovine lactoferrin-depleted serum was lyophilized and reconstituted exactly to the original volume. A control nonimmunoadsorbed FCS went through the same procedure using a CNBr-activated Sepharose without coupled antibody which caused no significant loss of CFU-GM.

RESULTS

The capacity of lactoferrin to inhibit the CFU-GM growth by decreasing the CSA production by the monocytes was first tested in an endogenously stimulated CFU-GM assay. Mononucleated marrow cells (3×10^5) were plated with iron-saturated lactoferrin at concentrations ranging from 10^{-18} to 10^{-8} M. In this assay, the marrow CFU-GM growth was stimulated by the endogenous monocytes present in the marrow sample. As shown in FIGURE 1, lactoferrin isolated from human milk failed to inhibit the CFU-GM growth of 14 normal marrows. In this experiment, 7 marrows were plated with the lactoferrin isolated in our laboratory and 7 other marrows were plated with the lactoferrin provided by Dr. Broxmeyer. As shown also on this figure, no inhibitory activity was observed no matter what batch of lactoferrin was used.

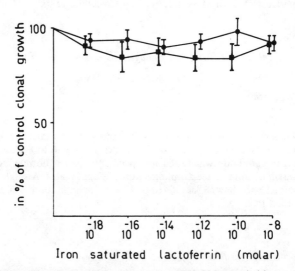

FIGURE 1. Effect of lactoferrin on the spontaneous CFU-GM growth (clusters and colonies). Results were expressed as the percentage of control growth of 14 marrows plated either with our lactoferrin ($n = 7$) (●) or with the lactoferrin provided by Dr. Broxmeyer ($n = 7$) (■). Vertical brackets represent ± 1 SEM. These 14 marrows produced 48–269 (median, 132) clones per 3×10^5 mononucleated cells.

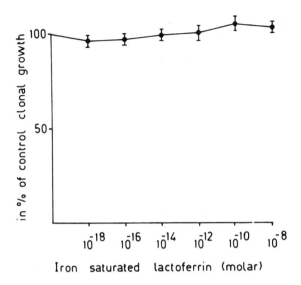

FIGURE 2. Effect of lactoferrin on the exogenously stimulated CFU-GM growth of five normal marrows depleted of adherent cells. CSA was produced by feeder layers of 0.5 or 1×10^6 normal mononucleated cells containing the different concentrations of lactoferrin. Vertical brackets represent $\pm$ 1 SEM. These five marrows produced 64-164 (median, 75) clones per 10^5 bone marrow cells depleted of adherent cells.

On the other hand, to investigate the effect of lactoferrin in an exogenously stimulated CFU-GM assay, a feeder layer assay was used. In this system the marrow CFU-GM growth was stimulated by CSA produced by 0.5 or 1×10^6 normal blood mononucleated cells present in a feeder layer containing either no lactoferrin or lactoferrin at concentrations ranging from 10^{-18} to 10^{-8} M. As shown in FIGURE 2, the CFU-GM growth of 10^5 nonadherent low-density marrow cells obtained from five normal subjects was not affected by including lactoferrin in the monocyte feeder layer; the results were the same whether clusters and colonies or colonies alone were considered. In two different experiments (not shown), lactoferrin was added to feeder layers of monocytes prepared in McCoy's 5 A medium. When McCoy's 5 A medium was used instead of Dulbecco's medium, no inhibitory activity of lactoferrin was observed for all the concentrations tested.

Indomethacin at 10^{-6} M was added to the feeder layers to inhibit the endogenous production of PGE_2 by the monocytes. As shown in FIGURE 3, monocytes incubated in feeder layers containing lactoferrin and indomethacin did not produce less CSA than controls without lactoferrin or without indomethacin.

The capacity of lactoferrin to inhibit the CSA production in conditioned medium was investigated by incubating 1×10^6 mononucleated peripheral blood cells with or without lactoferrin at 10^{-8} M for 3 days in liquid culture medium containing 20% fetal calf serum. As shown in TABLE 1, the stimulatory activity of five conditioned media incubated with lactoferrin was assayed on the CFU-GM growth of 1×10^5 normal nonadherent mononucleated marrow cells. In these five successive experiments, conditioned medium incubated with lactoferrin yielded for clusters and colonies, respectively, 101 and 124% of the control values.

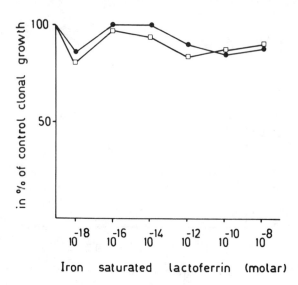

FIGURE 3. Effect of lactoferrin on the exogenously stimulated CFU-GM growth. CSA was produced by feeder layers of 0.5 or 1×10^6 normal peripheral mononucleated cells incubated with (●) or without (□) indomethacin at 1×10^{-6} M. This marrow produced 96 clones per 10^5 mononucleated cells.

To ascertain that the inhibitory effect of lactoferrin could not be modified by the method used to separate the low-density mononucleated cells, separation of the blood and marrow cells was carried out either on Ficoll-Hypaque or on bovine serum albumin (BSA). In one experiment (not shown), both methods of cell separation were tested on the same marrow cells. These two methods gave identical results, i.e., absence of inhibitory effect of lactoferrin at 10^{-8} M on the CFU-GM growth: 84 and 93% of the control growth were recovered when, respectively, Ficoll-Hypaque and BSA were used to separate the mononucleated cell population.

TABLE 1. Colony Stimulating Activity[a] of Five Different Conditioned Media (CM) Prepared by Incubating Mononucleated Blood Cells with Lactoferrin at 1×10^{-8} M

	Percentage of Control CM		
CM No.	Clusters	Colonies	Clusters & Colonies
1	108	96	105
2	99	115	106
3	100	153	117
4	106	113	108
5	95	124	105
Mean ± SEM:	101 ± 3	124 ± 9	109 ± 4

[a] 0.1 ml of CM was added to a normal marrow producing 321 clones per 10^5 nonadherent cells in the presence of control CM.

In three experiments, as shown in TABLE 2, when LIA obtained after incubation of leukemic blasts from three leukemic patients was added to the culture a significant inhibition of around 50% was observed for the three LIA samples tested.

The ability of lactoferrin to fix spontaneously to plastic was investigated since lactoferrin is known to have certain affinity to plastic compounds. A fixed amount of ^{125}I-labeled lactoferrin was mixed with various amounts of unlabeled lactoferrin in order to obtain concentrations of lactoferrin ranging from 10^{-11} to 10^{-8} M and incubated in Dulbecco's medium with 20% fetal calf serum in plastic tubes for 3 hr. As shown in TABLE 3, the fixation of lactoferrin to plastic never exceeded 1% of the amount of ^{125}I-lactoferrin placed for 3 hr in each tube no matter what amount of unlabeled lactoferrin was added. The fixation of lactoferrin did not exceed 3% when the time of incubation was increased up to 6 days.

In one experiment bovine lactoferrin was removed from FCS by affinity chromatography using a rabbit anti-bovine lactoferrin antibody. As shown in FIGURE 4, no inhibitory effect of lactoferrin at the two concentrations tested (10^{-14} and 10^{-8} M) was seen whether endogenous lactoferrin-depleted FCS or control FCS was used to culture nonadherent bone marrow cells.

TABLE 2. Leukemic Inhibiting Activity (LIA) on CFU-GM Growth

FAB Type of Leukemia[a]	Clones[b]		Inhibition (% of Control without LIA)	p^c
	Without LIA	With LIA		
M3	303 ± 13	117 ± 13	61	0.0006
M5	95 ± 11	47 ± 2	51	0.01
M4	233 ± 15	111 ± 7	52	0.002

[a] FAB: French-American-British classification of the acute leukemias.[27]

[b] Clusters and colonies (mean ± SEM) per 1×10^5 mononucleated cells plated of one normal marrow.

[c] *p*: Student's *t* test.

DISCUSSION

Mature granulocytes have been associated with feedback regulation of granulopoiesis *in vitro*. Two possible modes of action may be investigated to explain this inhibitory effect of mature polymorphonuclear cells (PMN) on the proliferation of the granulocyte-macrophage stem cells (CFU-GM). Agents produced by PMN could either inhibit directly the proliferation capacity of the CFU-GM, or abolish the production of CSA by the monocytes or other CSA-producing cells.[17-19] Recent studies have proposed that lactoferrin, an iron-binding glycoprotein isolated from milk but also present in the secondary granules of mature polymorphonuclears, was able to regulate the CSA production by acting on monocytes and macrophages.[8]

We have tested the effect of pure human lactoferrin at concentrations ranging from 10^{-18} to 10^{-8} M on the endogenously stimulated CFU-GM growth without observing any inhibitory effect of the two different batches of lactoferrin tested. The effect of lactoferrin was then tested on exogenously stimulated CFU-GM growth; the

CSA was produced in this assay either by feeder layers or in conditioned medium of normal peripheral monocytes incubated with or without lactoferrin. Using this system, lactoferrin at all the concentrations tested failed to inhibit the CFU-GM growth, thus probably to decrease the production of CSA by the monocytes present in the feeder layers.

To rule out the hypothesis that PGE_2, a known inhibitor of CFU-GM growth,[20] was masking the effect of lactoferrin by already maximally inhibiting the CFU-GM, the monocytes used for the preparation of CSA conditioned medium were incubated simultaneously in the presence of indomethacin, an inhibitor of prostaglandin synthetase. This hypothesis can be ruled out since even in the presence of indomethacin (at 10^{-6} M) an inhibiting effect of lactoferrin, as the one described by Broxmeyer, was not observed.

The discrepancy between our results and those of Broxmeyer is difficult to explain because the culture assay was the same. Experiments using McCoy's 5 A medium instead of Dulbecco's medium were carried out to exclude any masking effect due to the different compositions of these media, since Dulbecco's medium contains iron salts which are not present in McCoy's 5 A medium. Different cell separation methods were then compared to ascertain that the cell separation could not modify the cell physiology and mask the effect of lactoferrin by selecting a subpopulation of monocytes insensitive to lactoferrin. Indeed, Broxmeyer et al. have shown previously that lactoferrin acts only on a monocyte subpopulation carrying the Ia antigen; both Ia+ and Ia− monocytes are producing CSA, but Ia− monocyte subpopulation is not inhibited by lactoferrin.[21] The uniformly negative results, no matter what cell separation procedure was used, make it unlikely that a selection of monocytes had taken place.

As opposed to the complete absence of inhibition in the present study, Bagby et al. have observed an inhibitory effect of lactoferrin at low concentrations (10^{-17} to 10^{-11} M) but not at doses greater than 10^{-10} M.[11] This observation was explained by a possible aggregation or polymerization of lactoferrin molecules at high concentrations in the presence of Ca^{2+} (10 mM).[22] This hypothesis could not explain the discrepancy between our results and those of Broxmeyer seeing that (a) the Ca^{2+} concentration in the culture medium was within the physiological range around 1 mM thus 10 times lower than the Ca^{2+} concentration which induces lactoferrin aggregation, and (b) aggregation did not occur at lactoferrin concentrations lower than 10^{-10} M.

Bagby has proposed that lactoferrin could suppress the production or release by monocytes of factors which could stimulate T lymphocytes to produce CSA. In this

TABLE 3. Effect of Concentration and Incubation Time of Lactoferrin (LF) on Its Binding to Plastic Labware

Lactoferrin Concentration (M)	Incubation Time (hr)	^{125}I-LF Binding to Plastic	
		cpm	% of Total cpm
10^{-8}	3	242	0.1% of 59,211
10^{-9}	3	544	0.91
10^{-10}	3	538	0.90
10^{-11}	3	604	1.02
10^{-10}	24	1294	2.8% of 57,226
10^{-10}	48	1088	1.9
10^{-10}	96	1107	1.9
10^{-10}	144	1072	1.9

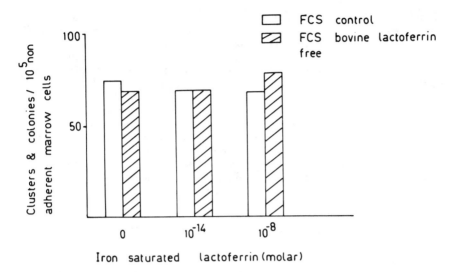

FIGURE 4. Comparison of the effects of lactoferrin on the growth of clusters and colonies in culture assays with or without lactoferrin-depleted fetal calf serum. When only colonies were considered, the results were similar (data not shown).

perspective, it is important to remember that all the experiments on monocyte CSA production in the present work were made on the mononuclear cell population, i.e., a mixture of monocytes and lymphocytes. Therefore, the proposed inhibiting activity of lactoferrin on monocytes, whether it acts on CFU-GM directly or via the T lymphocytes, should have been revealed by the experimental system used. This is particularly true for the endogenously stimulated system which was used in the first experiments since monocytes and lymphocytes were present in the same proportions as in the marrow *in vivo*.

To rule out the possibility that fixation of lactoferrin to plastic materials was suppressing the proposed physiological activity of lactoferrin in the culture assay used, the fixation of ^{125}I-labeled lactoferrin was investigated at four concentrations ranging from 10^{-11} to 10^{-8} M. The fixation of lactoferrin to plastic was very low (less than 3%) even after 6 days exposure and could not explain the absence of an inhibitory effect of lactoferrin in our culture assays.

None of our experiments support the alleged inhibitory activity of lactoferrin on human CFU-GM growth via monocyte CSA production. Moreover, knowing that the plasma concentration of lactoferrin[23] is around 0.5 to 1×10^{-8} M, a true physiological regulatory action of lactoferrin *in vivo* suppressing by approximately 50% the production of monocyte CSA at 1×10^{-8} M is difficult to understand. Indeed, since the same 50% inhibition was said to remain in the presence of considerably less lactoferrin, it is not seen how increased CFU-GM production can be obtained by fluctuation of the lactoferrin plasma level.

Taking into consideration that high concentrations of lactoferrin are reached in the serum,[23] one experiment was performed using a batch of fetal calf serum previously depleted of bovine lactoferrin by affinity chromatography. This experiment revealed two crucial observations: first, when lactoferrin-depleted FCS was used the CFU-GM growth was not increased as compared to a control experiment made with non-lactoferrin-depleted FCS; second, when exogenous human lactoferrin was added to human normal monocytes incubated on feeder layers containing FCS free of endogenous bovine lactoferrin, no inhibition of the CSA production was observed.

It has been emphasized recently that the inhibiting effect of lactoferrin on the CFU-GM could be masked in studies performed in the presence of leukemic inhibitory activity (LIA) which is known to inhibit the CFU-GM growth directly.[24] This leukemic inhibiting activity has been identified as acidic isoferritin and shown to be present also in tissues and in serum of normal subjects in lower concentrations however than in leukemic cells.[25,26] Thus normal acidic isoferritin present either in the conditioned medium or in the FCS used in our experiments could mask the effect of lactoferrin. It seems unlikely, however, that LIA was present in our culture system in sufficient amount to block colony formation and thereby mask the inhibiting effect of lactoferrin since the addition of exogenous LIA was regularly inhibiting our culture by 50%.

SUMMARY

Lactoferrin has been proposed recently as a physiological regulator of the granulocyte-monocyte progenitor (CFU-GM). This glycoprotein, when saturated with iron, has been said to limit the CFU-GM growth by decreasing production and release of colony stimulating activity by monocytes and macrophages.

Human milk lactoferrin saturated with iron, at concentrations ranging from 10^{-18} to 10^{-8} M, was added either to endogenously stimulated bone marrow cells or to mononucleated cells used as feeder layers for adherent cell-depleted marrow. Irrespective of the concentration of lactoferrin within the culture system used, no significant inhibition of the CFU-GM growth was observed. Moreover, the CFU-GM stimulating activity of medium conditioned by a 4 day incubation of 1×10^6 mononucleated blood cells in the presence or in the absence of lactoferrin was the same.

Various possible explanations for not confirming the reported inhibiting activity of iron-saturated lactoferrin were explored: (a) masking inhibition of the system by prostaglandin E_2 (PGE$_2$), (b) masking inhibition of the system by bovine lactoferrin present in the fetal calf serum, (c) preinhibition of the system by leukemic-associated inhibitory activity possibly present in the culture system, (d) the iron and calcium content of the culture medium used, (e) the fixation of lactoferrin to plastic compounds, (f) the source of the human lactoferrin used, and (g) the marrow cell separation methods used.

None of these factors was shown to play a role in vitro in the activity of lactoferrin and thus no evidence was found for a significant role of lactoferrin in the regulation of human granulopoiesis.

REFERENCES

1. GOLDE, D. W. & M. J. CLINE. 1972. Identification of the colony-stimulating cell in human peripheral blood. J. Clin. Invest. **51:** 2981.
2. CHERVENICK, P. A. & A. F. LoBUGLIO. 1972. Human blood monocytes: stimulators of granulocytes and mononuclear colony formation in vitro. Science **178:** 164.
3. RUSCETTI, F. W. & P. A. CHERVENICK. 1975. Release of colony-stimulating activity from thymus-derived lymphocytes. J. Clin. Invest. **55:** 520.

4. BURGESS, A. W., E. M. A. WILSON & D. METCALF. 1977. Stimulation by human placental conditioned medium of hemopoietic colony formation by human marrow cells. Blood **49:** 573.
5. BACKER, F. L., H. E. BROXMEYER & P. R. GALBRAITH. 1975. Control of granulopoiesis in man. III. Inhibition of colony formation by dense leukocytes. J. Cell. Physiol. **86:** 337.
6. HASKILL, J. S., R. D. MCKNIGHT & P. R. GALBRAITH. 1972. Cell-cell interaction in vitro: studies by density separation of colony forming, stimulating and inhibiting cells from human bone marrow. Blood **40:** 394.
7. PARAN, M., Y. TCHIKAWA & L. SACHS. 1969. Feedback inhibition of the development of macrophage and granulocyte colonies. II. Inhibition by granulocytes. Proc. Natl. Acad. Sci. USA **62:** 81.
8. BROXMEYER, H. E., A. SMITHYMAN, R. R. EGER, P. A. MEYERS & M. DE SOUSA. 1978. Identification of lactoferrin as the granulocyte-derived inhibitor of colony-stimulating activity production. J. Exp. Med. **148:** 1052.
9. GENTILE, P. & H. E. BROXMEYER. 1983. Suppression of mouse myelopoiesis by administration of human lactoferrin in vivo and the comparative action of human transferrin. Blood **6:** 982.
10. WINTON, E. F., J. M. KINKADE, W. R. VOGLER, M. B. PARKER & K. C. BARNES. 1981. In vitro studies of lactoferrin and murine granulopoiesis. Blood **57:** 574.
11. BAGBY, G. C., JR., V. D. RIGAS, R. M. BENNETT, A. A. VANDENBARK & H. S. GAREWAL. 1981. Interaction of lactoferrin, monocytes and T lymphocyte subsets in the regulation of steady-state granulopoiesis in vitro. J. Clin. Invest. **68:** 56.
12. BAGBY, G. C., E. MCCALL & D. L. LAYMAN. 1983. Regulation of colony-stimulating activity production. Interactions of fibroblasts, mononuclear phagocytes, and lactoferrin. J. Clin. Invest. **71:** 340.
13. BROXMEYER, H. E., E. GROSSBORD, N. JACOBSEN & M. A. S. MOORE. 1978. Evidence for a proliferative advantage of human leukemia colony-forming cells in vitro. J. Natl. Cancer Inst. **60:** 513.
14. QUERINJEAN, P., P. L. MASSON & J. F. HEREMANS. 1971. Molecular weight, single-chain structure and amino-acid composition of human lactoferrin. Eur. J. Biochem. **20:** 420.
15. MASSON, P. L., J. F. HEREMANS & E. SCHÖNNE. 1969. Lactoferrin, an iron-binding protein in neutrophilic leukocytes. J. Exp. Med. **130:** 643.
16. CASTELLINO, F. J., W. W. FISH & K. MANN. 1970. Structural studies on bovine lactoferrin. J. Biol. Chem. **245:** 4269.
17. PAUKOVITS, W. R., W. HINTERBERGER & J. B. PAUKOVITS. 1977. The granulocytic chalone. A specific inhibitor of granulopoiesis: molecular weight and chemical nature. Oncology **34:** 187.
18. HERMAN, S. P., D. W. GOLDE & M. J. CLINE. 1978. Neutrophil products that inhibit cell proliferation: relation to granulocytic "chalone." Blood **51:** 207.
19. BROXMEYER, H. E., P. RALPH, J. BOGNACKI, P. W. KINCADE & M. DESOUSA. 1980. A subpopulation of human polymorphonuclear neutrophils contains an active form of lactoferrin capable of binding to human monocytes and inhibiting production of granulocyte-macrophage colony stimulatory activities. J. Immunol. **125:** 903.
20. KURLAND, J. I., J. W. HADDEN & M. A. S. MOORE. 1977. Role of cyclic nucleotides in the proliferation of committed granulocyte-macrophage progenitor cells. Cancer Res. **37:** 4534.
21. BROXMEYER, H. E. 1979. Lactoferrin acts on Ia-like antigen-positive subpopulations of human monocytes to inhibit production of colony stimulatory activity in vitro. J. Clin. Invest. **64:** 1717.
22. BENNETT, R. M., G. C. BAGBY & J. DAVIS. 1981. Calcium-dependent polymerization of lactoferrin. Biochem. Biophys. Res. Commun. **101:** 88.
23. BENNETT, R. M. & C. MOHLA. 1976. A solid-phase radioimmunoassay for the measurement of lactoferrin in human plasma: variations with age, sex, and disease. J. Lab. Clin. Med. **88:** 156.
24. BROXMEYER, H. E. 1982. Acidic isoferritins and E-type prostaglandins in sources of colony stimulatory factors mask detection of cycling granulocyte-macrophage progenitor cells. Blood **60:** 1042.

25. BROXMEYER, H. E., J. BOGNACKI, M. H. DORNER & M. DE SOUSA. 1981. Identification of leukemia-associated inhibitory activity as acidic isoferritins. J. Exp. Med. **153:** 1426.
26. BROXMEYER, H. E., J. BOGNACKI, P. RALPH, M. H. DORNER, L. LU & H. CASTRO-MALASPINA. 1982. Monocyte-macrophage-derived acidic isoferritins: normal feedback regulators of granulocyte-macrophage progenitor cells in vitro. Blood **60:** 595.
27. BENNET, J. M., D. CATOVSKY, M. T. DANIEL, G. FLANDRIN, D. A. G. GALTON, H. R. GRALNICK & C. SULTAN. 1976. Proposals for the classification of the acute leukemias. Br. J. Haematol. **33:** 451.

DISCUSSION OF THE PAPER

M. MURPHY, JR. (*Hipple Cancer Research Center, Dayton, Ohio*): You showed us that when Dr. Broxmeyer's lactoferrin was assayed in your laboratory, it was noninhibitory. Was your lactoferrin ever assayed by Dr. Broxmeyer? If so, was it also found to be noninhibitory?

P. STRYCKMANS: We sent our lactoferrin to Dr. Broxmeyer and he found an inhibitory activity in his system.

P. J. QUESENBERRY (*St. Elizabeth's Hospital, Boston, Mass.*): I have two questions. (1) Could Dr. Broxmeyer's calf serum and other ingredients give him a basically different system? (2) Some of your graphs indicated that you got as much as 20% inhibitions at some concentrations. I gather you feel this was not significant. Is it possible that there would be a real decrease for some of your groups if you continued the experiments?

STRYCKMANS: Yes, we considered the 20% decreases occurring at individual points as not significant. One must also remember that there was a 24% increase in colonies when conditioned media were used. Concerning the materials used by Dr. Broxmeyer, one of my collaborators went to Dr. Broxmeyer's lab and returned with the calf serum, lactoferrin, and other materials used there. Despite our efforts, we still could not demonstrate an inhibitory activity.

Induction of Nonspecific Resistance and Stimulation of Granulopoiesis by Endotoxins and Nontoxic Bacterial Cell Wall Components and Their Passive Transfer

RENATE URBASCHEK AND BERNHARD URBASCHEK

Department of Immunology and Serology
Institute of Hygiene and Medical Microbiology
Klinikum Mannheim
University of Heidelberg
6800 Mannheim, Federal Republic of Germany

INTRODUCTION

The ability of endotoxins, the lipopolysaccharides of gram-negative bacteria, to enhance nonspecifically host resistance to bacterial infections was described in 1956.[1,2] Enhanced host resistance could also be demonstrated after 24 hr pretreatment with endotoxin in mice in which septicemia, due to gut-derived bacteria, was induced by cecal ligation and puncture.[3] Moreover, endotoxins have been shown to protect animals against the lethal effects of irradiation.[4,5] The stimulation of hematopoiesis by endotoxins,[6–8] first studied in the context of endotoxin-induced radioprotection,[9,10] is one of the mechanisms involved in enhanced nonspecific resistance.

Many attempts have been made to modify the lipopolysaccharide structure of endotoxins to eliminate their toxicity and pyrogenicity while retaining their beneficial activities.[11–15] We have demonstrated that a potassium methylated endotoxin[12] induced nonspecifically within 24 hr tolerance against the lethal effects of endotoxins of various gram-negative bacteria.[16,17] This preparation also prevented or mitigated severe disturbances of the microcirculation following endotoxin or burn trauma as observed by vitalmicroscopy.[18,19] The classic phenomenon of tolerance to the pyrogenic and lethal effects of endotoxin achieved by the injection of toxic endotoxins was recognized early to be mediated by nonspecific enhancement of reticuloendothelial system (RES) uptake of circulating endotoxin.[20] The complexity of endotoxin tolerance involving many target cells with generalized cytotoxicity and release of numerous mediators was recently reviewed.[21] Induction of nonspecific resistance to endotoxins and to lethal irradiation will be described here using several experimental models. These studies indicate the central role of the mediator-releasing activity of endotoxins in enhanced nonspecific host defense.

INDUCTION OF TOLERANCE IN ANIMALS
SENSITIZED TO ENDOTOXIN

Infection with *Mycobacterium bovis* BCG (bacillus Calmette-Guérin) results in an increased nonspecific resistance to bacterial infection[22,23] and at the same time, in an increased susceptibility to endotoxin.[24] The prolonged activated state of macrophages seems to be necessary for both effects. The infecting microorganisms, as well as endotoxins, are cleared more rapidly from the circulation. Endotoxins, however, elicit an increased cytotoxic effect on BCG-activated macrophages as demonstrated by Peavy *et al.*[25] This results in the release of macrophage mediators, some of which can produce locally destructive effects on adjacent tissue and cells. Among these are hydrolytic and proteolytic enzymes, vasoactive substances, and oxygen metabolites. In the case of Kupffer cells—the liver being the major organ to clear endotoxin—mediators may affect the endothelial lining and hepatocytes, thus provoking severe disturbances in their function as well as structural integrity. Together with McCuskey we were able

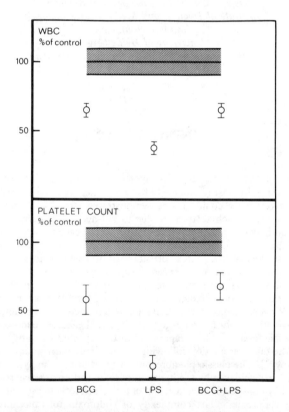

FIGURE 1. White blood cell (WBC) and platelet counts in NMRI mice 2 hr after i.v. injection of 5 μg endotoxin (LPS) (trichloroacetic acid (TCA) endotoxin was extracted in our laboratories from *Escherichia coli* 0111), 14 days after i.v. BCG infection (BCG) (5×10^7 CFU, *Mycobacterium bovis* BCG, Trudeau Institute, Saranac, N.Y.), and 2 hr after endotoxin injection of mice infected with BCG 14 days prior to the challenge with endotoxin (BCG+LPS).

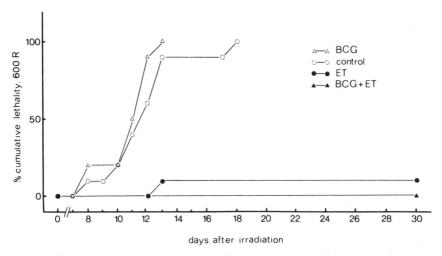

FIGURE 2. Lethality rate in NMRI mice following whole-body X irradiation without treatment (control), 14 days after i.v. BCG infection (BCG), and 24 hr after i.v. injection of 1 μg endotoxin without (ET) and with (BCG+ET) prior infection with BCG.

to demonstrate by high-resolution *in vivo* microscopy an accelerated phagocytic activity of Kupffer cells following BCG infection, as well as significantly delayed uptake and damage 2 hr after endotoxin injection in BCG-infected mice.[26]

An interesting observation in BCG-infected mice is that the characteristic endotoxin-induced drop in platelets and white blood cell counts fails to occur after endotoxin injection (FIGURE 1) although these animals die within hours thereafter. In regard to the radioprotective effect of endotoxins, BCG-infected mice were similar to mice not infected with BCG. The BCG treatment per se did not protect them from the consequences of lethal irradiation (FIGURE 2).

Two attempts were made to influence the hypersensitivity to endotoxin of BCG-infected mice. Several authors have studied the role of prostaglandins in the pathophysiology of endotoxemia and their prevention using prostaglandin synthesis inhibitors.[27,28] We injected mice 14 days after BCG infection with different endotoxin concentrations (0.05, 0.5, or 5.0 μg per mouse, i.v.). The endotoxin-concentration-dependent survival rate increased when 1.5 mg/kg i.v. indomethacin (Sigma, lot 75C-0261) was injected 45 min before the endotoxin challenge (FIGURE 3). These results are of interest in view of the role of macrophage mediators, which will be discussed later.

We also found that hyperreactivity to endotoxin could be reversed in BCG-infected mice by pretreatment with nonlethal minute concentrations of endotoxin administered 24 hr prior to the lethal challenge with endotoxin.[29] The tolerance produced with extremely low doses of endotoxin prior to the challenge may indicate that only a moderate effect is produced on the macrophages with the resulting release of small quantities of toxic substances which are insufficient to affect parenchymal cells. The possibility exists that other factors or mediators are produced also under these experimental conditions by the activated macrophages or hepatocytes which may have beneficial effects. C-reactive protein released from hepatocytes after injection of endotoxin[30] has recently been shown to act as an opsonin.[31] Several mediators from mac-

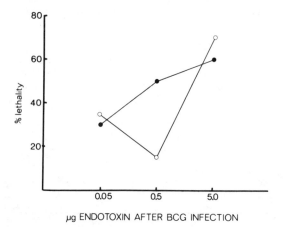

μg ENDOTOXIN AFTER BCG INFECTION

FIGURE 3. Lethality rate in BCG-infected NMRI mice after i.v. injection with different concentrations of endotoxin with (○) and without (●) pretreatment with indomethacin (1.5 mg/kg, Sigma, Munich, lot 75C-0261) injected i.v. 45 min before the challenge with endotoxin.

rophages of BCG-infected animals are released in large amounts *in vitro* and *in vivo* after endotoxin administration; these include tumor necrosis factor, interferon, colony stimulating factor (CSF), and interleukin 1.[32-35] The determination of mediators released *in vivo* from activated macrophages in BCG-infected mice after administration of the challenge dose of endotoxin in the tolerant as compared to the nontolerant animals may aid in elucidating those factors involved in the beneficial effects of low-level endotoxin stimulation.[36]

Some of these experiments on tolerance induction are summarized in TABLE 1. The status of tolerance lasted for 72 hr. Whereas 87.5% of BCG-infected mice died following an i.v. injection of 5 μg of endotoxin, the lethality rate was decreased to 37.5% when 10 ng of endotoxin was injected 72 hr before the lethal challenge. Pretreatment at 48 hr resulted in 12.5% lethality.

TABLE 1. Induction of Nonspecific Tolerance against Lethal Doses of Endotoxin in NMRI Mice 14 Days after BCG Infection

Pretreatment (i.v.)	Endotoxin (i.v.) Challenge 24 hr after Pretreatment (μg)	No. Dead/Total	Percentage Lethality
Endotoxin—0.1 μg	5.0	0/6	0
NaCl	5.0	9/9	100
Endotoxin			
0.1 μg	0.5	1/8	12.5
0.01 μg	0.5	1/8	12.5
0.001 μg	0.5	6/8	75.0
NaCl	0.5	6/8	75.0

RADIOPROTECTION AND STIMULATION OF HEMATOPOIESIS
BY BACTERIAL CELL WALL DERIVED SUBSTANCES

In continuation of the above-described studies on the induction of endotoxin tolerance by an endotoxin-derived preparation with reduced lethality,[16] we found in miniature pigs that many endotoxin-induced metabolic and hemodynamic changes failed to occur in the status of tolerance.[17] We were able to demonstrate that this detoxified endotoxin can also enhance nonspecific resistance to lethal irradiation exposure.[37,38] An increase in leukocyte count was observed[39] and bone marrow differentiation revealed an early hematopoietic recovery in detoxified pretreated, irradiated mice.[40]

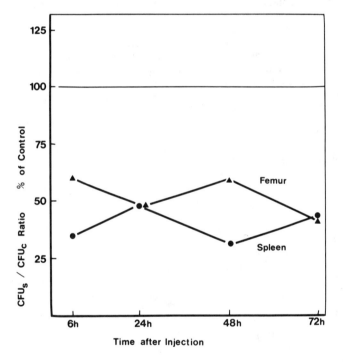

FIGURE 4. Femoral and splenic CFUs/CFUc ratio at different times after i.v. injection of 50 μg detoxified endotoxin in NMRI mice measured as a percentage of the control CFUs/CFUc ratio.

The techniques for the determination of pluripotent stem cells (CFUs),[41] granulocytic committed stem cells (CFUc), and colony stimulating factor (CSF)[42,43] were applied with modifications used in the department of Dr. Cronkite at Brookhaven National Laboratory, Upton, New York. A significant increase in endogenous colonies was observed following detoxified-endotoxin pretreatment in irradiated mice, similar to that known to occur following endotoxin injection.

Splenic CFUs were markedly increased with an unchanged f-fraction at 3 days as were blood CFUs at 6 hr and 3 days after injection of 50 μg of detoxified endotoxin. The granulopoietic stem cell compartment was stimulated to a much higher extent, expressed in an elevation of femoral CFUc and a much higher elevation of splenic CFUc.[44] Using hydroxyurea, known to be selectively lethal for cells in the phase of DNA synthesis during the cell cycle, we observed an increase in the number of CFUs and CFUc entering into active cell cycle following injection of detoxified endotoxins.[45] The CFUs/CFUc ratio (FIGURE 4) as compared to normal expresses the much higher increase of granulopoietic stem cells.

Although splenectomy does not exclude the significance of splenic CFUs and CFUc for survival and hematopoietic recovery in X-irradiated mice pretreated with detoxified endotoxin, we studied the survival and the status of the stem cells of bone marrow and blood after injection of detoxified endotoxin in splenectomized mice under the same experimental conditions. At the time of irradiation—4 weeks after splenectomy—the animals were not in the state of being more resistant to X irradiation (FIGURE 5). The pretreatment with detoxified endotoxin was as effective as in control mice. The larger increase in femoral CFUs (FIGURE 6) and CFUc suggests that the murine organism compensates for its auxiliary hematopoietic organ. It is interesting that the blood CFUs initially released from the bone marrow are increased much less than in nonsplenectomized mice. This may indicate that bone marrow-derived CFUs are released into the circulation to a high extent only when hematopoietic sites such as the spleen are present for sequestration.

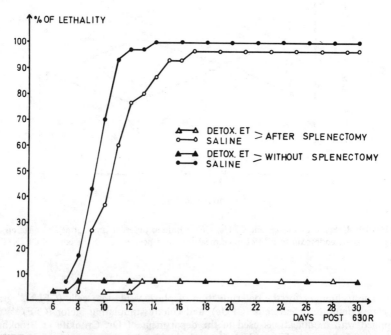

FIGURE 5. Cumulative lethality rate following whole-body X irradiation in NMRI mice 24 hr after pretreatment with 50 μg detoxified endotoxin with and without splenectomy and in control mice injected with saline.

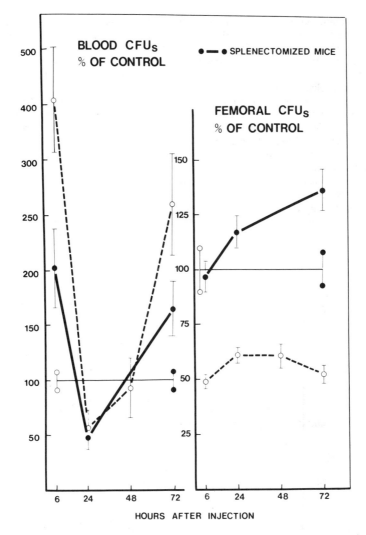

FIGURE 6. Number of blood and femoral CFUs at different times after i.v. injection of detoxified endotoxin in NMRI mice with (●) and without (○) splenectomy.

Considering the differential blood count (FIGURE 7), after an initial influx of band neutrophiles into the circulation an increase in monocytes is observed at 24 hr after injection of detoxified endotoxin. This is the time when lethal doses of endotoxins are tolerated.

The question as to whether the colony stimulating factor, CSF, necessary for *in vitro* proliferation and differentiation to form colonies of mature macrophages and/ or granulocytes, stimulates granulopoiesis *in vivo* remains to be answered. Serum CSF is known to be increased following injection of endotoxin[46–48] and detoxified endotoxin.[44,45,49] Experiments with anti-CSF to purified CSF suggested the role of CSF for *in vivo* granulopoiesis.[50] Using this antiserum we were able to suppress the endotoxin-induced elevation of splenic CFUc.[45] It is unknown why these results could not be reproduced later on.

Serum CSF levels decrease following injection of higher concentrations of detoxified endotoxin (FIGURE 8) in a manner similar to toxic preparations.[45] This is probably due to the release of CSF inhibitors. This phenomenon was never observed using a polysaccharide preparation extracted by C. Bona (Institute Pasteur, Paris, France) directly from the cell wall of *Salmonella typhimurium* according to the method of Freeman. This Freeman-type polysaccharide (FPS) was nontoxic, even in adrenalectomized mice, and nonmitogenic (Bona, personal communication). We found it to be nonpyrogenic. It was interesting to observe that FPS induced radioprotection (FIGURE 9) and stimulation of granulopoiesis.[45] Thus it seems evident, particularly using FPS, that some beneficial effects of lipopolysaccharides (LPS) are not necessarily due to their toxic components.

Nowotny *et al.*[49] have shown that a polysaccharide-rich, water-soluble fraction obtained by acid hydrolysis from extracted LPS enhanced CSF levels and the survival rate following X irradiation. A similar preparation used by Apte and Pluznik was not effective.[51]

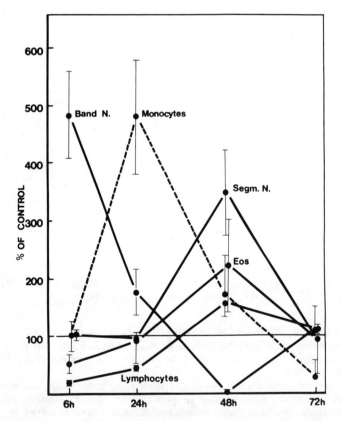

FIGURE 7. Differential blood count of NMRI mice at different times after i.v. injection of 50 μg detoxified endotoxin.

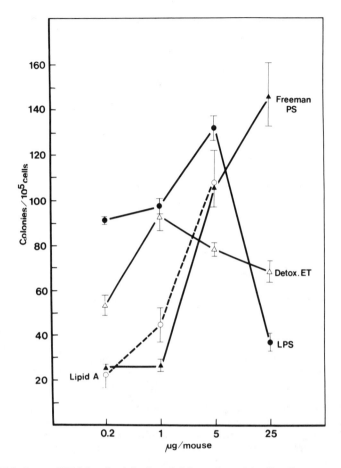

FIGURE 8. Serum CSF 2 hr after injection of different bacterial cell wall components (Lipid A, LPS (TCA endotoxin), Freeman-type polysaccharide, and detoxified endotoxin).

PASSIVE TRANSFER OF RADIOPROTECTION AND STIMULATION OF GRANULOPOIESIS BY POSTENDOTOXIN SERA FROM BCG-INFECTED MICE

The question arises whether increased CSF production and activation of hematopoiesis are induced through a direct effect or whether they occur secondarily. Initial mediators, such as the vasoactive substances histamine and serotonin, did not increase CSF levels.[52] Byron[53] has reported the stimulatory effect of 4-methyl-histamine on CFUs *in vitro*. We were unable to observe significant changes of splenic or femoral CFUs or CFUc after injection of histamine in mice.[52]

Subsequently, we studied whether other mediators—mainly of macrophage origin—are capable of stimulating granulopoiesis and nonspecific resistance to lethal

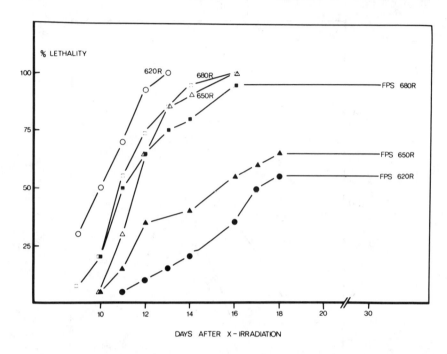

FIGURE 9. Cumulative lethality rate in NMRI mice after injection of 50 μg Freeman-type polysaccharide (FPS) following different doses of whole-body X irradiation.

irradiation. To approach this question a regimen for the release of these mediators was used, namely, the infection of mice with BCG prior to endotoxin challenge. Sera obtained after that treatment contain a myriad of mediators, mentioned above, with a peak at 2 hr after endotoxin injection. Many of these mediators have been extensively studied in the past years by several investigators.[54-56] We tested whether these post-endotoxin sera from BCG-infected mice could transfer radioprotection, comparing them with the effect of different control sera (TABLE 2). As detected with our kinetic *Limulus* amoebocyte lysate (LAL) microtiter test,[57,58] considerable amounts of endotoxin are present in such sera, which per se are sufficient to be effective. In post-endotoxin sera 380 ng/ml endotoxin was detected and in BCG/ET sera 140 ng/ml endotoxin was detected 2 hr after injection of 5 μg endotoxin. We found that 10 ng of endotoxin is sufficient to cause elevated CSF levels, when injected into endotoxin-susceptible mice. NMRI mice were protected against lethal irradiation by 60 ng of endotoxin: with pretreatment 6 out of 20 mice died within 30 days after 600 R whole-body X irradiation, whereas without pretreatment 23 out of 25 died. Therefore, to eliminate endotoxic effects and to study the activity of the humoral factors in BCG/ET sera, C3H/HeJ mice were used. This mouse strain is genetically resistant to endotoxic effects.[59] These mice cannot be protected against the consequences of irradiation by endotoxin,[38] and do not respond to endotoxin with elevated CSF or splenic CFUc.[60] BCG/ET sera induced marked radioprotection when they were injected into C3H/HeJ mice 24 hr before whole-body X irradiation (FIGURE 10). Similar protection was achieved with BCG/ET serum when it was injected 48 hr after irradiation. According to the literature, the optimal time to induce radioprotection with endotoxin in mice is 24 hr after pretreatment. Using detoxified endotoxin no protection could be induced when injected 24 or 48 hr after irradiation (unpublished observation). Whether the endotoxin-independent radioprotection by BCG/ET serum transfer is active in a different way than endotoxin, or whether C3H/HeJ mice respond in a different way than endotoxin-susceptible mice are questions which remain to be answered.

One of the humoral factors in BCG/ET sera that may be responsible for the enhanced nonspecific resistance is CSF.[34] The extent of radioprotection did not correlate with the CSF content or its fractions from zymosan-treated mice.[61] This does not exclude the essentiality of CSF for enhanced host defense, since the CSF content in the transferred serum is too low and less important than the capacity to induce elevated endogenous CSF production and release. We were able to demonstrate that BCG/ET serum induced increased serum CSF in C3H/HeJ mice 2 hr after injection followed by a significant increase in splenic CFUc after 3 days.[62] Fractions of these sera pooled after molecular sieving gave further evidence for the possibility that stimulation of endogenous CSF production correlates with radioprotection.[63] Two fractions that did not contain CSF were radioprotective and induced elevated serum

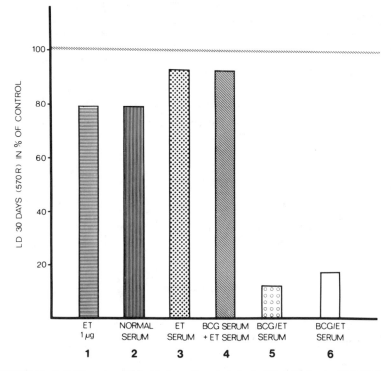

FIGURE 10. Lethality rates within 30 days after whole-body X irradiation in C3H/HeJ mice. Twenty-four hours before radiation exposure mice were pretreated with 1 μg of endotoxin (1), with 0.25 ml i.v. and 0.25 ml i.p. of normal mouse serum (2), of 2-hr postendotoxin serum (3), of a combination of postendotoxin serum plus serum obtained 14 days after BCG infection (4), or serum obtained 2 hr after endotoxin injection from BCG-infected mice (5). BCG/ET serum was injected 48 hr after irradiation (6).

CSF when injected into C3H/HeJ mice. One fraction that contained CSF was ineffective in both CSF production and radioprotection.

Besides the enhanced nonspecific resistance to radioprotection described here, Parant et al.[64] observed that BCG/ET serum enhanced nonspecific resistance to bacterial infections in C3H/HeJ mice. Further studies on endotoxin-mediated humoral factors capable of transferring these endotoxin-independent beneficial effects may shed some light on the underlying mechanisms. In this context the observation of Moore[65] is of interest that although interferon is considered to be antiproliferative, interferon-pretreated bone marrow cells had enhanced responsiveness to CSF. Kampschmidt and Pulliam demonstrated that leukocyte endogenous mediator (LEM)—probably identical to interleukin 1—had a protective effect against bacterial infection.[66] The interaction and cooperation of several of these endotoxin mediators on hematopoietic and immune cells express the complexity of increased host resistance.

TABLE 2. Sera Obtained from NMRI Mice[a]

Infection		Endotoxin (i.v.— 5 μg in 0.2 ml per mouse) Challenge (Time after Infection)	Blood Obtained: Time/After	Serum
Substance	Dose (i.v.) per Mouse			
BCG	5×10^7 CFU/0.2 ml	—	14 days/BCG	BCG serum
NaCl	0.2 ml	—	2 hr/NaCl	Control serum
NaCl	0.2 ml	14 days	2 hr/ET	ET serum
BCG	5×10^7 CFU/0.2 ml	14 days	2 hr/ET	BCG/ET serum

[a] BCG: *Mycobacterium bovis,* Trudeau Institute, Saranac, N.Y., Phipps, Strain 1029, 1.18×10^9 CFU/ml, lot A 14. ET—endotoxin.

ACKNOWLEDGMENT

The authors gratefully acknowledge the excellent technical assistance of Ms. Ruth Breunig.

REFERENCES

1. LANDY, M. & L. PILLEMER. 1956. J. Exp. Med. **104:** 383-409.
2. DUBOS, R. J. & R. W. SCHAEDLER. 1956. J. Exp. Med. **104:** 53-65.
3. URBASCHEK, B., B. DITTER, K.-P. BECKER & R. URBASCHEK. 1984. Circ. Shock **14:** 209-222.
4. MEFFERD, R. B., D. T. HENDEL & J. B. LOEFFER. 1953. Proc. Soc. Exp. Biol. Med. **85:** 54-56.
5. SMITH, W. W., M. ALDERMAN & R. E. GILLESPIE. 1957. Am. J. Physiol. **191:** 124-130.
6. CHERVENICK, P. A. 1972. J. Lab. Clin. Med. **79:** 1014-1020.
7. QUESENBERRY, P., A. MORLEY, F. STOHLMAN, K. RICKARD, D. HOWARD & M. SMITH. 1972. N. Engl. J. Med. **286:** 227-232.

8. MONETTE, F. C., B. S. MORSE, D. HOWARD, E. NISKANEN & F. STOHLMAN, JR. 1972. Cell Tissue Kinet. **5:** 121-129.
9. SMITH, W. W., G. BRECHER, S. FRED & R. A. BUDD. 1966. Radiat. Res. **27:** 710-717.
10. HANKS, G. E. & E. J. AINSWORTH. 1965. Radiat. Res. **25:** 195.
11. RIBI, E., K. C. MILNER & T. D. PERRINE. 1959. J. Immunol. **82:** 75-84.
12. NOWOTNY, A. 1963. Nature **197:** 721-722.
13. NOWOTNY, A. 1969. Bacteriol. Rev. **33:** 72-98.
14. MCINTIRE, F. C., M. P. HARGIE, J. R. SCHENCK, R. A. FINLEY, H. W. SIEVERT, E. T. RIETSCHEL & D. L. ROSENSTREICH. 1976. J. Immunol. **117:** 674-678.
15. SULTZER, B. M. 1971. Chemical modification of endotoxin. *In* Microbial Toxins. S. Kadis, G. Weinbaum & S. J. Ajl, Eds. **5:** 91-126. Academic Press, Inc. New York, N.Y.
16. URBASCHEK, B. & A. NOWOTNY. 1968. Proc. Soc. Exp. Biol. Med. **127:** 650-652.
17. URBASCHEK, B. & R. URBASCHEK. 1977. Some aspects of microcirculatory and metabolic changes in endotoxemia and in endotoxin tolerance. *In* Microbiology-1977. D. Schlesinger, Ed.: 286-292. American Society for Microbiology. Washington, D.C.
18. URBASCHEK, B., P.-I. BRÅNEMARK & A. NOWOTNY. 1968. Experientia **24:** 170.
19. URBASCHEK, B. 1971. Addendum—The effects of endotoxin in the microcirculation. *In* Microbial Toxins. S. Kadis, G. Weinbaum & S. J. Ajl, Eds. **5:** 261-275. Academic Press, Inc. New York, N.Y.
20. FREEDMAN, H. H. 1960. Ann. N.Y. Acad. Sci. **83:** 99-106.
21. GREISMAN, S. E. 1983. Induction of endotoxin tolerance. *In* Beneficial Effects of Endotoxins. A. Nowotny, Ed.: 149-178. Plenum Press. New York, N.Y.
22. DUBOS, R. J. & R. W. SCHAEDLER. 1957. J. Exp. Med. **106:** 703-715.
23. HOWARD, J. G., G. BIOZZI, B. N. HALPERN, C. STIFFEL & D. MOUTON. 1959. Br. J. Exp. Pathol. **40:** 281-290.
24. SUTER, E. & E. M. KIRSANOW. 1961. Immunology **4:** 354-365.
25. PEAVY, D. L., R. E. BAUGHN & D. M. MUSHER. 1979. Infect. Immun. **24:** 59-64.
26. MCCUSKEY, R. S., R. URBASCHEK, P. A. MCCUSKEY & B. URBASCHEK. 1983. Infect. Immun. **42:** 362-367.
27. FLETCHER, J. R. & R. W. RAMMWELL. 1977. J. Surg. Res. **24:** 154-160.
28. RIETSCHEL, E. T., U. SCHADE, O. LÜDERITZ, H. FISCHER & B. A. PESKAR. 1980. Prostaglandins in endotoxicosis. *In* Microbiology-1980. D. Schlesinger, Ed.: 66-72. American Society for Microbiology. Washington, D.C.
29. URBASCHEK, R. & B. URBASCHEK. 1982. Klin. Wochenschr. **60:** 746-748.
30. PATTERSON, L. T. & R. D. HIGGINBOTHAM. 1965. J. Bacteriol. **90:** 1520-1524.
31. MOLD, C., S. NAKAYAMA, T. J. HOLZER, H. GEWURZ & T. W. DU CLOS. 1981. J. Exp. Med. **154:** 1703-1708.
32. CARSWELL, W. A., L. J. OLD, R. L. KASSEL, S. GREEN, N. FIORE & B. WILLIAMSON. 1975. Proc. Natl. Acad. Sci. USA **72:** 3666-3670.
33. MÄNNEL, D. N., R. N. MOORE & S. E. MERGENHAGEN. 1980. Infect. Immun. **30:** 523-530.
34. URBASCHEK, R., R. K. SHADDUCK, C. BONA & S. E. MERGENHAGEN. 1980. Colony-stimulating factor in nonspecific resistance and in increased susceptibility to endotoxin. *In* Microbiology-1980. D. Schlesinger, Ed.: 115-119. American Society for Microbiology. Washington, D.C.
35. YOUNGER, J. S. & W. STINEBRING. 1965. Nature **208:** 456-458.
36. URBASCHEK, R., D. MÄNNEL, G. H. NORTHOFF, H. KIRCHNER, H.-G. LESER & B. URBASCHEK. In preparation.
37. URBASCHEK, B. 1967. Zur Frage des Wirkungsmechanismus bakterieller Endotoxine und seiner Beeinflussung. Habilitationsschrift, Med. Fakultät der Universität Heidelberg. Heidelberg, FRG.
38. URBASCHEK, R., S. E. MERGENHAGEN & B. URBASCHEK. 1977. Infect. Immun. **18:** 860-862.
39. URBASCHEK, B. & A. NOWOTNY. 1969. Endotoxin tolerance induced by endotoxoid. *In* La structure et les effets biologiques des produits bactériéns provenants de germes Gram-négatifs. L. Chedid, Ed. **174:** 357-365. Centre National de la Recherche Scientifique. Paris, France.
40. URBASCHEK, B. & R. H. RINGERT. 1975. The effect of detoxified endotoxin on bone marrow. *In* Gram-Negative Bacterial Infections and Mode of Endotoxin Ac-

tions—Pathophysiological, Immunological, and Clinical Aspects. B. Urbaschek, R. Urbaschek & E. Neter, Eds.: 200-205. Springer-Verlag. Vienna, Austria.
41. TILL, J. E. & E. A. McCULLOCH. 1961. Radiat. Res. **14**: 213-222.
42. PLUZNIK, D. H. & L. SACHS. 1965. J. Cell. Physiol. **66**: 319-324.
43. BRADLEY, R. R. & D. METCALF. 1966. J. Exp. Biol. Med. Sci. **44**: 287-300.
44. URBASCHEK, R. & B. URBASCHEK. 1977. Blut **35**: 357.
45. URBASCHEK, R. 1980. Effects of bacterial products on granulopoiesis. In Macrophages and Lymphocytes: Nature, Function and Interaction. Part B. M. R. Escobar & H. Friedman, Eds.: 51-64. Plenum Press. New York, N.Y.
46. CHERVENICK, P. A. 1972. J. Lab. Clin. Med. **79**: 1014-1020.
47. METCALF, D. 1971. Immunology **21**: 427-436.
48. QUESENBERRY, P., A. MORLEY, F. STOHLMAN, JR., K. A. RICHARD & D. HOWARD. 1972. N. Engl. J. Med. **286**: 227-232.
49. NOWOTNY, A., U. H. BEHLING & H. L. CHANG. 1975. J. Immunol. **115**: 199-203.
50. SHADDUCK, R. K., A. L. CARSTEN, G. CHIKKAPPA, E. P. CRONKITE & E. GERARD. 1978. Proc. Soc. Exp. Biol. Med. **158**: 542-549.
51. APTE, R. N. & D. H. PLUZNIK. 1976. In Progress in Differentiation Research. N. Müller-Bérat, Ed.: 493-500. North-Holland Publishing Co. Amsterdam, the Netherlands.
52. URBASCHEK, R. & B. URBASCHEK. 1980. The effect of endotoxic substances on granulopoiesis. In Natural Toxins. D. Eaker & T. Wadström, Eds.: 311-318. Pergamon Press. Elmsford, N.Y.
53. BYRON, J. W. 1977. Agents Actions **7**: 209-213.
54. SCHLESINGER, D. (Ed.). 1980. Endogenous mediators in host response to bacterial endotoxin. In Microbiology-1980. Pp. 3-167. American Society for Microbiology. Washington, D.C.
55. MÄNNEL, D. N., J. J. FARRAR & S. E. MERGENHAGEN. 1980. J. Immunol. **124**: 1106-1110.
56. MOORE, R. N., J. T. HOFFELD, J. J. FARRAR, S. E. MERGENHAGEN, J. J. OPPENHEIM & R. K. SHADDURCK. 1981. Lymphokines **3**: 119-148.
57. DITTER, B., K.-P. BECKER, R. URBASCHEK & B. URBASCHEK. 1982. Prog. Clin. Biol. Res. **93**: 385-392.
58. DITTER, B., K.-P. BECKER, R. URBASCHEK & B. URBASCHEK. 1983. Drug Res. **33**: 681-687.
59. SULTZER, B. M. 1968. Nature (London) **219**: 1253-1254.
60. APTE, R. N. & D. H. PLUZNIK. 1976. J. Cell. Physiol. **89**: 313-323.
61. ADDISON, P. D. & L. J. BERRY. 1981. J. Reticuloendothel. **30**: 301-311.
62. URBASCHEK, R. & B. URBASCHEK. 1983. Infect. Immun. **30**: 1488-1490.
63. URBASCHEK, R., S. E. MERGENHAGEN & B. URBASCHEK. 1983. Abstract B 167, p. 51, 83rd Annual Meeting of the American Society for Microbiology.
64. PARANT, M. A., F. J. PARANT & L. A. CHEDID. 1980. Infect. Immun. **28**: 654-659.
65. MOORE, R. N. & B. T. ROUSE. 1983. J. Immunol. **131**: 2374-2378.
66. KAMPSCHMIDT, R. F. & L. A. PULLIAM. 1975. J. Reticuloendothel. **17**: 162-169.

DISCUSSION OF THE PAPER

QUESTION: Dr. Urbaschek, what is the basis for the difference in susceptibility to endotoxin between C3H/HeJ and other mouse strains?

R. URBASCHEK: The resistance of C3H/HeJ mice to endotoxin is determined by a single mutation expressed as a cellular defect in response to endotoxin. Apparently, signaling from the cell membrane is lowered upon reaction with endotoxin.

The Role of Cholesterol and Its Biosynthesis in Lymphocyte Proliferation and Differentiation[a]

HANS-JÖRG HEINIGER, HARRY W. CHEN,[b] AND
GILBERT A. BOISSONNEAULT

The Jackson Laboratory
Bar Harbor, Maine 04609

MAX HESS AND HANS COTTIER

Department of Pathology
School of Medicine
University of Bern
Bern, Switzerland

RICHARD D. STONER

Department of Medicine
Brookhaven National Laboratory
Upton, New York 11913

FUNCTION OF CHOLESTEROL IN PLASMA MEMBRANES

Most membranes of eucaryotes contain sterols with 27 to 30 carbon atoms. In mammalian cells the major membrane sterol is cholesterol (5-cholesten-3β-ol). The physiochemical role of this molecule has been investigated intensively and is today fairly well understood, although some details still require further study. This subject has been reviewed extensively[1-10] and therefore we restrict ourselves to briefly summarizing the present state of knowledge on the role of membrane sterol in lymphocyte function.

The relative distribution of the major membrane constituents in mammals, proteins, phospholipids, and cholesterol, varies considerably according to the types of membranes and cells. Nuclear, mitochondrial, and ergastoplasmic membranes contain relatively small amounts of cholesterol whereas the plasma membrane contains phos-

[a] The writing of this article and the experimental work reported herein were supported by Grant CA 19305 from the National Cancer Institute, U.S. National Institutes of Health.

[b] Present address: Central Research and Development, Du Pont Experimental Station, Wilmington, Del. 19898.

111

pholipids and cholesterol in comparable molar concentrations. As an example of the differences between cell types it may be noted that hamster lymphocytes[11] have a cholesterol/phospholipid ratio (CPR) of 0.92 and human thymocytes[12] one of 0.75.

Phospholipid bilayers, such as those found in cell membranes, undergo characteristic temperature-dependent phase transitions from the L-β-crystalline phase to the L-α-liquid-crystalline phase. In pure lipid species (i.e., membranes containing only one type of fatty acid in the phospholipids) the transition occurs at a well-defined temperature. The longer the acyl chains they have and the fewer double bonds they contain the higher the temperature has to be to initiate the transition.[13] Cholesterol, if added to such phospholipid bilayers, interferes with their phase transition,[13-15] and at molar concentrations of more than 33 mol% the phase transition vanishes.[15] Thus cholesterol in such phospholipid bilayers has the dual effect of making phospholipid mixtures more fluid at lower temperature and of condensing (solidifying) them at higher temperatures. A cholesterol-containing phospholipid bilayer is therefore in a state of intermediate fluidity or gel state.[5]

The first in-depth considerations of phospholipid-cholesterol interactions were made almost 30 years ago by Finean[16] and were then further developed by others.[5,17-19] Some chemical details are still under investigation but there is a general consensus today that the 3β-hydroxy group of the sterol interacts with the polar head of the phospholipid, since the interaction does not take place with the 3α-configuration (epicholesterol).[20] Darke et al.[21] and also Stoffel et al.[22] have very elegantly depicted the specific interactions of cholesterol with the phospholipids. The solidifying effect of the sterol (i.e., prevention of a complete crystalline $\rightarrow$ liquid transition) seems to be confined to a region corresponding to carbon atoms 4 to 8 in the fatty acid chains, whereas the liquefying effect (i.e., induction of greater molecular movement of the fatty acid chains) appears to take place distal of carbon atom 10 toward the core of the bilayer, imposing on it the intermediate gel-type fluidity.[5] FIGURE 1 is a simplified sketch of such a membrane model.

Some functional aspects of plasma membranes appear to be altered when the concentration of cholesterol changes (for review see References 8, 23-25) including ion transport and permeability,[26-28] lateral diffusion of receptors,[29,30,31] transmembrane modulation of signals, cell-to-cell interaction, and specific mechanical deformation of the cell surface.[32,33] Since the temperature in mammals is maintained at a constant level, we postulated[23] that the modulation of fluidity in mammalian membranes is of a chemotropic rather than thermotropic nature.

The additional presence of proteins in the plasma membranes greatly complicates their structure. Wallach and Zahler and Changeux et al.[34,35] pioneered mosaic models based mainly on structural considerations of membrane proteins. Later the widely quoted Singer-Nicolson model[36] was formulated. In both cases the role of cholesterol did not receive much attention. However, Wallach has reviewed[37,38] critically and comprehensively the structure and function of mammalian membranes and further refined the membrane lattice hypothesis presented by Changeux et al.[34] It would be impossible in the context of this section to discuss this highly complex model. Suffice it to emphasize some of the implications of these hypotheses as they may be relevant to our subject matter:

Mammalian membranes represent a heterogeneous mixture of molecular species, such as phospholipids and cholesterol, which interact with each other and with proteins. Such cooperative interactions may occur at short- and long-range intervals between protomers.[27,39,40] Specific proteins, such as enzymes, may require highly specific microenvironments (boundary layers) of lipids to be able to function, as seen with Ca^{2+}-ATPase and Na^+-K^+-ATPase.[27,39,40] In general, it appears that cholesterol is excluded from such microenvironments allowing for specific cooperative interactions of phospholipids or sphingomyelins with the protein.[23,37,38] It is reasonable to assume that for each species of protein specific lipid-protein interactions occur in discrete areas which are critical for the function of a membrane protein at any given time. These microdomains appear to be in a highly dynamic state and multiple in nature. Those lipid domains which are temporarily not interacting with proteins may best be pictured as being in an intermediate gel state whose fluidity is modulated by cholesterol. We speculate that membranes change constantly according to the cell cycle phase and to the degree of functional differentiation. Because of the short duration of cooperative lipid-lipid and lipid-protein interactions, lateral diffusion of proteins through entire membrane domains is likely, and the speed of such movement can be expected to vary greatly according to the specific proteins in question. Indeed, available data for a vast number of different proteins differ from one another by a factor of more than 10,000,[24] meaning that some membrane proteins are considerably restricted in their lateral movements, whereas others diffuse rapidly in the plane of the membrane (for further details see References 10, 24, 41, and 42).

The enormous complexity of mammalian membranes has to be kept in mind, especially when one attempts to understand the functions of lymphocytes which are capable of displaying rather dramatic rapid changes in their cell surfaces, as is evident by capping phenomena, appearance and disappearance of microvilli, display of specific membrane antigens, secretion of antibodies, endocytosis, and specific effector-target cell interactions (for a review see Reference 43).

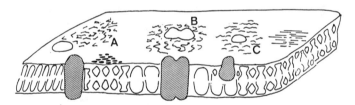

FIGURE 1. Simplified illustration of three areas in a hypothetical section of plasma membrane. (A) An area pictured containing phospholipids in a solid state (β-crystalline phase) which are represented by the symbols ⋔. A monomeric transmembrane protein is represented by a hatched area. To its right is pictured an area containing only cholesterol (◇◇). (B) Area around a dimeric protein consisting of phospholipid molecules in the α-liquid-crystalline state (⌒). (C) An area of the intermediate gel state is depicted where phospholipids and cholesterol interact (⌒◇⌒). The sizes of the various components are roughly drawn to scale to each other. The areas occupied by single species of membrane proteins vary greatly (not accounted for in this sketch).

STEROL BIOSYNTHESIS AND ITS REGULATION
IN LYMPHOCYTES

Most studies of sterol biosynthesis have not used lymphocytes, but rather established cultured cell types. Two excellent reviews have been written recently on the corresponding metabolic pathway,[25,44] so we thus confine our summary of present knowledge to that relevant to the following discussion of the effects of cholesterol and its oxygenated derivatives on the functions of lymphocytes.

Cholesterol is the major product of the biosynthetic pathway of isoprenoid compounds and of its key regulatory enzyme 3-hydroxy-3-methylglutaryl-CoA reductase

(HMG-CoA reductase; EC 1.1.1.34) (FIGURE 2). This pathway also yields the other minor cellular products dolichol, coenzyme Q (ubiquinone), and isopentenyl-adenosine.

It was originally believed, based on feeding experiments, that cholesterol regulates its own biosynthesis via suppression of the synthesis of HMG-CoA reductase. However in 1973, Kandutsch and Chen made the important discovery that chemically pure cholesterol is unable to suppress the enzyme activity in cultured L cells[45,46] whereas certain oxygenated sterols (diols) are powerful inhibitors of HMG-CoA reductase in nanomolar concentrations. The structural requirements for such an inhibitory action[47-50] are a hydroxyl function (in β configuration) in the three position, an intact side chain, and an additional oxygen (hydroxyl or ketone) function in position 6, 7, 14, 15, 20, 22, 24, 25, or 32 (FIGURE 3). Oxygenation of any of the carbon atoms in the first ring (A ring) of the molecule seems to be ineffective (A. A. Kandutsch, personal communication), whereas the presence of an oxygen function in any of the other ring positions or in the side chain may yield an inhibitory molecule, although the inhibitory strength varies greatly.[51,52] Most of these diols are easily generated from cholesterol by simple, noncatalytic autoxidation[25] which occurs in the presence of oxygen, and thus are potential, although minor, components of the human diet.[53]

The mechanism of the inhibition of HMG-CoA reductase is still not adequately understood. It is clear that it does not involve competitive inhibition of the enzyme,

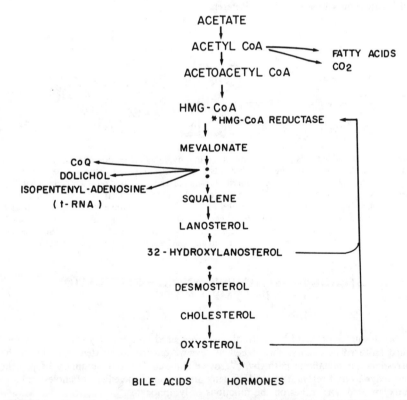

FIGURE 2. Biosynthetic pathway of isoprenoid compounds with the feedback regulation of the activity of the key enzyme in the pathway, HMG-CoA reductase.

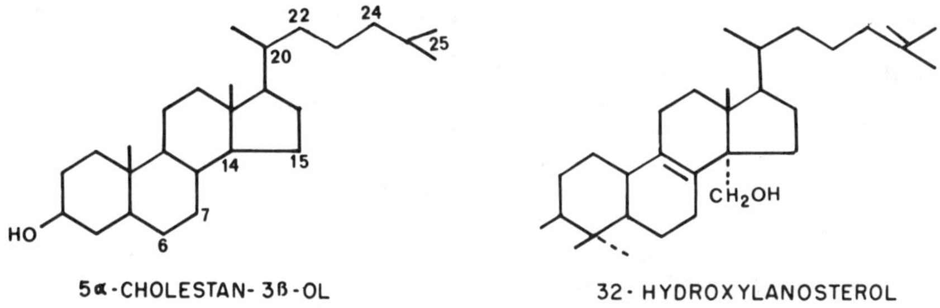

5α-CHOLESTAN- 3β-OL   32- HYDROXYLANOSTEROL

FIGURE 3. Left: Products of cholesterol autoxidation which are known inhibitors of sterol biosynthesis. A hydroxyl or ketone function on any of the designated carbon atoms yields an inhibitory molecule. Molecules that are oxidized in more than two positions are either weak inhibitors or do not inhibit HMG-CoA reductase at all. Right: 32-Hydroxylanosterol is a physiologic precursor of cholesterol.

nor is there convincing evidence for any direct effect of the oxygenated sterol on the enzyme. Experiments using metabolic inhibitors of RNA and protein synthesis and the use of enucleated cytoplasts[54] suggest strongly that the inhibition occurs at the transcriptional level involving the synthesis of the enzyme or its degradation, or both.

The oxygenated sterols, which inhibit sterol biosynthesis, not only occur spontaneously as a result of cholesterol autoxidation but also as natural metabolites in bile acid (7α-hydroxycholesterol) and steroid hormone (20α-hydroxycholesterol, 22-hydroxycholesterol) production.[25,48] 32-Hydroxylanosterol, an obligatory precursor of cholesterol, may be present in all mammalian cells.[47,50] Most experimental data available today, especially results obtained in mutant clones of cultured Chinese hamster cells,[51,55,56] suggest that all oxygenated sterols act through a common mechanism in inhibiting sterol biosynthesis. These cell lines were not only resistant to all these sterols but also to serum and to lipoproteins.[57] These results suggested that the ability of serum and lipoproteins to inhibit sterol synthesis might be due to the contaminating oxysterol in lipoproteins.

Even though the mechanism of action of oxygenated sterols is not clear at present, several recent studies suggest it may involve the binding to cytosolic (and perhaps nuclear) proteins.[58,59]

A variety of fungal metabolites, the most prominent of which is compactin (ML236B), have been found to be potent competitive inhibitors of HMG-CoA reductase.[60,61] Although these compounds have been proven to be of great experimental value in unraveling the complexity of the regulation of sterol biosynthesis and also may be of future therapeutic importance,[62] they are most probably not present in mammals under normal physiological conditions and are unlikely common contaminants of the diet.

In general, the synthesis of cholesterol appears to be regulated in lymphocytes in a way analogous to that in other mammalian cells. The lymphoid cells, however, seem to display some particular features which may be related to their specific physiologic functions and to their exposure to very different environments such as the interstitial space in various tissues vs. the serum of the vascular bloodstream. Nonstimulated lymphocytes synthesize cholesterol at very low rates.[63-66] The significance of this low rate of endogenous synthesis of cholesterol, which is also observed *in vivo,* is not understood but appears to be real. In our laboratory we have incubated splenic lymphocytes simultaneously with [^{14}C]acetate (to measure *de novo* cholesterol synthesis) and [³H]cholesterol (to monitor uptake of exogenous cholesterol) and established the ratio of the isotope in the digitonin-precipitable sterol fraction after extraction of the lipids from the cells. The $^{14}C/^3H$ ratio increases continuously over time in favor of [¹⁴C]acetate incorporation independent of serum concentration in the culture medium. These preliminary findings imply that a low rate of sterol synthesis may be of critical importance for the lymphocytes, and that cellular sterols cannot entirely be substituted by exogenous supply. This relative refractiveness of the lymphocytes to exogenous sterol concentration is at variance with results obtained in established tissue culture cells, whose rate of sterol synthesis is definitively dependent on the concentration of exogenous serum sterols.[23,67]

In contrast, lymphocytes stimulated by lectins[68-72] in mixed lymphocyte reactions[73] or by antibodies[74,75] synthesize cholesterol at a high rate. In phytohemagglutinin (PHA)- and concanavalin (Con A)-stimulated lymphocytes, a discrete peak of sterol synthesis distinctly precedes the cycle of DNA synthesis (FIGURE 4). It is of interest to mention here that these stimulated lymphocytes seem to be sensitive to very small doses of oxygenated sterols. In fact, they appear to show the highest sensitivity out of a large variety of cells analyzed.

Leukemic cells, from mice, guinea pigs, and humans,[63,66,76,77] display an excessively high rate of sterol synthesis, i.e., elevated up to 150-fold in comparison to normal lymphoid cells. In the case of leukemic cells from AKR mice this high rate of sterol synthesis is even enhanced further when the cells are exposed to small doses of PHA.[78] The mechanisms and causes of this excessive increase in sterol synthesis in leukemic cells remain unknown. It does not appear to be correlated with the concentration of sterols in the serum nor does the effect seem to be due to a loss of feedback regulation since sterol synthesis in leukemic cells is suppressed when they are exposed to oxygenated sterols.[66,78] (For further discussion of regulation of sterol synthesis in tumor cells see Reference 23.)

Relatively few studies have been done on the regulation of sterol synthesis in lymphocytes *in vivo*. This is experimentally difficult, due to the cellular heterogeneity of lymphoid organs. In the homeostatic steady state, i.e., in animals which have not been overtly challenged with specific exogenous antigens, it was found that lymphoid tissues, such as spleen, synthesize a relatively small amount of sterol as compared to the total amount synthesized by all other tissues.[79]

BIOLOGICAL EFFECTS OF OXYGENATED STEROLS ON LYMPHOCYTE FUNCTIONS

Effects on DNA Synthesis and the Proliferation of Lymphocytes

In 1975 we reported that a distinct peak of sterol synthesis preceded the cycle of DNA synthesis in PHA-stimulated lymphocytes[68] (FIGURE 4). When these cells were incubated with 25-hydroxycholesterol or 20α-hydroxycholesterol, their sterol synthesis was depressed. The dose required for total suppression was 0.75 μg/ml. DNA synthesis was inhibited by 80% at a dose of 25-hydroxycholesterol of 1 μg/ml. Fatty acid synthesis and CO_2 production (cellular respiration) were unaffected by the oxygenated sterols. Furthermore, DNA synthesis was only inhibited when the oxygenated sterols were present in the medium before or during the peak of sterol synthesis; if added at a later time interval they did not affect the DNA synthesis. These observations have since been confirmed by several laboratories using lymphocytes from a variety of species including man.[69,70,72,78,80] It was reestablished that inhibition of sterol synthesis by oxygenated sterols prevented the initiation of DNA synthesis, whereas hydroxyurea, which inhibits DNA synthesis directly, did not affect sterol synthesis. Interestingly enough, serum also inhibited to some degree both sterol and DNA synthesis of lectin-stimulated lymphocytes[68] as did the addition of low-density lipoprotein (LDL) in a dose-dependent fashion.[81,82] The latter two findings provoked the suspicion that the

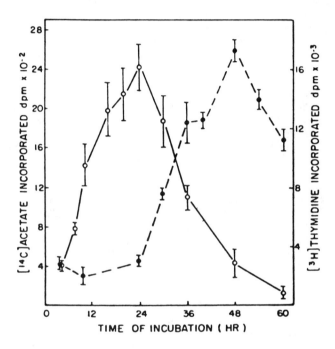

FIGURE 4. Time course of PHA stimulation of the syntheses of sterol and DNA. PHA was added at the beginning of the experiment and radioactive acetate or thymidine was added 2 hr before the end of the experiment. In experiments concerned with sterol synthesis (○) 0.5 ml of blood was cultured in a total volume of 5 ml. In those concerned with DNA synthesis (●) 0.05 ml of blood was cultured in a total volume of 0.5 ml. Triplicate samples were analyzed; points and ranges represent mean ± SEM. Data for control cultures without PHA are not shown; however, both sterol and DNA radioactivity counts were very low and were linear over the entire incubation period. (Reprinted with permission from Proc. Natl. Acad. Sci. USA **72** (1975): 1950.)

inhibitory components in these proteins may indeed be oxygenated sterols. Schuh *et al.*[83] provided evidence for this, although their report fell short of presenting definitive proof, due to technical problems related to the detection and identification of small, putative amounts of oxygenated sterols. However, it was concluded that an oxidized lipid was the inhibitory agent in the lipoprotein.

The relationship between sterol synthesis and DNA synthesis was further analyzed in our laboratory in mixed lymphocyte reactions (MLRs) involving an allogeneic difference at the major histocompatibility locus H-2 (H-2^b → H-2^d). The time course of the sterol synthesis and DNA synthesis was found to be somewhat different from the situation encountered in lectin-stimulated cultures. In primary cultures the onset of sterol synthesis slightly preceded DNA synthesis but then increased further, up to day 5, at which time also DNA synthesis peaked. Cytotoxic titers in these cultures were highest between days 5 and 7 and then declined steadily between days 7 and 12.[84,85] Several factors may account for this difference compared to lectin-stimulated lymphocytes: PHA- or Con A-stimulated T cells appear to exhibit a high degree of synchronization, at least during the first cell cycle, in which most experiments are made. In contrast, mixed lymphocyte cultures consist of asynchronous populations of proliferating cells with some of them exerting helper functions and others differentiating into cytotoxic effector cells.[86] The observed rates of sterol synthesis and DNA synthesis over time may thus reflect the average synthetic activity of the entire culture at any one time rather than reflecting distinct phases of the cell cycle of a given cell population. However, the initial increase of sterol synthesis in these cultures, preceding DNA synthesis, may be directly related to the first proliferative cell cycle of a cell population which responds initially to the allogeneic stimulation and thus may be directly compared to the situation observed in lectin-stimulated lymphocytes. The continuing elevated rate of sterol synthesis between days 4 and 8 trails the bulk of DNA synthesis and may represent an activity only partially related to proliferation. We propose that it is related to the actual induction and maintenance of the differentiated cytotoxic state of the effector cells.

Mixed lymphocyte cultures (MLCs) are extremely sensitive to oxygenated sterols: 25-hydroxycholesterol suppressed sterol synthesis to 30% at a dose of 0.05 μg/ml medium, and at a dose of 0.1 μg/ml (2.5 × 10^{-7} M) it completely abolished the sterol production. Consequently DNA synthesis was suppressed by 90% in the same cultures, extending the previously discussed observations in PHA- or Con A-stimulated lymphocytes. The effect of the oxygenated sterol on the MLR was observed as early as 6 hr after addition of the inhibitory sterol, suggesting an urgent need for *de novo* synthesized cholesterol and an absence of any sizable pool of free cholesterol in these cells.

Simultaneous addition of mevalonic acid, the product of HMG-CoA reductase, prevented the 25-hydroxycholesterol-mediated suppression of DNA synthesis for 24 to 48 hr thus arguing against direct effects of the oxysterol on the cells other than the depression of their HMG-CoA reductase activity for sterol biosynthesis.

It is appropriate to mention here the findings of Yachnin's group[80,87] that certain oxygenated sterols interfere, possibly by their insertion into the lipid bilayer, with certain membrane phenomena such as T-cell E-rosette formation, or that they provoke erythrocyte echinocytosis. Such direct effects of some oxygenated sterols on the cell membrane are not related to their interference with sterol synthesis, and no good correlation exists, for the sterols tested, between the potencies of their effects on sterol synthesis and the direct membrane effect of the compounds.[51,80,87] Most importantly, 25-hydroxycholesterol displayed no such direct membrane effects even at concentrations much higher than 1 μg/ml medium, and it is known that only minimal amounts can insert into the plasma membrane.[88]

The effects of oxygenated sterols on B cells, to our knowledge, have not been studied extensively. Humphries and McConnell[75] have exposed B-cell precursor cells during antigenic stimulation to 25-hydroxycholesterol and found that their plaque-forming ability was inhibited. They interpreted this to be due to the inhibition of proliferation, i.e., expansion of the antibody-producing clone.

The need for an enhanced rate of sterol synthesis preceding DNA synthesis and cell division in stimulated lymphocytes may be explained in several ways: (a) the cell needs cholesterol for the synthesis of new plasma membranes required for the two daughter cells resulting from cellular division, even in the presence of extracellular cholesterol (serum); (b) modulation of membrane fluidity may be required during the cell cycle as a mechanism for altering ion transport and other membrane-related biochemical events and may be accomplished by varying the concentration of membrane cholesterol via changes in the rate of sterol synthesis (chemotropic regulation of fluidity); and/or (c) the inhibition of DNA synthesis could also be related to a depressed synthesis of dolichol. However, we are of the opinion that substantial evidence for this last possibility is still lacking, since the synthesis of cholesterol has to be completely inhibited before an effect on dolichol synthesis becomes apparent.[89] Furthermore, the nature of the relationship between cell surface glycosylation and DNA replication is not known at present. The possibility that the availability of mevalonic acid (MVA), isopentenyl-adenosine (IPA), or coenzyme Q (CoQ) may be critical for DNA synthesis cannot be excluded. A direct effect of MVA or one of its products on cellular proliferation has been postulated in established tissue culture cells.[90–92] One group of investigators also reported that IPA exhibited a stimulatory action on lymphocytes[93] similar to the mitogenic effect of lectins. We have so far not been able to reproduce these results in our laboratory and feel that the possibility that MVA, IPA, or CoQ is responsible for the regulation of DNA synthesis is an interesting issue which, however, awaits further experimental evidence. All these interpretations are simplifications insofar as they focus on the proliferation of lymphocytes and ignore the fact that these cells simultaneously also differentiate from an immunologically inactive state into specifically functioning immunocytes, e.g., T-cell precursors into cytotoxic effector cells and B-cell precursors into antibody-producing cells.

Effects on Lymphocyte Differentiation and Function

We have used two experimental systems to analyze the role of sterol synthesis for lymphocyte function: the allogeneic mixed lymphocyte reaction and the polyclonal induction of cytotoxic T cells. Exposure of mixed lymphocyte cultures to micromolar concentrations of oxygenated sterols, such as 25-hydroxycholesterol, 20α-hydroxy-cholesterol, or 7-ketocholesterol, abolished the cytotoxic titers in these cultures as determined by the ^{51}Cr assay.[73] Cytotoxicity was abolished when the oxygenated sterols were present for 12 to 24 hr prior to the cytotoxicity assay. We excluded the possibility that the inhibition of cytotoxicity was caused by interference with the initial lymphocyte-target binding (doublet formation), since addition of PHA, a manipulation which is known to overcome allogeneic mismatching, was unable to restore the cytotoxicity of the effector cells. The presence of 25-hydroxycholesterol, even in high doses, during the cytotoxicity assay did not affect the test, thus excluding a direct effect of the oxygenated sterol on the function of the plasma membrane. To exclude the possibility that oxygenated sterols affect the formation of cytotoxic effector cells solely by inhibiting proliferation, i.e., expansion of specific clones of T-cell precursors, we used 11-day-old primary MLCs which were restimulated either by allogeneic cells or by supernatants from secondary MLCs.[73] It had previously been demonstrated that cytotoxic titers in such cultures rise rapidly within the first 24 hr after restimulation in the absence of DNA synthesis, i.e., even in the presence of potent inhibitors of DNA synthesis such as cytosine-arabinoside-C (ara-C).[94,95] We demonstrated that sterol synthesis increases dramatically shortly after restimulation of such cultures and parallels the increase in cytotoxic titers.[73] As summarized in TABLE 1, sterol synthesis

TABLE 1. Sterol Synthesis, Fatty Acid Synthesis, CO_2 Production, and Cytotoxicity 24 hr after Induction of Secondary CTLS[a]

Culture	$^{14}CO_2$ Production (dpm/10^6 cells)	Percentage of Control	Fatty Acid Synthesis (dpm/10^6 cells)	Percentage of Control	Sterol Synthesis (dpm/10^6 cells)	Percentage of Control	LU/10^6 Cells	Percentage of Control	Percentage Recovery of Cells (%)
Unstimulated cultures	14,556 ± 772	61	5,166 ± 313	19	1,215 ± 298	5	11	10	66
Unstimulated cultures + allogeneic cells (control)	23,960 ± 5,430	100	43,687 ± 9,260	100	23,582 ± 6,033	100	111	100	47
Unstimulated cultures + allogeneic cells + 25-OH-cholesterol	19,780 ± 8,047	83	23,247 ± 5,669	53	609 ± 54	2.5	<1	<1	44

[a] Cells recovered from C57BL/6 anti-DBA/2 long-term primary MLC were restimulated with irradiated allogeneic spleen cells (DBA/2) or MLC supernatant alone or in the presence of 25-OH-cholesterol at 2 µg/ml. After 24 hr of incubation, some of the cells were used in a 3-hr ^{51}Cr release assay on P-815 (DBA/2) target cells to determine the cytolytic activity and the remainder of the cells were used to determine $^{14}CO_2$ production, fatty acid synthesis, and sterol synthesis. The values represent means ± SEM from three cultures. (Data from Proc. Natl. Acad. Sci. USA 75 (1978): 5683.)

was up 20-fold and cytotoxic titers 10-fold, 24 hr after restimulation of the primary cultures. This occurred in the absence or presence of ara-C. When oxygenated sterols, such as 25-hydroxycholesterol, were added to the cultures in doses of 0.5-3 $\mu g/ml$ at the moment of restimulation, the cytotoxic titers were not only prevented from increasing but the residual titers of day 11 disappeared. The rather dramatic effects of the oxygenated sterols on the cytotoxic effector cells could be partially prevented by simultaneous addition of relatively large doses of MVA or cholesterol, an effect similar to the one observed for DNA synthesis. Altogether these results provided initial evidence, since then confirmed by others,[70] that an adequate supply of cholesterol is critical for T cells to acquire and maintain their cytotoxic function besides being a requirement for DNA synthesis and cellular proliferation. *De novo* synthesis seems to be necessary, at least to some degree, since exogenous supply of MVA or cholesterol appears to be unable to completely overcome the effects of oxygenated sterols.

The findings on MLR have since been further corroborated in our laboratory, as well as by other investigators, using polyclonally activated T cells.[70,71] These studies reaffirm the hypothesis that oxygenated sterols interfere with both the proliferation and the differentiation of these cells by limiting the supply of endogenous cholesterol through inhibition of its biosynthesis. In addition, using polyclonally activated T cells, we were able to demonstrate that differentiation occurs in these cells, even in the absence of DNA synthesis as long as they are allowed to go through a normal cycle of sterol synthesis.[71] Thus, it appears to be established that the availability of cholesterol through a combination of endogenous and exogenous sources is essential for the physiological functions of lymphocytes; nevertheless, the nature of the specific function of cholesterol in the plasma membrane of these highly specialized cells remains unknown.

The role of cholesterol for B-cell function has not been as extensively investigated. Some studies[74,75] have, as mentioned, suggested that it affects the production of antibody mainly by inhibiting the proliferation of the relevant clone. However, more experiments appear to be necessary to support this statement. Since the molecular structures of the gamma globulin chains and their RNA precursors are now known,[96–101] it will be of great interest to analyze the structural requirements of the lipid moiety of the plasma membrane of B cells in relation to the functioning of B-cell receptors and/ or the secretion of antibodies.

Finally, we want to mention here that the function of circulating human natural killer cells (NK cells) was not affected by exposure to oxygenated sterols (Heiniger and Cerottini, unpublished results). This finding requires further investigation, but may be due to the fact that such circulating "lymphoid" cells may not exhibit any appreciable rate of sterol synthesis. If this is indeed the case, then the experiment merely reemphasizes our conclusion that oxygenated sterols act specifically via inhibition of sterol synthesis.

Effects of Oxygenated Sterols on Immune Phenomena in Vivo

Since oxygenated sterols are potential contaminants of the human diet[102] it would be of great interest to know their effects on the immune system *in vivo* if they are ingested. So far it is known that feeding of oxysterols to mice inhibits their appetite, temporarily suppresses sterol synthesis in intestine and liver, and interferes with the growth of young animals.[103] Other investigators[104] analyzed the cholesterol ÷ phospholipid ratio (CPR) in the plasma membranes of lymphocytes obtained from immunized and nonimmunized rats and found that in the cells from immune animals the CPR was lower due to a relative decrease of cholesterol, implying that these lymphocytes may have a more fluid plasma membrane.

Recently Peng et al.[105] demonstrated in squirrel monkeys that radioactively labeled 25-hydroxycholesterol fed in a single dose (in a marshmallow which the monkeys devoured avidly), preferentially accumulated in the very low density lipoprotein (VLDL) and low density lipoprotein (LDL) fractions of the serum lipoproteins. The same authors also stated that they found oxygenated sterols in many components of the human diet such as pancake mix, cheeses, lard, and concentrated milk formulas. Smith similarly reported the presence of such sterols in various foodstuffs.[102] These findings of course prompted the suspicion that lymphocytes, as rapidly circulating cells, may be exposed to such sterols.

Experiments are presently under way in our laboratory to analyze the effect of orally administered oxygenated sterols on the immune response against tetanus toxin. Inbred mice, mainly C57BL/6J females, were subdivided into the following groups, each consisting of 10-20 animals: (a) control group receiving standard mouse diet, (b) experimental group receiving a diet containing 0.25% 7-ketocholesterol (this amount of oxygenated sterol does not contribute significantly to the caloric value of the diet), and (c) experimental group receiving 1% cholesterol in the diet. After a primary immunization via both hind footpads, the animals were kept for 28 days. Half the animals of each group were killed to determine primary titers against tetanus toxoid. One hour prior to sacrifice, the mice were given a pulse of [^{3}H]thymidine for an estimate of the proliferative activity in their lymphatic tissues. Liver, spleen, and popliteal lymph nodes were removed and incubated in vitro with [^{14}C]acetate in order to determine the rates of sterol synthesis.

The remaining animals of each group were reimmunized with tetanus toxoid. Secondary immune antitoxin responses were measured at days 2, 4, and 5 after restimulation, and at these time intervals the mice were processed precisely as described above.

The partial evaluation of some of the experiments as far as completed, indicates the following:

1. Sterol synthesis is demonstrable in all lymphoid tissues.
2. The diet containing 0.25% 7-ketocholesterol only moderately influences the primary immune response, but appears to have a suppressive effect on the secondary response (FIGURE 5).

At this point experimental results are insufficient for firm statements regarding the biological effects of the oxygenated sterols in vivo on cellular and humoral defenses. The clinical significance of major efforts in that direction is evident.

CONCLUSIONS

Some years ago only a few laboratories were interested in the biosynthetic pathway of cholesterol. The discovery of the biological activity of oxygenated sterols brought about a dramatic change. This area of research is rapidly expanding because of the obvious significance of the synthetic pathway of isoprenoid compounds in many areas of biomedical research, such as immunology, cancer, and atherosclerosis research, to name but a few examples.

The bulk of the data collected on lymphocytes in vitro indicates that unstimulated lymphocytes synthesize cholesterol at a low rate, which, however, appears to be real and not simply the reflection of methodological shortcomings (high background, etc.). Upon stimulation, lymphocytes display a high rate of sterol synthesis, apparently linked to both their proliferative cycle and their functional differentiation, such as the acquisition of cytotoxic activity by T cells. The high rate of sterol synthesis is abolished upon exposure of the cells to nanomolar concentrations of oxygenated sterols, but chemically pure cholesterol does not affect the biosynthetic activity. Prevention of lymphocytes from entering the cycle of sterol synthesis upon stimulation not only abolishes cell division but also specific immunological functions. The regulation of cholesterol synthesis in these cells appears to be far more complex than originally conceived and understanding it remains a challenge for future investigations.

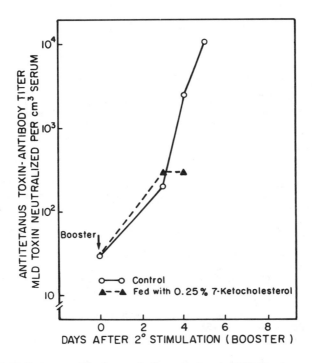

FIGURE 5. Preliminary results from a feeding experiment. C57L/J mice were fed a diet containing 0.25% (W/W) 7-ketocholesterol or normal pulverized chow for the entire observation period. Each point represents the tetanus antitoxic titer of pooled sera from two to five mice. Uptake of oxysterol appeared to have no influence on primary responses, but secondary antitoxin titers were depressed.

ACKNOWLEDGMENTS

We wish to express our appreciation to Drs. D. L. Coleman and P. W. Rossow for their critical review of this paper. The work would not have been possible without the professional assistance of Ms. Jan D. Marshall.

REFERENCES

1. BRETSCHER, M. S. 1973. Membrane structure: some general principles. Science **181:** 622.
2. CHAPMAN, D. 1968. Biological Membranes. Physical Fact and Function. Academic Press, Inc. New York, N.Y.
3. CHAPMAN, D. 1973. Some recent studies of lipids, lipid-cholesterol and membrane systems in biological membranes. *In* Biological Membranes. D. Chapman & D. F. H. Wallach, Eds. **2:** 91. Academic Press, Inc. New York, N.Y.
4. CRONAN, J. E. & E. P. GELMANN. 1975. Physical properties of membrane lipids: biological relevance and regulation. Bacteriol. Rev. **39:** 232.
5. DEMEL, R. A. & B. DE KRUYFF. 1976. The function of sterols in membranes. Biochim. Biophys. Acta **457:** 109.
6. GREEN, D. E. 1972. Membrane structure and its biological applications. Ann. N.Y. Acad. Sci. **195:** 5.
7. MCCONNELL, H. M. 1975. Role of lipid in membrane structure and function. *In* Cellular Membranes and Tumor Cell Behavior. (A collection of papers presented at the 28th Annual Symposium of Fundamental Cancer Research.) Williams & Wilkins. Baltimore, Md.
8. NICHOLSON, G. L., G. POSTE & T. H. JI. 1977. The dynamics of cell membrane organization. *In* Dynamic Aspects of Cell Surface Organization. G. Poste & G. L. Nicholson, Eds.: 1. Elsevier/North-Holland Biomedical Press. Amsterdam, the Netherlands.
9. BROCKENHOFF, H. 1974. Model of interaction of polar lipids, cholesterol, and proteins in biological membranes. Lipids **9:** 645.
10. SHAMOO, A. E. 1975. Carriers and channels in biological systems. Ann. N.Y. Acad. Sci. **264:** 1.
11. SCHMIDT-ULLRICH, R., D. F. H. WALLACH & F. D. G. DAVIS. 1976. Membranes of normal hamster lymphocytes and lymphoid cells neoplastically transformed by simian virus 40. I. High-yield purification of plasma membrane fragments. J. Natl. Cancer Inst. **57:** 1107.
12. ALLAN, D. & M. J. CRIMPTON. 1972. Isolation and composition of human thymocyte plasma membrane. Biochim. Biophys. Acta **274:** 22.
13. CHAPMAN, D. 1975. Phase transitions and fluidity characteristics of lipids and cell membranes. Q. Rev. Biophys. **9:** 195.
14. KROES, J., R. OSTWARD & A. KEITH. 1972. Erythrocyte membranes: compression of lipid phases by increased cholesterol content. Biochim. Biophys. Acta **274:** 71.
15. LADBRROKE, B. D., R. M. WILLIAMS & D. CHAPMAN. 1968. Studies on lecithin-cholesterol-water interactions by differential scanning calorimetry and x-ray differentiation. Biochim. Biophys. Acta **150:** 133.
16. FINEAN, J. B. 1953. Phospholipid-cholesterol complex in the structure of myelin. Experientia **9:** 17.
17. HUANG, C.-H. 1976. Roles of carbonyl oxygens at the bilayer interface in phospholipid-sterol interaction. Nature (London) **259:** 242.
18. LUCY, J. A. 1968. Theoretical and experimental models for biological membranes. *In* Biological Membranes. D. Chapman, Ed.: 233. Academic Press, Inc. New York, N.Y.
19. VANDENHEUVEL, F. A. 1963. Study of biological structure at the molecular level with stereomodel projections. I. The lipids in the myelin sheath of the nerve. J. Am. Oil Chem. Soc. **40:** 455.
20. KRUYFF, G., R. A. DE DEMEL & L. L. M. VAN DEENEN. 1972. The effect of cholesterol and epicholesterol incorporation on the permeability and on the phase transition of intact *Acholeplasma laidlawii* cell membranes and derived liposomes. Biochim. Biophys. Acta **255:** 331.
21. DARKE, A., E. G. FINER, A. G. FLOOK & M. C. PHILLIPS. 1972. Nuclear magnetic resonance of lecithin-cholesterol interactions. J. Mol. Biol. **63:** 265.
22. STOFFEL, W., B. D. TUNGGAL, O. ZIERENBERG, E. SCHREIBER & E. BINCZEK. 1974. ^{13}C-nuclear magnetic resonance studies of lipid interactions in single and multi-component lipid vesicles. Hoppe-Seyler's Z. Physiol. Chem. **355:** 1367.

23. CHEN, H. W., A. A. KANDUTSCH & H.-J. HEINIGER. 1978. The role of cholesterol in malignancy. *In* Progress in Experimental Tumor Research. F. Homburger, Ed. **22:** 275. Karger. Basel, Switzerland.

24. CHERRY, R. J. 1976. Protein and lipid mobility in biological and model membranes. *In* Biological Membranes. D. Chapman & D. F. H. Wallach, Eds. **3:** 47. Academic Press, Inc. New York, N.Y.

25. KANDUTSCH, A. A. 1980. Biological effects of some products of cholesterol autooxidation. *In* Autooxidation in Food and Biological Systems. M. G. Simic & M. Karel, Eds.: 589. Plenum Press. New York, N.Y.

26. BALDASSARE, J. J., Y. SAITO & D. F. SILBERT. 1979. Effect of sterol depletion on LM cell sterol mutants. Changes in the lipid composition of the plasma membrane and their effects on 3-O-methylglucose. J. Biol. Chem. **254:** 1108.

27. CHEN, H. W., H.-J. HEINIGER & A. A. KANDUTSCH. 1978. Alteration of ^{86}Rb$^+$ influx and efflux following depletion of membrane sterol in L cells. J. Biol. Chem. **253:** 3180.

28. SINENSKY, M., F. PINKERTON, E. SUTHERLAND & F. R. SIMON. 1979. Rate limiting of (Na$^+$ + K$^+$)-stimulated adenosine triphosphatase by membrane acyl chain ordering. Proc. Natl. Acad. Sci. USA **76:** 4893.

29. FAHEY, P. F., D. E. KIPELL, L. S. BARAK, D. E. WOLF, E. L. ELSON & W. W. WEBB. 1976. Lateral diffusion in planar lipid bilayers. Science **195:** 305.

30. SCHLESSINGER, J., D. AXELROD, D. E. KOPELL, W. W. WEBB & E. L. ELSON. 1976. Lateral transport of a lipid probe and labeled proteins on a cell membrane. Science **195:** 307.

31. SCHLESSINGER, J., D. E. KOPELL, D. AXELROD, K. JACOBSON, W. W. WEBB & E. L. ELSON. 1976. Lateral transport on cell membranes: mobility of concanavalin A receptors of myoblasts. Proc. Natl. Acad. Sci. USA **73:** 24.

32. HEINIGER, H.-J., A. A. KANDUTSCH & H. W. CHEN. 1976. Depletion of L-cell sterol depresses endocytosis. Nature (London) **263:** 515.

33. HEINIGER, H.-J. & J. D. MARHSALL. 1979. Pinocytosis in L-cells: its dependence on membrane sterol and the cytoskeleton. Cell Biol. Int. Rep. **3:** 409.

34. CHANGEUX, J.-P., J. THIERY, Y. TUNG & C. KITTEL. 1969. On the cooperativity of biological membranes. Proc. Natl. Acad. Sci. USA **57:** 1552.

35. WALLACH, D. F. H. & H. P. ZAHLER. 1966. Protein conformations in cellular membranes. Proc. Natl. Acad. Sci. USA **56:** 1552.

36. SINGER, S. J. & G. L. NICHOLSON. 1972. The fluid mosaic model of the structure of cell membranes. Science **175:** 720.

37. WALLACH, D. F. H. 1976. Membrane abnormalities of neoplastic cells. Med. Hypoth. **2**(No. 6): 241.

38. WALLACH, D. F. H. (Ed.). 1979. Plasma Membrane and Disease. Academic Press, Inc. New York, N.Y.

39. KIMELBERG, H. K. & D. PAHAHADJOPOULOS. 1972. Phospholipid requirements for (Na$^+$ and K$^+$)-ATPase activity: head-group specificity and fatty acid fluidity. Biochim. Biophys. Acta **282:** 277.

40. WARREN, G. B., M. D. HOUSLAY, J. C. METCALFE & N. J. M. BIRDSALL. 1975. Cholesterol is excluded from the phospholipid annulus surrounding an active calcium transport protein. Nature New Biol. **255:** 684.

41. HYNES, R. A. 1976. Cell surface proteins and malignant transformation. Biochim. Biophys. Acta **458:** 73.

42. KLEEMAN, W. & H. M. MCCONNELL. 1976. Interactions of proteins and cholesterol with lipids in bilayer membranes. Biochim. Biophys. Acta **419:** 206.

43. LOOR, R. 1977. Structure and dynamics of the lymphocyte surface. *In* B and T Cells in Immune Recognition. F. Loor & G. Roelants, Eds.: 153. G. E. Wiley and Sons. Chichester, England.

44. SCHROEPFER, G. 1981. Sterol biosynthesis. Annu. Rev. Biochem. **50:** 585.

45. KANDUTSCH, A. A. & H. W. CHEN. 1973. Inhibition of sterol synthesis in cultured mouse cells by 7α-hydroxycholesterol, 7β-hydroxycholesterol and 7-ketocholesterol. J. Biol. Chem. **248:** 8403.

46. KANDUTSCH, A. A. & H. W. CHEN. 1974. Inhibition of sterol synthesis in cultured mouse cells by cholesterol derivatives oxygenated in the side chain. J. Biol. Chem. **249:** 6057.

47. GIBBONS, G. F., C. R. PULLINGER, H. W. CHEN, W. K. CAVENEE & A. A. KANDUTSCH. 1980. Suppression of cholesterol biosynthesis in cultured cells by probable precursor sterols. J. Biol. Chem. **255**: 295.

48. KANDUTSCH, A. A., H. W. CHEN & H.-J. HEINIGER. 1978. The biological activity of some oxygenated sterols. Science **201**: 498.

49. SCHROEPFER, G. J., JR., R. A. PASCALL, JR., R. SHAW & A. A. KANDUTSCH. 1978. Inhibition of sterol biosynthesis by 14α-hydroxymethyl sterols. Biochem. Biophys. Res. Commun. **83**: 1024.

50. TABACIK, C., S. ALTAN, B. SERROU & A. CRASTES DE PAULET. 1981. Post HMG CoA reductase regulation of cholesterol biosynthesis in normal human lymphocytes: lanosten-3-β-ol-32-al, a natural inhibitor. Biochem. Biophys. Res. Commun. **101**: 1087.

51. CAVENEE, W. K., G. F. GIBBONS, H. W. CHEN & A. A. KANDUTSCH. 1979. Effects of various oxygenated sterols on cellular sterol biosynthesis in Chinese hamster lung cells resistant to 25-hydroxycholesterol. Biochim. Biophys. Acta **575**: 225.

52. KANDUTSCH, A. A. & H. W. CHEN. 1978. Inhibition of cholesterol synthesis by oxygenated sterols. Lipids **13**: 704.

53. SIMIC, M. G. & M. KAREL (Eds.). 1980. Autooxidation in Food and Biological Systems. Plenum Press. New York, N.Y.

54. CAVENEE, W. K., H. W. CHEN & A. A. KANDUTSCH. 1981. Regulation of cholesterol biosynthesis in enucleated cells. J. Biol. Chem. **256**: 2675.

55. CHEN, H. W., W. K. CAVENEE & A. A. KANDUTSCH. 1979. Variant Chinese hamster lung cells selected for resistance to 25-hydroxycholesterol: cross resistance to 7-keto-cholesterol, 20α-hydroxycholesterol and serum. J. Biol. Chem. **254**: 615.

56. SINENSKY, M., G. DUWE & F. PINKERTON. 1979. Defective regulation of 3-hydroxy-3-methylglutaryl coenzyme A reductase in a somatic cell mutant. J. Biol. Chem. **254**: 4482.

57. BROWN, M. S. & J. L. GOLDSTEIN. 1975. Receptor-mediated control of cholesterol metabolism. Science **191**: 150.

58. KANDUTSCH, A. A., H. W. CHEN & E. P. SHOWN. 1977. Binding of 25-hydroxycholesterol and cholesterol to different cytoplasmic proteins. Proc. Natl. Acad. Sci. USA **74**: 2500.

59. KANDUTSCH, A. A. & E. B. THOMPSON. 1980. Cytosolic protein(s) that bind oxygenated sterols: cellular distribution, specificity and some properties. J. Biol. Chem. **255**: 10813.

60. ENDO, A., K. KURODA & K. TANZAWA. 1976. Competitive inhibition of 3-hydroxy-3-methylglutaryl coenzyme A reductase by ML-236 A and ML-236 B fungal metabolites having hypocholesteremic activity. FEBS Lett. **72**: 323.

61. KANEKO, I., Y. HAZAMA-SHIMADA & A. ENDO. 1978. Inhibitory effects of lipid metabolism in cultured cells of ML-236 B, a potent inhibitor of 3-hydroxy-3-methylglutaryl coenzyme A reductase. Eur. J. Biochem. **87**: 313.

62. BROWN, M. S., P. T. KOVANEN & J. L. GOLDSTEIN. 1981. Regulation of plasma cholesterol by lipoprotein receptors. Science **212**: 628.

63. CHEN, H. W. & H.-J. HEINIGER. 1974. Stimulation of sterol synthesis by human lymphocytes and monocytes. J. Lipid Res. **20**: 379.

64. FOGELMAN, A. M., J. SEAGER, M. HOKOM & P. A. EDWARDS. 1979. Separation of and cholesterol synthesis by human lymphocytes and monocytes. J. Lipid Res. **20**: 379.

65. O'DONNELL, V. J., P. OTTOLENGHI, A. MALKIN, O. F. DENSTEDT & R. D. H. HEARD. 1958. The biosynthesis from acetate-1-^{14}C of fatty acids and cholesterol in formed blood elements. Can. J. Biochem. **36**: 1125.

66. PHILIPPOT, J. R., A. G. COOPER & D. F. H. WALLACH. 1976. 25-Hydroxycholesterol and 1,25-dihydroxycholecalciferol are potent inhibitors of cholesterol biosynthesis by normal and leukemic (L_2C) guinea pig lymphocytes. Biochem. Biophys. Res. Commun. **72**: 1035.

67. CHEN, H. W. & A. A. KANDUTSCH. 1985. Cholesterol requirement for cell growth: endogenous synthesis vs. exogenous sources. *In* The Nutritional Requirements of Vertebrate Cells in Vitro. R. G. Ham & C. Waymouth, Eds. University of Cambridge Press. London, England.

68. CHEN, H. W., H.-J. HEINIGER & A. A. KANDUTSCH. 1975. Relationship between sterol synthesis and DNA synthesis in phytohemagglutinin-stimulated mouse lymphocytes. Proc. Natl. Acad. Sci. USA **72**: 1950.

69. CHEN, S. S. H. 1979. Enhanced sterol synthesis in concanavalin A-stimulated lymphocytes: correlation with phospholipid synthesis and DNA synthesis. J. Cell. Physiol. **100:** 147.
70. DABROWSKI, M. P., W. E. PEEL & A. E. R. THOMPSON. 1980. Plasma membrane cholesterol regulates human lymphocyte cytotoxic function. Eur. J. Immunol. **10:** 821.
71. HEINIGER, H.-J. & J. D. MARSHALL. Oxygenated derivatives of cholesterol and lymphocyte function: sterol synthesis in polyclonally activated cytotoxic spleen cells and its requirement for differentiation and proliferation. In preparation.
72. PRATT, H. P. M., P. A. FITZGERALD & A. SAXON. 1977. Synthesis of sterol and phospholipid induced by the interaction of phytohemagglutinin and other mitogens with human lymphocytes and their relation to blastogenesis and DNA synthesis. Cell. Immunol. **32:** 160.
73. HEINIGER, H.-J., K. T. BRUNNER & J.-C. CEROTTINI. 1978. Cholesterol is a critical cellular component for T-lymphocyte cytotoxicity. Proc. Natl. Acad. Sci. USA **75:** 5683.
74. HUMPHRIES, G. M. K. 1981. Compactin and oxidized cholesterol, both known to inhibit cholesterol biosynthesis, differ in their ability to suppress in vitro immune responses. Cancer Res. **41:** 3789.
75. HUMPHRIES, G. M. K. & H. M. McCONNELL. 1979. Potent immunosuppression by oxidized cholesterol. J. Immunol. **122:** 121.
76. CHEN, H. W., A. A. KANDUTSCH, H.-J. HEINIGER & H. MEIER. 1973. Elevated sterol synthesis in lymphatic leukemia cells from two inbred strains of mice. Cancer Res. **33:** 2774.
77. HEINIGER, H.-J., H. W. CHEN, O. L. APPLEGATE, L. P. SCHACTER, B. Z. SCHRACTER & P. N. ANDERSON. 1976. Elevated synthesis of cholesterol in human leukemia cells. J. Mol. Biol. **1:** 109.
78. CHEN, H. W., H.-J. HEINIGER & A. A. KANDUTSCH. 1977. Stimulation of sterol and DNA synthesis in leukemic blood cells by a low concentration of phytohemagglutinin. Exp. Cell Res. **109:** 253.
79. TURLEY, S. D., J. M. ANDERSON & J. M. DIETSCHY. 1981. Rates of sterol synthesis and uptake in the major organs of the rat in vivo. J. Lipid Res. **22:** 551.
80. YACHNIN, S. & R. HSU. 1980. Inhibition of human lymphocyte transformation by oxygenated sterol compounds. Cell. Immunol. **51:** 42.
81. HAGMANN, J., I. WEILER & E. WAELTI. 1979. Effects of low density lipoproteins on lymphocyte stimulation. FEBS Lett. **97:** 230.
82. MORSE, J. H., L. D. WITTE & P. S. GOODMAN. 1977. Inhibition of lymphocyte proliferation stimulation by lectins and allogeneic cells by normal lipoproteins. J. Exp. Med. **146:** 1791.
83. SCHUH, J., A. NOVOGRODSKY & R. H. HASCHEMEYER. 1978. Inhibition of lymphocyte mitogenesis by autooxidized low-density lipoprotein. Biochem. Biophys. Res. Commun. **84:** 763.
84. CEROTTINI, J.-C., H. D. ENGERS, H. R. MACDONALD & K. T. BRUNNER. 1974. Generation of cytotoxic T lymphocytes in vitro. I. Response of normal and immune mouse spleen cells in mixed leukocyte culture. J. Exp. Med. **140:** 703.
85. ENGERS, H. D. & H. R. MACDONALD. 1976. Generation of cytolytic T lymphocytes in vitro. *In* Contemporary Topics in Immunobiology. W. Weigel, Ed. **5:** 145. Plenum Press. New York, N.Y.
86. RYSER, J. E. & H. R. MACDONALD. 1979. Limiting dilution analysis of alloantigen-reactive T lymphocytes. I. Comparison of precursor frequencies for proliferation and cytolytic responses. J. Immunol. **122:** 1691.
87. YACHNIN, S., R. A. STREULI, L. J. GORDON & R. C. HSU. 1979. Alteration of peripheral blood cell membrane function and morphology by oxygenated sterol, a membrane hypothesis. Curr. Top. Hematol. **2:** 245.
88. HSU, R. C., J. R. KANOFSKY & S. YACHNIN. 1980. The formation of echinocytes by the insertion of oxygenated sterol compounds into red cell membranes. Blood **56:** 109.
89. JAMES, M. J. & A. A. KANDUTSCH. 1979. Interrelationship between dolichol and sterol synthesis in mammalian cell cultures. J. Biol. Chem. **254:** 8442.
90. HABENICHT, A. J. R., J. A. GLOMSET & R. ROSS. 1980. Relation of cholesterol and mevalonic acid to the cell cycle in smooth muscle and Swiss 3T3 cells stimulated to divide by platelet-derived growth factor. J. Biol. Chem. **255:** 5134.

91. QUESNEY-HUNEEUS, V., M. H. WILEY & M. D. SIPERSTAIN. 1979. Essential role for mevalonate synthesis in DNA replication. Proc. Natl. Acad. Sci. USA **76:** 5056.
92. QUESNEY-HUNEEUS, V., M. H. WILEY & M. D. SIPERSTEIN. 1980. Isopentenyladenine as a mediator of mevalonate-regulated DNA replication. Proc. Natl. Acad. Sci. USA **77:** 5842.
93. GALLO, R. C., J. WANG-PENG & S. PERRY. 1969. Isopentenyladenosine stimulates and inhibits mitosis of human lymphocytes treated with phytohemagglutinin. Science **165:** 400.
94. MACDONALD, H. R., H. D. ENGERS, J.-C. CEROTTINI & K. T. BRUNNER. 1974. Generation of cytotoxic T lymphocytes in vitro. J. Exp. Med. **140:** 718.
95. MACDONALD, H. R., H. D. ENGERS, J.-C. CEROTTINI & K. T. BRUNNER. 1975. Generation of cytotoxic T lymphocytes in vitro. J. Exp. Med. **142:** 622.
96. ALT, F. W., A. L. M. BOTHWELL, M. KNAPP, E. SIDEN, E. MATHER, M. KOSHLAND & D. BALTIMORE. 1980. Synthesis of secreted and membrane-bound immunoglobulin μ chains is directed by mRNAs that differ at their 3' ends. Cell **20:** 293.
97. BERGMAN, Y., C. BLATT, Z. ESHAR & J. HAIMOVICH. 1979. The differences in structure between secreted and cell surface membrane immunoglobulins. *In* Cell Biology and Immunology of Leukocyte Function. M. R. Quastel, Ed.: 245. Academic Press, Inc. New York, N.Y.
98. LUI, C.-P., P. W. TUCKER, J. F. MUSHINSKI & F. R. BLATTNER. 1980. Mapping of heavy chain genes for mouse immunoglobulins M and D. Science **209:** 1348.
99. MOSHMANN, T. R. & A. R. WILLIAMSON. 1980. Structural mutations in a mouse immunoglobulin light chain resulting in failure to be secreted. Cell **20:** 283.
100. ROGERS, J., P. EARLY, C. CARTER, K. CALAME, M. BOND, L. HOOD & R. WALL. 1980. Two mRNAs with different 3' ends encode membrane-bound and secreted forms of immunoglobulin μ chain. Cell **21:** 303.
101. SAKANO, H., R. MAKI, Y. KUROSAWA, W. ROEDER & S. TONEGAWA. 1980. Two types of somatic recombination are necessary for the generation of complete immunoglobulin heavy chain genes. Nature **286:** 676.
102. SMITH, L. L. 1980. The autoxidation of cholesterol. *In* Autooxidation in Food and Biological Systems. M. G. Simic & M. Karel, Eds.: 119. Plenum Press. New York, N.Y.
103. KANDUTSCH, A. A., H.-J. HEINIGER & H. W. CHEN. 1977. Effects of 25-hydroxycholesterol and 7-ketocholesterol, inhibitors of sterol synthesis, administered orally to mice. Biochim. Biophys. Acta **486:** 260.
104. SMITH, W. I., C. T. LADOULIS, D. N. MISRA, T. J. GILL III & H. BAZIN. 1975. Lymphocyte plasma membranes. III. Composition of lymphocyte plasma membranes from normal and immunized rats. Biochim. Biophys. Acta **383:** 505.
105. PENG, S. K., B. C. TAYLOR, E. H. MOSBACH, W. Y. HUANG, J. HILL & B. MIKKELSON. 1982. Distribution of 25-hydroxycholesterol in plasma lipoproteins and its role in atherogenesis. A study in squirrel monkeys. J. Atherosclerosis **41:** 395.

Regulation of Human Erythroid Proliferation *in Vitro* by Leukocyte Surface Components[a]

NICHOLAS DAINIAK AND CARL M. COHEN[b]

Departments of Medicine and Biomedical Research
St. Elizabeth's Hospital of Boston
Boston, Massachusetts 02135

Departments of Medicine and [b]Molecular Biology and Microbiology
School of Medicine
Tufts University
Boston, Massachusetts 02155

INTRODUCTION

Given appropriate conditions, mammalian erythroid cells will multiply and synthesize hemoglobin in primary tissue culture. Although the complicated *in vivo* behavior that results in the production of mature, functional erythrocytes is more readily understood by examining erythropoiesis *in vitro* using chemically defined growth media,[1-3] cellular and molecular complexities of seeded hematopoietic tissue obscure the nature of specific requirements for erythroid growth. Thus, while it is apparent that cellular interactions are one important determinant of optimal erythropoiesis,[4,5] little is known about how hematopoietic and other cells communicate to support erythropoiesis *in vitro,* and even less information is available regarding such regulation within the local bone marrow environment. Leukocytes represent one cell type located in proximity to developing erythroid cells *in vivo.* They impart to tissue culture medium a growth factor that is essential for survival and proliferation of erythroid burst forming units (BFU-Es).[6] We approached the characterization of one type of cellular interaction, the leukocyte-erythroid interaction, by asking how circulating leukocytes might release growth promoting molecules.

When considering the manner in which mammalian cells release biologically active materials into liquid medium during incubation, three potential mechanisms come to mind (see FIGURE 1). First, they may eject macromolecules that have been packaged in intracellular vesicles by the process of vesicle fusion with the surface membrane (exocytosis). Second, they may shed or exfoliate membrane components from the cell surface in the form of vesicles that may contain small quantities of cytoplasmic

[a]This work was supported by National Institutes of Health Research Grants AM31060 and AM27071 to Dr. Dainiak.

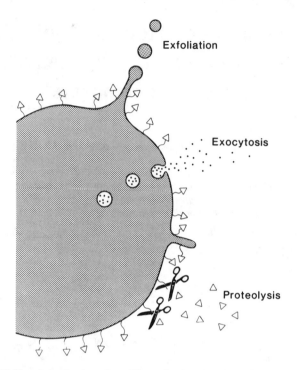

FIGURE 1. Highly schematic view of possible mechanisms involved with the release of cellular material into liquid culture medium during incubation.

material. And third, critical surface components of the plasma membrane may be cleaved during the process of proteolysis. In this paper we will review data suggesting that release of erythroid burst promoting activity from leukocytes involves exfoliation of surface components.[7]

STIMULATION OF ERYTHROID BURST FORMATION BY CELL MEMBRANE-DERIVED VESICLES

The formation of BFU-E-derived colonies in tissue culture requires the presence of unknown growth factors in serum or other factors that may replace serum.[8] The latter activity, termed erythroid burst promoting activity (BPA) appears in liquid medium after incubation with a variety of cell types, including unstimulated circulating leukocytes.[6,9] We collected lymphocyte-rich fractions of peripheral blood cells by separation over Ficoll-Paque (Pharmacia Fine Chemicals, Piscataway, N.J.) followed by mixture with carbonyl iron (Technicon Instruments Corporation, Tarrytown, N.Y.) to remove the majority of macrophages. Greater than 98 and 95% of these cells are viable after 1 and 2 days, respectively, of incubation in serum-free alpha medium (Flow Laboratories, Englewood, Calif.) at 37°C, 5% CO_2. We found that relative to alpha medium incubated in the absence of cells, cell "conditioned" medium stimulated erythroid burst formation by human bone marrow cells that were nonadherent to nylon or polyester in fibrin clot cultures established at the threshold serum concentration of 4.5% fetal calf serum (FCS).[7]

We reasoned that one simple way to evaluate leukocyte conditioned medium for the presence of insoluble or partially soluble, bioactive, cell-derived macromolecules was to subject it to high-speed centrifugation, and to determine whether BPA is pelletable. Thus, following centrifugation at $40,000 \times g$ for 30 min, conditioned medium was separated into supernatant and pellet fractions. FIGURE 2 shows that both fractions supported erythroid burst formation over a wide range of erythropoietin concentrations. While the amount of BPA present in either fraction alone was less than that present in unseparated conditioned medium, reconstitution of washed pellets in the original volume of supernatant resulted in full recovery of activity (data not shown). Since approximately one-half of the BPA present in conditioned medium was

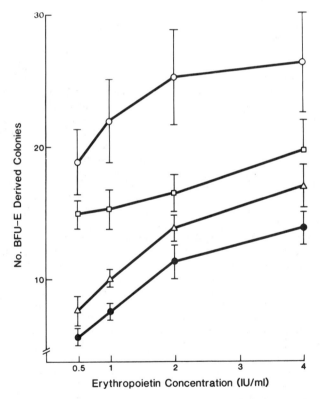

FIGURE 2. Support of BFU-E proliferation by unseparated conditioned medium (○) and its pellet (□) and supernatant (△) fractions. Cultures contained the indicated erythropoietin concentrations (International Units (IU)/ml) plus 9.0% (v/v) unseparated medium, supernatant, or pellet washed in 5 mM Na phosphate and resuspended in NCTC-109 (Microbiological Associates, Bethesda, Md.) or NCTC-109 alone (●).

pelletable, it was of interest to examine the pellets microscopically for the presence of particulate material.

Phase contrast microscopy showed the pellets contain abundant refractile, particulate material. Freeze-fracture electron microscopy of the pellet revealed the presence of a heterogeneous population of unilamellar membrane vesicles ranging in size from 0.1 to 0.4 μm in diameter. FIGURE 3 displays electron micrographs of a typical pellet prepared from conditioned medium. When washed vesicles were resuspended at increasing protein concentrations in NCTC-109 and tested in culture, BPA increased in a saturable pattern (data not shown). Taken together, these studies provide strong evidence that vesicular material in leukocyte conditioned medium expresses BPA in tissue culture.

CHARACTERIZATION OF VESICLES IN
CONDITIONED MEDIUM

Since it is possible that vesicles in conditioned medium are released from leukocyte surfaces, we labeled leukocyte plasma membrane glycoproteins with ^{125}I-wheat germ agglutinin (^{125}I-WGA). We observed that at both 4 and 25°C whole-cell-associated ^{125}I activity diminished with time, while activity in unseparated conditioned medium gradually increased (see FIGURE 4). Some of the cell surface-derived ^{125}I-WGA was found in the high-speed leukocyte conditioned medium (LCM) pellet showing that some of the pelletable material was derived from the leukocyte plasma membranes. Furthermore, when we compared the glycoprotein composition of vesicles to that of partially purified leukocyte plasma membranes, we found that substantial amounts of ^{125}I-WGA-binding glycoproteins in vesicles co-migrated with major glycoproteins of the membranes.[7] These findings strongly support the contention that the origin of medium-derived vesicles is the plasma membrane.

To examine the mode of action of vesicles, we considered that they might contain molecules sealed within them. To determine whether vesicles were impermeable to macromolecules, we tested whether they could respond osmotically to 70,000 molecular weight dextran. We centrifuged vesicles to equilibrium on continuous gradients of dextran T70 ($\rho = 1.005-1.1$) prepared in either isotonic saline or a hypotonic medium. In isotonic saline the vesicles equilibrated at $\rho = 1.03$, while in hypotonic medium they were found closer to $\rho = 1.005$ (see FIGURE 5). BPA co-migrated with vesicle-containing fractions of the gradients in both cases (see FIGURE 6). This shows that vesicles respond osmotically to 70,000 molecular weight dextran and must be impermeable to it, and to similarly sized molecules which might be trapped within them. Thus it is possible that vesicles contain trapped soluble bioactive molecules which diffuse out during incubation and act to support erythroid burst proliferation.

The following observations, however, support the surface origin of vesicular BPA. First, physical disruption of the vesicles by alternate freezing-thawing or distilled water lysis did not release BPA from the vesicles. Second, incubation of the vesicles for 24-48 hr in liquid culture medium did not release BPA into the medium. Third, when cultured in a two-layer fibrin clot system, vesicles expressed BPA only when placed in proximity to marrow target cells. Therefore, our findings suggest that vesicular surface rather than intravesicular molecules contain components that express BPA.

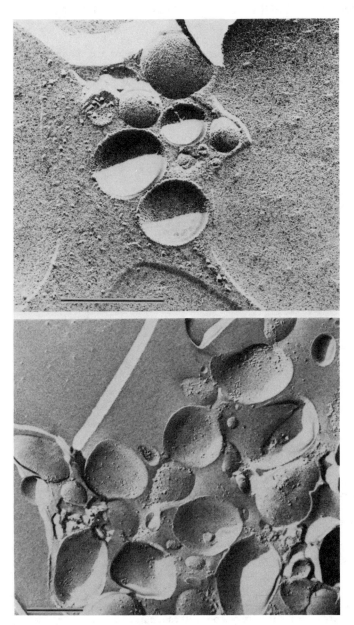

FIGURE 3. Freeze-fracture electron micrographs of washed conditioned medium-derived pellets resuspended in 5 mM Na phosphate and frozen by immersion in liquid-N_2-cooled freon-22. The lower panel shows vesicles containing protrusions thought to be intramembrane particles. Vesicles in the upper panel are predominantly smooth in appearance. Bars: 0.25 μm.

IMMUNOGENICITY OF LEUKOCYTE PLASMA MEMBRANES

The suggestion that plasma membranes or plasma membrane-derived materials may stimulate hematopoietic cell differentiation or growth was made over a decade ago.[10] Indeed, surface membranes have been shown to generate colony stimulating

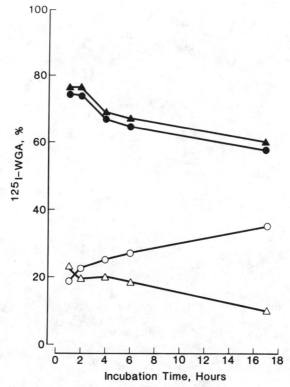

FIGURE 4. Release of cell surface components into liquid medium. Leukocytes were prelabeled with submitogenic quantities of ^{125}I-WGA and incubated at 25 (●) or 4°C (▲) for the indicated times. Percentage radioactivity remaining on cells after the indicated time in culture at 25°C (●, ▲). Percentage radioactivity in supernatant after the indicated time in culture at 25°C (○). Percentage radioactivity in LCM pellets relative to whole LCM after the indicated time in culture at 25°C (△).

activity.[11,12] With these earlier observations in mind and with our evidence suggesting that vesicular BPA most likely has a plasma membrane origin, we measured the effects of leukocyte subcellular fractions on erythroid burst formation. We observed that both crude and purified plasma membrane fractions express significantly more BPA per microgram protein than do the whole cell homogenate or other cellular fractions, including nuclear and mitochondrial pellets and high-speed cytosol supernates.[7] We therefore explored the well-known immunogenic properties of cell membranes as a potential mechanism to generate anti-BPA antibodies.

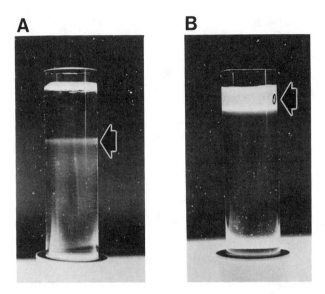

FIGURE 5. Photograph of vesicles spun to equilibrium on dextran gradients. Washed pellets were resuspended in 0.3 mM Na phosphate and layered on 5-ml continuous (ρ = 1.005-1.10) gradients of dextran T70 in either (A) isotonic saline or (B) 0.3 mM Na phosphate. Gradients were centrifuged at 200,000 $\times$ g for 17 hr in a Beckman SW51 rotor. The major band of vesicles (arrows) equilibrated at either (A) ρ = 1.03 or (B) at the top of the gradient (ρ = 1.005).

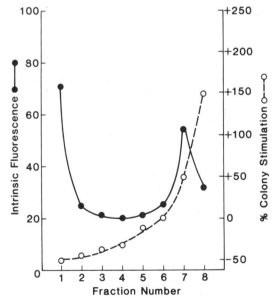

FIGURE 6. BPA assays of dextran gradient fractions. Vesicles were centrifuged in a dextran gradient as described in the caption for FIGURE 5B and located within the gradient fractions by intrinsic fluorescence. High fluorescence at the bottom of the gradient reflects the high dextran concentration in this portion of the gradient. Note that primarily those fractions with increased amounts of vesicles express BPA.

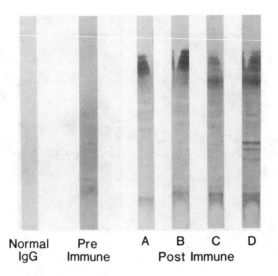

FIGURE 7. Electroblots of human leukocyte membrane proteins incubated with rabbit IgG. Membrane proteins were electrophoresed on 5-15% acrylamide gels and transferred to nitrocellulose paper by the electroblot technique. Blots were incubated with IgG and stained with peroxidase-conjugated second antibody to test for cross-reactivity. A-D: IgG purified from sera of four different rabbits.

Leukocytes were obtained from the American Red Cross as by-products of platelet pheresis residues. Following plastic adherence, approximately 85-90% of cells were identified as lymphocytes from which plasma membranes were isolated by a modification of the method of Jett et al.[13] Approximately 100-350 μg of partially purified leukocyte plasma membrane protein emulsified with Freund's complete adjuvant was injected intradermally into four rabbits. Rabbit IgG fractions were precipitated with ammonium sulfate, purified on DEAE-cellulose, and tested for cross-reactivity with plasma membrane vesicles using the electroblot technique. FIGURE 7 shows that whereas normal rabbit IgG and preimmune IgG show little or no cross-reactivity with membrane proteins, IgG from postimmune sera stained with peroxidase-conjugated second antibody shows multiple proteins that are reactive. Preliminary experiments suggest that antibodies cross-react not only with vesicle-containing pellets but also with vesicle-free supernatants of conditioned medium (data not shown). In addition to these findings, pilot experiments appear to indicate that IgG from postimmune rabbits neutralizes BPA present in both unseparated conditioned medium and its fractions (manuscript in preparation).

POSSIBLE PHYSIOLOGIC SIGNIFICANCE OF VESICULAR BPA

While the physiologic role of BPA has not been determined, reports of increased levels of this growth factor(s) in serum and urine of anemic individuals suggest that BPA may possibly serve as a physiologic regulator of erythropoiesis.[14,15] We have recently investigated the pathogenesis of severe anemia (hemoglobin level of 4 g/dl) in an adult male with marked erythroblastopenia of the bone marrow and B-cell chronic lymphocytic leukemia. The monoclonal lymphocytes were Ia positive and Fc receptor positive; they expressed surface mu-lambda immunoglobulin. Whereas serum from this individual stimulated erythroid burst proliferation by normal bone marrow cells, an atypical pattern of BPA expression was observed in alpha medium conditioned by patient circulating E-rosette-depleted lymphocytes. FIGURE 8 shows that the amount of BPA expressed by unseparated medium incubated for 24 hr with patient lymphocytes was less than that expressed by medium incubated with normal donor lymphocytes. Separation of the culture medium into supernatant and pellet provided an unexpected result. Whereas supernatant derived from patient cell conditioned medium contained a similar amount of BPA as found in supernatant from normal donor cell conditioned medium (see FIGURE 8), patient cell-derived vesicles did not express BPA (see FIGURE 9).

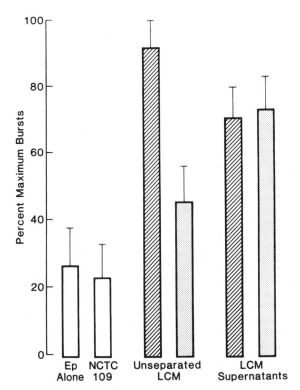

FIGURE 8. Effects of unseparated media and supernatants on colony formation. Circulating mononuclear cells from a normal donor and a severely anemic patient with erythroblastopenia and chronic lymphocyte leukemia were washed three times in alpha medium and resuspended at a density of 5×10^6 cells/ml in tissue culture flasks. Conditioned medium was harvested after 24 hr incubation and freed of cells by centrifugation at $280 \times g$ for 20 min. Nine percent (v/v) unseparated media and medium supernatants were added to cultures of normal human marrow cells as described previously. All cultures contained 2.0 IU/ml erythropoietin (Ep). Means ± 1 SEM are displayed for results obtained using medium conditioned by normal donor (hatched bars) and patient (stippled bars) cells.

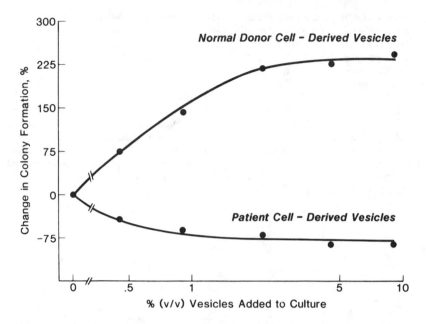

FIGURE 9. Effects of medium-derived vesicles on colony formation. Pellets obtained following high-speed centrifugation of media prepared as described in the caption to FIGURE 8 were washed in 5 mM Na phosphate, resuspended to 200 μl in NCTC-109, and added to cultures of normal human marrow cells to achieve the concentrations denoted in the figure. Cultures with no added vesicles contained 100 μl NCTC-109. All cultures contained 2.0 IU/ml erythropoietin.

Several possibilities are raised by these findings. First, it is possible that B lymphocytes from normal individuals do not express vesicular BPA. To test this, we performed several experiments with medium conditioned by Ig-positive and E-rosette-positive cells derived from macrophage-depleted circulating lymphocytes of healthy donors. Lymphocytes were passed over a 10-ml Sephadex G-200 anti-human (Fab)$_2$ immunoabsorbent column at a flow rate of 1 ml/min. Adherent Ig-positive cells were eluted with alpha medium containing human gamma globulin. In other cases, lymphocytes were incubated for 45 min at 37°C in a 3-ml nylon wool column from which they were removed by gentle agitation. Lymphocytes from the same donor collection were also incubated with 2-aminoethylisothiouronium bromide (AET)-treated sheep erythrocytes and rosetted cells were recovered from pellets formed after centrifugation over a cushion of Ficoll-Paque by ammonium chloride lysis. Conditioned medium was prepared from each cell population, fractionated in the usual fashion, and assayed for BPA.

As outlined in TABLE 1, vesicles derived from media conditioned by Ig-bearing cells consistently expressed BPA (mean of 1.96-fold enhancement in 10 studies relative to cultures containing NCTC-109 alone). In contrast, vesicles from E-rosette-forming cells showed no BPA (mean of 1.05-fold enhancement). Although these studies suggest that vesicles derived from B lymphocytes express BPA, they do not necessarily suggest that vesicles derived from T lymphocytes do not express this activity. Since attachment of lymphocytes to sheep erythrocytes may of itself result in a broad range of surface architectural changes in both cell types,[16,17] and because AET treatment may also significantly alter lymphocyte surfaces,[18] failure to express vesicular BPA may represent an *in vitro* artifact. Therefore, additional approaches to positive selection of T cells must be taken (experiments in progress).

Second, it is possible that exfoliation of membrane components from leukemia B-lymphocyte surfaces is quantitatively different from exfoliation of normal B-lympho-cyte surface components. Since the patient described above expired before additional material could be obtained, quantitative measurements based on protein concentration were not made, although medium-derived pellets appeared by inspection to be of equal size to those obtained from similar volumes of medium conditioned by normal B lymphocytes.

Third, it is possible that leukemia B lymphocytes shed qualitatively abnormal vesicles. For example, it has been suggested that surface membranes of chronic lym-phocytic leukemia lymphocytes may lack certain cell surface proteins.[19,20] Moreover, Van Blitterswijk *et al.* have found significant differences in the phospholipid com-position of shed membrane vesicles from leukemic mouse lymphocytes relative to normal mouse lymphocytes.[21] It is possible that qualitative changes that resulted in impaired BPA release may have also existed in vesicles derived from our patient's cells.

CONCLUDING REMARKS

While cellular interactions are known to influence the differentiation and prolif-eration of hematopoietic stem cells *in vitro,* little is known of the molecular mechanisms

TABLE 1. BPA Assays of Vesicles Derived from Media Conditioned by Ig+ or E-Rosette+ Cells

Adherence Technique	Burst Promoting Activity[a]	
	Ig+ Cell Pellets	E-Rosette+ Cell Pellets
Nylon	1.7 (86%)	1.0
Nylon	1.8 (66%)	0.9
Nylon	2.1 (79%)	1.1
Nylon	1.9 (97%)	0.8
Nylon	1.8 (88%)	1.2
Sephadex	1.8 (91%)	1.1
Sephadex	2.0 (99%)	1.0
Nylon	1.7 (90%)	0.9
Nylon	2.1 (82%)	1.4
Sephadex	2.7 (99%)	1.1
Mean ± SD:	1.96 ± 0.3	1.05 ± 0.2

[a] Burst promoting activity was assayed as fold stimulation relative to cultures of nonadherent marrow cells containing NCTC-109. Ig+ cell pellets: These pellets were derived from media conditioned by Ig-bearing lymphocytes which were separated by adherence to either Nylon wool or Sephadex anti-human Fab columns. Numbers in parentheses are the percentage Ig+ cells in the eluted cell fraction. E-rosette+ cell pellets: These pellets were derived from media conditioned by rosetting lymphocytes obtained from the same donor and prepared concurrently with those from the Ig+ cells.

by which such events occur. Our approach has been to investigate mechanisms by which cells impart growth factors to tissue culture medium. Our findings suggest that exfoliation or shedding of cell surface components is one mechanism by which mononuclear cells release the erythropoietic growth factor BPA. It is probable that other mechanisms such as exocytosis are also involved in BPA release. Our preliminary findings that antimembrane IgG cross-reacts with and neutralizes soluble BPA suggest that soluble BPA may share antigenic determinants with plasma membranes. Although release *in vitro* of bioactive surface-derived molecules by proteolysis is also possible, studies with protease inhibitors suggest that this is a less likely mechanism of BPA release.[7] Of potentially great interest is that our findings may have relevance to physiologic control of erythropoiesis. Moreover, they raise numerous questions regarding the molecular mechanisms involved in regulating extracellular vesiculation.

ACKNOWLEDGMENTS

We are grateful to Catherine Korsgren and Sandra Kreczko for their excellent technical assistance and to Dr. A. Najman, Hôpital Saint-Antoine, Paris, France, for providing patient specimens for study.

REFERENCES

1. TEPPERMAN, A. D., J. E. CURTIS & E. A. McCULLOCH. 1974. Blood **44:** 659-669.
2. GUILBERT, L. J. & N. N. ISCOVE. 1976. Nature **263:** 594-595.
3. ISCOVE, N. N., L. J. GUILBERT & C. WEYMAN. 1980. Exp. Cell Res. **126:** 121-126.
4. CLINE, M. J. & D. W. GOLDE. 1979. Nature **277:** 177-181.
5. ZANJANI, E. D. & M. E. KAPLAN. 1979. Prog. Hematol. **11:** 173-191.
6. AYE, M. T. 1977. J. Cell. Physiol. **91:** 69-78.
7. DAINIAK, N. & C. M. COHEN. 1982. Blood **60:** 583-594.
8. ISCOVE, N. N. 1978. *In* Hematopoietic Cell Differentiation. D. W. Golde, M. J. Cline, D. Metcalf & C. F. Fox, Eds. **10:** 37-52. Academic Press, Inc. New York, N.Y.
9. ZUCKERMAN, K. S. & M. HAAK. 1983. Br. J. Haematol. **55:** 145-153.
10. RUBIN, S. H. & D. H. COWAN. 1973. Exp. Hematol. **1:** 127-131.
11. PRICE, G. B. & E. A. McCULLOCH. 1978. Semin. Hematol. **15:** 283-300.
12. PRICE, G. B., E. A. McCULLOCH & J. E. TILL. 1975. Exp. Hematol. **3:** 227-233.
13. JETT, M., T. M. SEED & G. A. JAMIESON. 1977. J. Biol. Chem. **252:** 2134.
14. NISSEN, C., N. N. ISCOVE & B. SPECK. 1979. *In* Experimental Hematology Today. S. J. Baum & G. D. Ledney, Eds.: 79-87. Springer-Verlag. New York, N.Y.
15. DUKES, P. P., D. MEYETES, A. MA, G. DIROCCO, J. A. ORTEGA & N. A. SHORE. 1978. *In* Hematopoietic Cell Differentiation. D. W. Golde, M. J. Cline, D. Metcalf & C. F. Fox, Eds. **10:** 119-128. Academic Press, Inc. New York, N.Y.
16. ZALEUSKI, P. D. & J. J. FORBES. 1979. Clin. Exp. Immunol. **36:** 536-546.
17. RENAU-PIQUERRAS, J. & J. CERVERA. 1979. Acta Haematol. **62:** 185-190.
18. PELLIGRINO, M. A., S. FERRONE & J. THEOFILPOULOS. 1976. J. Immunol. Methods **11:** 273-279.
19. SIMMONDS, M. A., G. SOBCZAK & S. P. HAUPTMAN. 1981. J. Clin. Invest. **67:** 624-631.
20. MENDELSOHN, J. & J. NORDBERG. 1979. J. Clin. Invest. **63:** 1124-1132.
21. VAN BLITTERSWIJK, W. J., G. DE VEER, J. H. KROL & P. EMMELOT. 1982. Biochim. Biophys. Acta **688:** 495-504.

DISCUSSION OF THE PAPER

R. K. SHADDUCK (*Montefiore Hospital, Pittsburgh, Pa.*): Most people use mitogens to enhance the release of growth-promoting molecules from monocytes and lymphocytes. Did you simply incubate the white cells or were they mitogen stimulated?

N. DAINIAK: They were not mitogen stimulated. You are quite right, most people do use PHA, but PHA induces tremendous aggregation that would severely distort the surface architecture of the cells and that was the reason we did not use it. Several investigators have shown and we have confirmed that PHA is not needed for the release of BPA activity. (AYE, M. T. 1977. Erythroid colony formation in cultures of human marrow: effect of leukocyte conditioned medium. J. Cell. Physiol. **91:** 69-78; DAINIAK, N. & C. M. COHEN. 1982. Surface membrane vesicles from mononuclear cells stimulate erythroid stem cells to proliferate in culture. Blood **60:** 583-594.)

QUESTION: Is the BPA activity produced on a continuous basis? If one added puromycin or cycloheximide or other similar compounds to inhibit protein synthesis, would BPA release be prevented? My guess is, it would not, if only a loss of vesicles from the cell surface were involved.

DAINIAK: I have not done those studies, but they are under way. I would guess, as you have, that we would not see any difference in BPA release. Another question is whether the vesicles are released from specific domains of the lymphocyte surface. I have shown a diagram suggesting that they are exfoliated from the villi. We certainly do not know this for certain, but there is some evidence for it. Van Blitterswijk has suggested that specific domains may be involved in cell surface exfoliation (VAN BLITTERSWIJK, W. J., G. DE VEER, J. H. KROL & P. EMMELOT. 1982. Biochim. Biophys. Acta **688:** 495-504). At another level, the cytoskeleton may be important (EMERSON, S. G. & R. E. CONE. 1979. Differential effects of colchicine and cytochalasins on the shedding of murine B cell membrane IgM and IgD. Proc. Natl. Acad. Sci. USA **76:** 6582-6586).

K. R. RAI (*Long Island Jewish-Hillside Medical Center, New Hyde Park, N.Y.*): Dr. Dainiak, several years ago you and Ron Hoffman published a paper that has become quite famous about T-cell CLL accompanied by a pure red cell anemia (HOFFMAN, R., S. KOPEL, S. D. HSU, N. DAINIAK & E. D. ZANJANI. 1978. T cell chronic lymphocytic leukemia: presence in bone marrow and peripheral blood of cells that suppress erythropoiesis *in vitro*. Blood **22:** 255-260). How do the data you presented today relate to the anemia seen in some cases of CLL?

DAINIAK: The data are certainly compatible with the same mechanism, i.e., cellular interaction resulting in impaired erythroid colony formation. One question is whether cells actually contact target cells, such as progenitor cells, or whether vesiculation mediates the contact. Along these lines, we have reported that most patients with myelophthisic anemia have normal erythroid burst formation (DAINIAK, N., V. KULKARNI, D. HOWARD, M. KALMANTI, M. C. DEWEY & R. HOFFMAN. 1983. Mechanisms of abnormal erythropoiesis in malignancy. Cancer **51:** 1101-1106). However, we had three patients with reduced colony formation and all three had B-cell neoplasms.

G. CHIKKAPPA (*Veterans Administration Medical Center, Albany, N.Y.*): You call it erythroblastopenia; we call it pure red cell aplasia associated with CLL. However, we are clearly talking about the same thing. Mangan published several papers claiming that the T cell is responsible for the suppression of erythropoiesis in these patients (MANGAN, K. F., G. CHIKKAPPA, L. Z. BIELER, W. B. SCHARFMAN & D. R. PARKINSON. 1982. Regulation of human blood erythroid burst-forming unit (BFU-E) proliferation by T-lymphocyte subpopulations defined by Fc receptors and monoclonal antibodies. Blood **59:** 990-996; MANGAN, K. F., G. CHIKKAPPA & P. C. FARLEY. 1982. T gamma (T) cells suppress growth of erythroid colony-forming units *in vitro* in the pure red cell aplasia of B-cell chronic lymphocytic leukemia. J. Clin. Invest. **70:** 1148-1156). In your patient a B lymphocyte failing to release a stimulator appears to be involved. Have you studied the T cells in this patient and can you exclude the possibility that they inhibited erythropoiesis?

DAINIAK: This is a good question. I knew it would be asked. Unfortunately, the patient died before we could do the study. As you know, it is now accepted that there is collaboration between lymphocytes, perhaps T cells, and monocytes that results in the expression of BPA activity. Such collaboration could have taken place in our studies since we cannot be sure we removed all monocytes. I can thus not be certain what cell type was ultimately responsible for the lack of BPA expression. It could have been due to a collaboration between cells rather than a single cell type.

Direct Morphological and Functional Examination of Murine Pluripotent Hemopoietic Stem Cells[a]

D. W. VAN BEKKUM,[b] J. W. M. VISSER,

J. G. J. BAUMAN, A. H. MULDER, J. F. ELIASON,

AND A. M. DE LEEUW

Radiobiological Institute TNO
Rijswijk, the Netherlands

INTRODUCTION

The incidence of murine pluripotent hemopoietic stem cells (PHSC) in adult mouse bone marrow is estimated to be between 0.2 and 0.7%.[1] Therefore, this cell type cannot be examined by direct methods without preenrichment. In 1971, van Bekkum et al.[2] described a method for 10- to 40-fold enrichment of CFU-S (colony forming unit–spleen[3]) involving equilibrium density centrifugation of the bone marrow from nitrogen mustard-treated mice. Examination of the enriched suspensions by electron microscopy revealed that the enrichment for CFU-S strongly correlated with the enrichment for a morphologically distinct cell type which was different from the known more mature cells in the marrow. The incidence of this cell type, the candidate stem cell or CMOMC (Cell Meeting Our Morphological Criteria), as observed directly in electron microscope preparations of enriched stem cell fractions from mouse and rat bone marrow, was half that of the calculated number of PHSC.[1,4] In 1981, Visser and Bol[5] described a method for 60- to 100-fold enrichment of CFU-S from mouse bone marrow combining equilibrium density centrifugation with light-activated cell sorting for wheat germ agglutinin (WGA)-positive cells. These highly enriched suspensions behaved normally with respect to their homing and their ability to protect lethally irradiated mice.[6] For further purification of PHSC, this method has now been combined with light-activated cell sorting for H-2k antigen-positive cells, which are known to contain the CFU-S.[7,8] This combination of separation steps yielded a 135-fold enrichment of predominantly day 12 CFU-S and a similar enrichment of the cell type that provides radioprotection.

These enriched suspensions were employed for direct examination of the mor-

[a] This investigation was supported by a program grant from the Netherlands Foundation for Medical Research (FUNGO), which is subsidized by the Netherlands Organization for the Advancement of Pure Research (ZWO). J. F. Eliason was the recipient of a National Research Service Award (No. AF 32 AM 06110) from the National Institute of Arthritis, Metabolism and Digestive Diseases, Bethesda, Md.

[b] Author to whom correspondence should be addressed: Prof. Dr. D. W. van Bekkum, Radiobiological Institute TNO, 151 Lange Kleiweg, 2288 GJ Rijswijk, the Netherlands.

phology by light and electron microscopy and of the function at the earliest steps of hemopoietic differentiation by *in vitro* culture methods.

EXPERIMENTAL METHODS AND RESULTS

Bone marrow cells from 7-week-old BC_3 mice were separated by equilibrium density centrifugation on a discontinuous metrizamide gradient and simultaneously labeled with WGA conjugated to fluorescein isothiocyanate (WGA-FITC). The low-density cells ($p < 1.078$ g·cm^{-3}) were analyzed by a light-activated cell sorter (FACS II). Fluorescent cells with medium forward light scatter (FLS) and low perpendicular light scatter (PLS) intensities were sorted using electronic selection windows as described previously.[5] This fraction constituted 4 to 6% of all nucleated low-density cells. The enrichment for CFU-S obtained by this method (TABLE 1) was similar to that reported previously.[5,6] The sorted cells were incubated with the competitive sugar, N-acetyl-D-glucosamine, to remove WGA-FITC and subsequently with anti-H-2K^k-biotin and avidin-FITC. The latter labeling method was developed to avoid interference with homing, which is a disadvantage of other antibody-staining procedures. The cells were again analyzed by the FACS and two major subpopulations of cells could be distinguished on the basis of fluorescence intensity differences. The most brightly fluorescent cells (30 ± 5% of the total remaining population) were sorted and assayed for CFU-S. The various steps in the purification are depicted in FIGURE 1.

Colonies were counted 8 and 12 days after transplantation (TABLE 1). The number of day 12 CFU-S in the sorted fraction was about 3-fold higher than the number of day 8 CFU-S, suggesting that the sorting procedure selects for delayed-type CFU-S.[9] The day 12 CFU-S were enriched 3- to 4-fold by the additional H-2k sorting step, reaching a final enrichment of a factor of 135. The overall recovery of day 12 CFU-S averaged 40%.

The ability of the sorted cells to protect lethally irradiated mice was determined by the 30-day survival assay using graded numbers of cells. It was found that (3.1 ± 0.7) × 10^4 unfractionated bone marrow cells versus 170 ± 30 sorted cells were

TABLE 1. CFU-S Enrichment by Combining Density Separation and Light-Activated Cell Sorting after WGA and H-2K Labeling[a]

| | CFU-S/10^5 Cells | | Enrichment Factor for | Percentage Recovery | |
| | | | | | |
Cells	Day 8	Day 12	Day 12 CFU-S	Nucleated Cells	Day 12 CFU-S
Unfractionated bone marrow cells	38 (19-77)	49 (21-96)	1	100	100
Sorted WGA$^+$ low-density cells	1600 (710-2300)	2100 (800-3000)	42	1.0 (0.7-1.2)	50
Sorted WGA$^+$ and H-2K$^+$ low-density cells	2000 (690-4000)	6600 (1900-13,000)	135	0.3 (0.2-0.4)	40

[a] Figures represent the mean and range (in parentheses) of between 5 and 14 experiments.

CFU–S ENRICHMENT PROCEDURE

mouse bone marrow suspension (BC$_3$)

$\downarrow$ 2×10^8

WGA–FITC labeling during density cut

$\downarrow$ 2×10^7

FACS CFU–S window: fls, pls, WGA–FITCfl

$\downarrow$ 10^6

N–acetyl–D–glucosamine incubation

$\downarrow$ 10^6

anti H–2K–biotin labeling

$\downarrow$ 10^6

avidine – FITC labeling

$\downarrow$ 10^6

FACS CFU–S window: fls, H2K–FITCfl

$\downarrow$ 3×10^5

CFU–S, etc., assays

FIGURE 1. Flow sheet of purification steps employed for mouse marrow PHSC. Abbreviations: BC$_3$, C57BL/Rij $\times$ C3H F1 hybrid; WGA-FITC, wheat germ agglutinin-fluorescein isothiocyanate; FACS, fluorescence-activated cell sorter; CFU-S, colony forming unit-spleen; WGA-FITCfl, WGA-FITC fluorescence.

required to protect 50% of the animals, indicating an average enrichment of 180-fold. The number of day 12 CFU-S required for 50% radioprotection was 14.9 $\pm$ 1.3 for grafts of unfractionated bone marrow cells and 10.6 $\pm$ 1.4 for sorted cells. Since the average enrichment factor for day 12 CFU-S in these experiments was 130, it seems that a minority of the protective stem cell population are day 8 CFU-S.

The morphology of the sorted cells was examined by light microscopy after May-Grünwald-Giemsa staining and by electron microscopy. All cells could be classified as undifferentiated blasts by light microscopy. Electron microscopy of these preparations revealed two predominant cell types in the sorted fraction: between 43 and 59% of the cells resembled the candidate stem cell described by van Bekkum *et al.*[2] (FIGURE 2a) and 24 to 43% were similar except for somewhat more cytoplasm and deeper nuclear indentations (FIGURE 2b); the remaining 15 to 17% of the cells were clearly more differentiated.

These observations suggested 85% purity of the stem cell concentrates. Since the presence of two morphologically slightly different types of stem cells in the concentrates might be due to PHSC being in different stages of the cell cycle, DNA content was assessed on fixed sorted cells by staining with propidium iodide (PI) and analysis by the FACS.[10] The fluorescence histograms, however, showed that 98 to 100% of the sorted cells contained 2n DNA. Therefore, these cells were either in the G_0 or in the G_1 phase of the cycle.

Routinely, some of the cells were deposited by the FACS at one cell per well in Terasaki trays during the last (H-2k) separation step. This automated cloning facilitates the tracing of single cells for direct monitoring of the first events of hemopoietic differentiation from the beginning of culture. The colony stimulating activity (CSA)

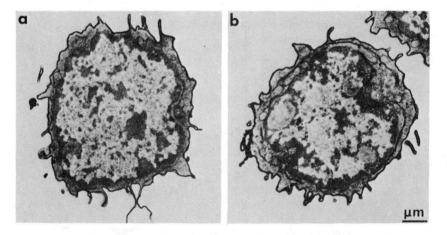

FIGURE 2. Electron microscope pictures of cells from the sorted suspension. (a) Typical example of the CMOMC. (b) Typical example of the cell type closely resembling the CMOMC.

and enhancing factors used were specific for culturing myeloid cells, i.e., pregnant mouse uterus extract (PMUE) and 18-hr postendotoxin serum (PES).[11,12] Thirty percent of the sorted cells could be triggered to produce progeny *in vitro*. It is envisaged that this percentage can be increased by using a more complete set of stimulating factors and by improving culture conditions.

When small colonies (2-32 cells) at day 3 of culture were stained with May-Grünwald-Giemsa, cells were classified as undifferentiated blast cells. Only after 2 weeks of culture when the wells contained 10^2-10^4 cells, could fully differentiated monocytes and granulocytes be observed. This suggests that a very early hemopoietic cell type is being detected by this culture technique. The fact that some of the PHSC would produce colonies in this medium is probably due to the presence of slight amounts of stem cell activity factor in the PES.

DISCUSSION

The results of both the CFU-S and the 30-day survival assays indicated that 120- to 200-fold enrichment for PHSC can be achieved by our new combination of separation methods. In the three experiments with the highest enrichment, an average of 10 ± 1 day 12 spleen colonies were observed per 100 injected sorted cells. This demonstrates that the seeding efficiency of sorted CFU-S to the spleen (the f-factor) is at least 2-fold higher than 0.05, which is the value of the f-factor as obtained by "classical" retransplantation experiments.[1,13,14] The latter method determines in reality the f-factor of a second transplantation of CFU-S and therefore applies to the distribution of cycling PHSC. Lahiri and van Putten[15] have demonstrated that within hours after a first transplantation the quiescent CFU-S become proliferating cells. Monette and DeMello[16] have provided evidence that the f-factor of CFU-S in the S, G_2, and M phases of the cell cycle is only half that of CFU-S in G_0 or G_1. From the two observations it can be concluded that the f-factor of quiescent CFU-S in the first transplantation is twice that of the (proliferating) CFU-S in the second transplantation. Therefore, an incidence of 10 spleen colonies per 100 injected cells is in agreement with 100% pure spleen colony forming cells. Using the f-factor of 0.1, the average purity of the PHSC in the series of enrichment experiments reported here was 65% and the range in 15 experiments was 35-110%.

Electron microscopic examination of the purified preparations revealed that two morphologically similar cell types may both give rise to spleen colonies. One of these types strictly resembles the candidate stem cell (CMOMC) described by van Bekkum *et al.*[2] and the other contains more cytoplasm and somewhat deeper nuclear indentations. The incidence of the first type in the sorted suspensions was generally somewhat higher than that of the latter type. These results may be explained by the hypothesis that both cell types are PHSC, one type, the CMOMC, being quiescent PHSC in the G_0 phase of the cell cycle, and the other type PHSC in the G_1 phase of the cell cycle. This hypothesis is supported by the late appearance of the sorted CFU-S. The sorting procedure yielded PHSC which formed three times more spleen colonies at 12 days than at 8 days after infusion. Baines and Visser[17] recently demonstrated that the day 12 CFU-S can largely be separated from day 8 CFU-S by light-activated cell sorting after labeling with the supravital DNA stain H33342. Those experiments suggested that the day 12 spleen colonies arise from quiescent PHSC in the G_0 phase of the cell cycle, whereas day 8 colonies originate from proliferating PHSC. Our present findings with the sorted cells are in agreement with this hypothesis. The morphologically predominant cell type in the sorted suspension, which is identical to the CMOMC, then would be the quiescent PHSC giving rise to day 12 colonies and the other cell type would give rise to day 8 spleen colonies.

The Terasaki tray culture system combined with the FACS single-cell sorting facility is of great importance for direct examination of the functional characteristics of PHSC at the earliest events of hemopoietic differentiation. In addition, liquid cultures instead of semisolid ones can be used for quantitation of *in vitro* plating efficiency in such systems. The liquid cultures facilitate the manipulation of progeny for further functional analysis. This feature of the cloning system may have great possibilities for quantitation of human PHSC. Until now, no reproducible clonogenic assay for human PHSC was available. Automated cloning of FACS-selected cells from human bone marrow in liquid culture facilitates replating of divided cells during the first few days after cloning to identify the daughter cells as BFU-e, GM-CFU, etc., by reproducible culture systems. In addition, a computer memory can store the optical features of each sorted cell together with the position of the well so that later on, after examination of the offspring, the optical characteristics and, concomitantly, a number of cyto-physical and cytochemical features of the progenitor cells can be determined. Application of such a system is only limited now due to a scarcity of specific markers for very early hemopoietic cells in men.

SUMMARY

Pluripotent hemopoietic stem cells (PHSC) were isolated from adult mouse bone marrow by a combination of equilibrium density centrifugation and light-activated cell sorting for WGA-positive and H-2k antigen-positive cells.

The sorted cells gave rise to 2 spleen colonies per 100 injected cells at 8 days and 6.6 colonies per 100 cells at 12 days after transplantation into lethally irradiated syngeneic recipients. The average enrichment factor for day 12 CFU-S (colony forming unit-spleen) equalled 135 (range, 90-230; $n = 15$). Enrichment for the cell type that provides radioprotection was equal to 180 $\pm$ 70, indicating that PHSC and CFU-S are identical. Evidence is provided that the spleen seeding efficiency (the f-factor) of these cells was 0.10 and, therefore, that the average purity of the sorted PHSC was 65% (range in 15 experiments, 35-110%). The sorted cells were all in the G_0 or G_1 phase of the cycle. They appeared to be undifferentiated blasts by morphological criteria, the majority of the cells being similar in structure to the PHSC previously identified in less purified concentrates. Electron microscopy revealed that the sorted cells consisted primarily of two cell types, possibly representing G_0 and G_1 cells.

The FACS was used to deposit single selected cells into individual microwells of Terasaki trays. Thirty percent of the sorted cells could be induced to form progeny *in vitro*. This procedure facilitates direct examination of the first events of hemopoietic regulation.

ACKNOWLEDGMENTS

We are greatly indebted to Miss I. D. Kooijman and Mrs. M. Hogeweg-Platenburg for their assistance.

REFERENCES

1. VAN BEKKUM, D. W., G. J. VAN DEN ENGH, G. WAGEMAKER, S. J. L. BOL & J. W. M. VISSER. 1979. Structural identity of the pluripotent hemopoietic stem cell. Blood Cells 5: 143.
2. VAN BEKKUM, D. W., M. J. VAN NOORD, B. MAAT & K. A. DICKE. 1971. Attempts at identification of hemopoietic stem cell in mouse. Blood 38: 547.
3. TILL, J. E. & E. A. MCCULLOCH. 1961. A direct measurement of the radiation sensitivity of normal mouse bone marrow cells. Radiat. Res. 14: 213.
4. VAN BEKKUM, D. W. 1977. The appearance of the multipotential hemopoietic stem cell.

In Experimental Hematology Today. S. J. Baum & G. D. Ledney, Eds.: 3-10. Springer. New York, N.Y.

5. VISSER, J. W. M. & S. J. L. BOL. 1981. A two-step procedure for obtaining 80-fold enriched suspensions of murine pluripotent hemopoietic stem cells. Stem Cells **1:** 240.

6. VISSER, J. W. M. & J. F. ELIASON. 1983. In vivo studies on the regeneration kinetics of enriched populations of haemopoietic spleen colony forming cells from normal bone marrow. Cell Tissue Kinet. **16:** 385.

7. VAN DEN ENGH, G. J., J. L. RUSSELL & D. DECICCO. 1978. Surface antigens of hemopoietic stem cells: the expression of BAS, Thy-1, and H-2 antigen of CFU-S. *In* Experimental Hematology Today. S. J. Baum & G. D. Ledney, Eds.: 9-15. Springer. New York, N.Y.

8. TRASK, B. & G. J. VAN DEN ENGH. 1980. Antigen expression of CFU-S determined by light activated cell sorting. *In* Experimental Hematology Today. S. J. Baum, G. D. Ledney & D. W. van Bekkum, Eds.: 299-307. Karger. Basel, Switzerland.

9. MAGLI, M. C., N. N. ISCOVE & N. ODARTCHENKO. 1982. Transient nature of early haemopoietic spleen colonies. Nature **295:** 527.

10. MARTENS, A. C. M., G. J. VAN DEN ENGH & A. HAGENBEEK. 1981. The fluorescence intensity of propidium iodide bound to DNA depends on the concentration of sodium chloride. Cytometry **2:** 24.

11. VAN DEN ENGH, G. J. 1974. Quantitative *in vitro* studies on stimulation of murine haemopoietic cells by colony stimulating factor. Cell Tissue Kinet. **7:** 537.

12. VAN DEN ENGH, G. J. & S. BOL. 1975. The presence of a CSF enhancing activity in the serum of endotoxin-treated mice. Cell Tissue Kinet. **8:** 579.

13. LAHIRI, S. K., H. J. KEIZER & L. M. VAN PUTTEN. 1970. The efficiency of the assay for haemopoietic colony forming cells. Cell Tissue Kinet. **3:** 355.

14. MATIOLI, G., H. VOGEL & H. NIEWISCH. 1968. The dilution factor of intravenously injected hemopoietic stem cells. J. Cell. Physiol. **72:** 229.

15. LAHIRI, S. K. & L. M. VAN PUTTEN. 1969. Distribution and multiplication of colony forming units from bone marrow and spleen after injection in irradiated mice. Cell Tissue Kinet. **2:** 21.

16. MONETTE, F. C. & J. B. DEMELLO. 1979. The relationship between stem cell seeding efficiency and position in cell cycle. Cell Tissue Kinet. **12:** 161.

17. BAINES, P. & J. W. M. VISSER. 1983. Analysis and separation of murine bone marrow stem cells by H33342 fluorescence-activated cell sorting. Exp. Hematol. **11:** 701-708.

Early Hemopoietic Progenitor Cells: Direct Measurement of Cell Cycle Status[a]

C. CILLO,[b,c,d] R. P. SEKALY,[e,f] M. C. MAGLI,[b,d] AND
N. ODARTCHENKO[b]

[b]Swiss Institute for Experimental Cancer Research
1066 Epalinges, Switzerland

[e]Ludwig Institute for Experimental Cancer Research
Lausanne Branch
1066 Epalinges, Switzerland

Recent years have been marked, in the field of somatic cell differentiation, by the development of assay systems for clonogenic cells, particularly for hemopoietic tissues (see Reference 1 for a review). The technology and methodology used have been constantly improving, thus allowing progressively deeper insights into precursor cells and their regulatory factors. The present state of research in what concerns hemopoiesis is well reviewed by Quesenberry and Levitt[2] and the basic uncertainties concerning the most controversial concept of this and similar fields, that of stem cells as progenitors, are reviewed and thoroughly discussed for normal tissues by Lajtha[3] and by Potten et al.,[4] and for leukemias by Cronkite.[5]

Ever since clones of all types of blood cells were first produced from genetically marked single cells, in systems such as the classic spleen colony assay of Till and McCulloch,[6] the mode of regulation of relative numbers of cells belonging to various blood lineages has been the subject of many investigations.

All cells belonging to various lineages are derived from relatively small numbers of progenitor cells through a series of intermediate precursors that become progressively more restricted in the types of blood cells they can generate. Large numbers of mature blood cells are produced by amplification and maturation of the appropriate committed precursor cells. One explanation implies that the cellular microenvironment[7] has an instructive or determinative role involving, for example, cell-cell interactions or short-range acting "inducers." An alternative view sees regulation of proliferation and differentiation as being a purely random genetic process,[8] possibly involving some kind of DNA rearrangements.[9] It has been argued that in spleen colonies the relative numbers of various types of the earliest precursors (CFU-S,

[a]Supported in part by the Swiss National Foundation for Scientific Research and the Swiss League Against Cancer.

[c]Work done while on leave of absence from I Istituto di Chimica Biologica, II Facoltá di Medicina Universitá di Napoli, Via S. Pensini 5-80131, Naples, Italy.

[d]Present address: Ontario Cancer Institute, 500 Sherbourne Street, Toronto, Ontario M4X 1K9, Canada.

[f]Present address: Laboratory of Immunogenetics, NIAID, NIH, Bethesda, Md. 20205.

BFU-E)[g] are markedly correlated, irrespective of colony size or of cell morphology.[10] Our own recent results are also opposed to an instructive role of tissue microenvironment acting at the commitment stage. Using the classic spleen colony assay, we have shown that the colonies containing mixed cell types after 11-12 days are not in the same positions as early (7-8 days) erythroid colonies and that only late colonies contain precursors capable of proliferating in culture giving rise to mixed-type colonies.[11] This not only argues against a determinative role of the splenic environment on differentiation pattern during colony growth, but also means that a number of conclusions about hemopoietic progenitors, essentially based on early colony counts, will need to be reassessed.

In continuously renewing cell systems, such as the hemopoietic system, in which functionally mature cells are derived from progenitor cells or stem cells through proliferation and differentiation, the proliferative status of hemopoietic precursors is an essential parameter which any further studies will have to take into account. This has prompted us to use direct measurement methods for its evaluation. Different approaches have been used previously. Cell "suicide" experiments using tritiated thymidine have shown that most colony forming cells appear to either have a long generation time or remain in the quiescent G_0 phase.[12,13] Similar results have been obtained using other approaches such as treatment with hydroxyurea, which is selectively lethal for cells in the S phase of the cell cycle,[14] and physical separation techniques such as discontinuous density gradients[15] or velocity sedimentation.[16] However, the results of these experiments have remained inconclusive since it has not been possible to work with homogeneous populations of progenitor cells, let alone with fully synchronized cells.[1,12] Recently, following the demonstration of markers specific for hemopoietic progenitors, cell separation procedures were used[17,18] to obtain subpopulations of bone marrow cells which are highly enriched in progenitor cells.

In the present report, we have studied the proliferative status of bone marrow hemopoietic progenitors. To circumvent the difficulties encountered in conventional synchronization techniques, we have used the recently described[19] Hoechst 33342 bisbenzimidazole dye, which stains cells quantitatively according to their DNA content without affecting viability, and a fluorescence-activated cell sorter (FACS) to obtain pure populations of G_0/G_1 and $S-G_2+M$ cells. It appears that the vast majority of multipotential cells (CFU-S) and of both types of committed progenitor cells (GM-CFU and BFU-E) are located in the G_0/G_1 phase of the cell cycle.

MATERIALS AND METHODS

Mice

Adult inbred mice of strains Balb/c, C57Bl/6, C3H, and DBA/2 from the mouse colony of the Swiss Institute for Experimental Cancer Research were used throughout these experiments. The original breeding pairs were obtained from the Jackson Laboratory, Bar Harbor, Maine.

---

[g]Abbreviations: BFU-E, burst forming unit-erythroid; BPA, burst promoting activity; BSA, bovine serum albumin; CFC, colony forming cell; CFU-S, colony forming unit-spleen; FBS, fetal bovine serum; FLS, forward light scatter; GM-CFU, granulocytic macrophage-colony forming unit; GM-CSA, granulocytic macrophage-colony stimulating activity; IMDM, Iscove modified Dulbecco's medium; PLS, perpendicular light scatter; WEHI-3, Walter Eliza Hall-Institute-3.

Cell Preparation and DNA Staining

Female mice, 10-13 weeks old, were sacrificed by cervical dislocation. Bone marrow cells were then flushed into Iscove modified Dulbecco's medium (IMDM). A dispersed cell suspension was prepared by gentle pipetting. Red blood cells were lysed by incubation with a buffered solution of 0.15 M ammonium chloride (Tris-NH$_4$Cl), pH 7.5, for 10 min at 37°C. Following incubation, cells were washed three times with IMDM and then counted in a hemocytometer. Cell counts were adjusted to 1×10^6 cells/ml in IMDM containing 5% fetal bovine serum (FBS) and 6 µg/ml Hoechst 33342 (a gift from Dr. H. Loewe, Hoechst AG, Frankfurt, FRG). After 90 min incubation at 37°C, cells were again washed three times and resuspended in cold IMDM for analysis and sorting. In one series of experiments, regenerating bone marrow was studied. Marrow regeneration was induced by injecting intravenously 2.5×10^7 nucleated marrow cells into mice irradiated (800 rad) previously.[20] Bone marrow cells were collected 6 days after injection as described above.

Flow Cytometry and Light Scatter Cell Sorting

Flow cytometric analysis was performed using a Spectra-Physics laser (Spectra-Physics, Mountain View, Calif.; 500-mW output at 488 nm) and a conventional FACS II electronic system modified to allow three-parameter sorting.[19] Viable bone marrow cells were routinely gated by a combination of narrow angle forward light scatter (FLS) and perpendicular light scatter (PLS).[17,18] For each analytical determination 10,000-40,000 gated events were accumulated. Before sorting cells, the sample tubing of the FACS was flushed sequentially with detergent, sterile distilled water, and 96% ethanol. The tubing was then rinsed for a minimum of 30 min with a solution of gentamicin (50 µg/ml) in phosphate-buffered saline which was also used throughout the sorting procedure. Enriched populations of colony forming cells (CFC) were then obtained by sorting cells according to their FLS and PLS.[17,18] A high proportion of blast cells (large cells with nearly spherical nuclei, containing prominent nucleoli and a thin rim of basophilic cytoplasm) was found in this fraction. The selected populations were collected in sterile plastic tubes whose interiors were coated with sterile FBS. The flow rate of viable cells being sorted was generally 2×10^3 gated events/sec. Depending on the sample, between 4×10^5 and 2×10^6 cells were collected.

DNA Content Analysis and Sorting

DNA analysis and sorting of cells according to their DNA content were performed using an argon ion laser (50-mW output at 351-363 nm). Bone marrow cells were stained with Hoechst 33342 and first sorted according to light scatter as described above. Hoechst fluorescence was detected without any intervening optical filters. A minimum of 50,000 cells were accumulated for each DNA histogram. G_0/G_1 and $S-G_2+M$ subpopulations were then sorted on the basis of their fluorescence intensity and collected as described above. Cell viability, determined by Trypan blue exclusion, was at least 90% in all experiments. Once collected, cells were immediately diluted in culture medium. Cell counts provided by the FACS were used to determine the cell concentrations in suspensions and dilutions were made accordingly. Percentages of cells in G_1, S, and G_2 + M were calculated as previously described.[19]

In Vitro *Culture Assays and Scoring of Hemopoietic Precursors*

Erythroid and granulocytic colonies were obtained using the method of Iscove.[20] Briefly, 10^4 to 10^5 nucleated cells collected from whole bone marrow or from the different sorted fractions were plated in 35-mm plastic petri dishes (Greiner, Nürtingen, FRG) in a 1-ml volume of IMDM containing 15% (vol/vol) FBS and 0.8% (w:vol) methylcellulose (Dow Chemical, 4000 mPa · s, premium grade). Delipidated and deionized bovine serum albumin (BSA) at a concentration of 10 mg/ml was also added to the cultures as well as transferrin 2Fe (300 μg/ml), soybean lipid and cholesterol (250 μg/ml), and α-thioglycerol (10^{-4} M). Erythropoietin (Step III, Connaught, Willowdale, Ontario, Canada) was added to the culture medium at a final concentration of 2 μg/ml. Conditioned medium from the WEHI-3 myelomonocytic cell line was also added to the medium at a 10% (vol/vol) concentration as a source of burst promoting activity (BPA)[21] and granulocytic macrophage-colony stimulating activity (GM-CSA).[22] Cultures were incubated at 37°C with 5% CO_2 in a water-saturated incubator. Granulocytic colonies (GM-CFU) composed of more than 50 cells and erythroid colonies (BFU-E) containing more than 200 cells were scored, respectively, at days 7 and 10 following initial plating, using a phase-contrast inverted microscope (Diavert, Leitz, Wetzlar, FRG) at 40× magnification.

Spleen Colony Assays

CFU-S assays were performed according to the procedure of Magli *et al.*[11] Briefly, syngeneic Balb/c mice, 8-12 weeks old, were given 800 rad total-body irradiation. (The X-ray machine was operated at 250 kW, 15 mÅ with 0.2 mm Cu filter, 50 cm focal skin distance under full backscatter conditions at a rate of 242 rad/min.) Cells collected after sorting were injected through the tail vein into irradiated mice. Six mice were used per cell sample (10^4 or 10^3 fractionated cells in 0.5 ml per animal). After 8 days, spleens were removed and colonies were counted with a dissecting microscope (11× magnification). In addition, six lethally irradiated mice were injected with cell-free medium as controls. Under the latter conditions, no endogenous colonies were observed.

RESULTS AND DISCUSSION

Bone marrow cells from 2-month-old Balb/c mice were supravitally stained with the DNA-specific dye Hoechst 33342. The results (FIGURE 1) confirmed that the majority of cells in all bone marrow are located in the G_0/G_1 phase of the cell cycle.[17] A fraction of marrow cells was obtained by sorting with a high narrow angle forward light scatter and a low perpendicular scatter since it has been previously shown that these cells are highly enriched in CFC.[17,18] When these cells were plated in methyl-cellulose in the presence of the appropriate hemopoietic stimulators, or injected into lethally irradiated mice, a 5-fold enrichment in myeloid, erythroid, and multipotential precursors was noted (FIGURE 2). It is known that these cells constitute 10% of the marrow cells; about 80% of hemopoietic precursors were recovered in this fraction. This is in agreement with results previously obtained by Nicola et al.[17] and Visser et

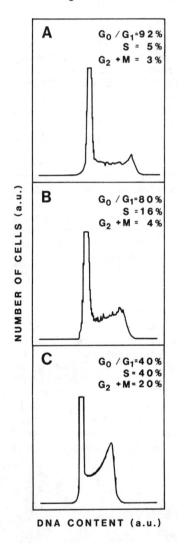

FIGURE 1. DNA distribution of different Balb/c bone marrow cell populations. Cells obtained from normal whole bone marrow (A), from the fraction of bone marrow cells with high forward light scatter and low perpendicular light scatter (B), and from a regenerating bone marrow (C), were stained with Hoechst 33342 (6 µg/ml for 90 min at 37°C) and run on a FACS II gated to exclude nonviable cells. Percentages of cells in G_0/G_1, S, and G_2+M phases of the mitotic cycle were calculated as previously described.[19] (a.u. = arbitrary units.)

al.[18] In order to evaluate the cell cycle status of cells obtained from this fraction, cells that had already been stained with Hoechst 33342 prior to the light scatter sorting were subsequently excited at an appropriate wavelength (351-363 nm). When this blast cell fraction was compared to the whole bone marrow cell population a 3-fold enrichment of S-phase cells (16%) was observed (FIGURE 1B).

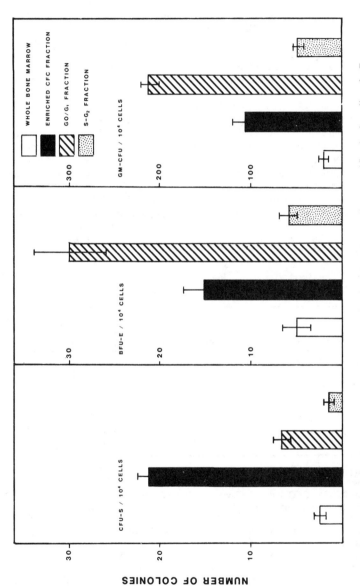

FIGURE 2. Hemopoietic progenitor cell content of mouse bone marrow fractions sorted according to position in the cell cycle. Bone marrow cells from Balb/c mice (10-13 weeks old) were obtained and stained with Hoechst 33342 as detailed in the caption to FIGURE 1. A fraction of bone marrow cells with high forward light scatter and low perpendicular light scatter was obtained by light scatter sorting. This population was subsequently fractionated according to position of cells in the cell cycle. Colony assays for GM-CFU, CFU-S, and BFU-E were performed as detailed under Materials and Methods. The percentage of all CFC occurring in sorted fractions was obtained as in TABLE 1 from five separate experiments for GM-CFU and BFU-E, and from two experiments for CFU-S.

In an attempt to selectively increase the number of progenitor cells belonging to different hemopoietic lineages, cells in the blast fraction were sorted again according to their position in the cell cycle. Two fractions were collected: (1) cells with a diploid DNA content which were considered G_0/G_1 cells (G_0 and G_1 cells could not be distinguished from one another), and (2) cells with a markedly higher content of DNA which were considered S-G_2+M cells. These fractions were subsequently placed in culture in the presence of the proper hemopoietic stimulators. The cloning efficiency of bone marrow cells was not affected after staining with Hoechst 33342 (data not shown). A slight increase in the frequency of both erythroid and granulocytic progenitors was noted when G_0/G_1 cells were compared to the total blast cell fraction (TABLE 1). It should also be noted that the absolute yield or recovery of GM-CFU and BFU-E in the G_0/G_1 fraction was 20-fold higher than that in the S-G_2+M population. These data were reproduced in a series of five experiments (FIGURE 3) with a mean recovery of 95% for GM-CFU and BFU-E in the G_0/G_1 fraction and of 5% in S-G_2+M. The latter two fractions were also injected into lethally irradiated syngeneic mice. The recovery of CFU-S 8 days after injection of the sorted population from G_0/G_1 cells was 20-fold higher than that from S-G_2+M cells (TABLE 1). In contrast to GM-CFU and BFU-E, the absolute recovery of CFU-S was low (36%) as shown in FIGURE 3. This cannot be due to the fact that CFU-S were separated in another light scatter fraction since other sorted subpopulations yielded no CFU-S (data not shown). One possible explanation for this low recovery is the fact that the sorting period exceeded 2-3 hr, in order to get enough cells for the *in vivo* assays, possibly resulting in cell death.

TABLE 1. Progenitor Cell Content in Relation to Cell Cycle[a]

Cell Population	Total Cells	Precursors/10^4 Viable Cells			Total Precursors		
		GM-CFU[b]	BFU-E[b]	CFU-S[c]	GM-CFU	BFU-E	CFU-S
	Input					Input	
Enriched CFC fraction[d]	119,168 (100%)	105	15	14	1246	179	169
	Recovered[e,f]					Recovered[g]	
G_0/G_1	64,493 (88%)	141	21	9	911	135	59
S-G_2+M	8,794 (12%)	48	7	3	42	6	3

[a]These data represent the results of a typical experiment, in which 10^7 total bone marrow cells were processed as detailed under Materials and Methods.

[b]Colony counts for GM-CFU and BFU-E were performed, respectively, at day 7 and day 10 of culture. All fractions were cultured at 10^4 and at 10^3 cells per plate. All plates were done in duplicate.

[c]Colony counts for CFU-S were performed 8 days after injection of 10^4 or 10^3 cells per mouse. Each group contained six mice.

[d]Enriched populations of CFC were sorted according to their forward light scatter and perpendicular light scatter as described by Nicola et al.[17] and Visser et al.[18]

[e]Total number of cells recovered in each sorted fraction. The total represents 61.4% of the starting cell population.

[f]Percentage of cells recovered in each cell fraction normalized to 100% of total.

[g]Total number of colonies recovered in each cell fraction. For GM-CFU, the total number of colonies recovered from the G_0/G_1 and the S-G_2+M sorted fractions represents 70% of the total input, while the recoveries for BFU-E and CFU-S are, respectively, 79.2 and 36%.

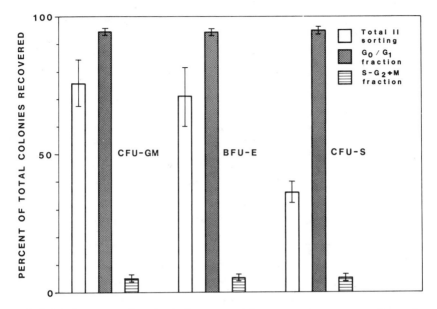

FIGURE 3. Percentage of total colonies recovered from mouse bone marrow after sorting according to position in the cell cycle. G_0/G_1 and $S-G_2+M$ cells were sorted as described in FIGURE 2. The mean percentage of CFC recovered in the G_0/G_1 and $S-G_2+M$ sorted fractions was normalized to 100% of total obtained from the first sorting in five separate experiments for GM-CFU and BFU-E, and in two experiments for CFU-S.

The same experimental protocol was repeated with three different age groups of Balb/c mice (3, 8, and 18 months). The results shown in TABLE 2 indicate no age-related differences in the cycling status of progenitor cells from bone marrow, since the cell cycle distribution of blast cells appears identical in all three age groups analyzed with a majority of cells in G_0/G_1. A 3-fold enrichment of cells in S phase was obtained in the blast cell fraction and the recovery of BFU-E and GM-CFU was always 20-fold higher in G_0/G_1 blast cells than in the $S-G_2+M$ fraction.

Four other strains of adult mice (CBA, DBA/2, C3H, and C57Bl/6) have been compared to Balb/c using the same experimental conditions. DNA histograms of blast cell fractions obtained from CBA, DBA, and C3H mice confirmed that the majority of the cells (80%) were in G_0/G_1 (TABLE 2). The recovery of GM-CFU and BFU-E was 20-fold higher in the G_0/G_1 fraction than in the $S-G_2+M$ fraction. When C57Bl/6 blast cells were analyzed for their cell cycle distribution, a 3-fold higher percentage of cells in $S-G_2+M$ was observed (TABLE 2) as compared to the other strains studied. Only a 3-fold difference in recovery of GM-CFU between G_0/G_1 and $S-G_2+M$ cells could be observed in this strain. In three experiments, $S-G_2$ cells obtained from C57Bl/6 yielded no BFU-E. These data are in agreement with results from Suzuki and Axelrod[23] who found that BFU-E were not killed by high-specific-activity [³H]thymidine in C57Bl/6 mice.

These experiments were repeated using a regenerating bone marrow. DNA histograms of bone marrow cells obtained 6 days after reconstitution of sublethally irradiated mice (FIGURE 1C) were consistent with what would be expected of an exponentially growing population with 40% of cells in G_0/G_1, 40% in S, and 20%

in G_2+M. In agreement with previous reports,[20,24] a 5-fold enrichment in $S-G_2+M$ cells is observed as compared to normal bone marrow. G_0/G_1 and $S-G_2+M$ cells were sorted following staining with Hoechst 33342 and placed in culture in the presence of appropriate stimulators. Results shown in TABLE 2 indicate that there is a 2-fold-increased recovery of GM-CFU and BFU-E in the G_0/G_1 as compared to the $S-G_2+M$ fraction. This is in contrast to the 20-fold difference obtained previously with control, untreated cells, and confirms that in regenerating bone marrow a large number of progenitor cells do enter cycle.

Various reports indicate that the proportion of multipotential progenitors in cycle is lower than that of committed progenitor cells of the granulocytic macrophage and the erythroid lineages. With the exception of the results of Dicke and van Bekkum,[25] a higher suicide rate for GM-CFU or BFU-E (35-85%) than for spleen colony forming cells (5-20%) has been reported,[23,26,27] indicating that under normal conditions GM-

TABLE 2. Proliferative Status of Hemopoietic Progenitor under Different Experimental Conditions

Mice	Percentage $G_0/G_1{}^a$	Percentage $S-G_2+M^a$	GM-CFU/10^7 Cells Processed		BFU-E/10^7 Cells Processed	
			$G_0/G_2{}^b$	$S-G_2+M^b$	$G_0/G_2{}^b$	$S-G_2+M^b$
Balb/c, 3 months[c]	88	12	911	42	135	6
Balb/c, 8 months	86	14	843	38	152	7
Balb/c, 18 months	84	16	939	46	163	7
DBA	87	13	1007	43	167	7
CBA	85	15	736	38	127	6
C3H	84	16	923	52	149	8
C57Bl/6[d]	60	40	683	246	151	9
Reg. Balb/c[e]	40	60	382	179	59	31

[a]Enriched CFC fractions of bone marrow cells were obtained as described in TABLE 1 and then sorted into G_0/G_1 and $S-G_2+M$ cells as previously described.
[b]Total number of colonies recovered in each cell fraction (i.e., TABLE 1).
[c]This is a typical experiment. (See FIGURE 3 for means and standard deviations on each fraction.)
[d]Average data from four separate experiments each using two replicate cultures of each fraction.
[e]Regenerating bone marrow was obtained as detailed under Materials and Methods.

CFU and BFU-E proliferate more rapidly than CFU-S. We were not able to show such differences, since we consistently obtained 20-fold more hemopoietic progenitors with a G_0/G_1 DNA content than with an $S-G_2 + M$ DNA content. These discrepancies may be due to the fact that previously reported results were obtained in vivo or in vitro using conventional synchronization techniques such as [3H]thymidine suicide or hydroxyurea treatment. It should be recognized, however, that results obtained using these two methods are characterized by a wide variability. These discrepancies may be related to the doses of drugs used,[28,29] to secondary effects of drugs on progenitor cells, or to third-party cells involved in hemopoiesis.[30] Marked variations in the susceptibility of individual mice to cytotoxic drugs have also been reported.[31,32] The use of different hemopoietic stimulators constitutes another potential source of variability in the size of the proliferative compartment of progenitor cells.[24] Physical methods such as velocity sedimentation and discontinuous BSA density gradients[15,16] have also been used. However, these methods allow only partial synchronization of the hemo-poietic precursors.[33] Using supravital DNA staining and flow cytometry we have directly achieved synchronization of a fraction of bone marrow cells enriched in all three types of hemopoietic precursors. It should be noted that in our experiments we underestimate the proportion of cells in cycle since it is not possible through the use of Hoechst 33342 dye to distinguish between G_0 and G_1 cycling cells. Since the number of cells in $S-G_2 + M$ is proportional to the total number of cells in cycle, the proportions obtained should be regarded as relative and not absolute figures.

Our results reproducibly indicate that the majority of hemopoietic precursors are in the G_0/G_1 phase of the cell cycle. It should be possible to repeat these studies using highly purified populations of stem cells obtained by three-parameter cell sorting.[17,18] The use of specific markers combined with cell sorting could also allow further investigation of the kinetics of bone marrow precursors and of their interactions with purified growth factors.[19]

SUMMARY

We have investigated the cell cycle status of murine hemopoietic progenitors using vital DNA staining and flow sorting. Suspended Balb/c bone marrow cells were stained with Hoechst 33342 dye and separated first on light scattering properties; this procedure allowed a 5-fold enrichment in progenitor cells. A second sorting based on DNA content indicated that 80% of these cells were in G_0/G_1 and 20% in $S-G_2 + M$. When G_0/G_1 and $S-G_2 + M$ cells were assayed separately in methylcellulose cultures, or with the *in vivo* colony forming assay, the G_0/G_1 cells were shown to be markedly enriched in CFU-S, BFU-E, and GM-CFU as compared to $S-G_2 + M$ cells with the final recovery increased 20-fold. Comparison of different strains or age groups yielded results identical to those obtained with Balb/c with the exception of C57B1/6. In the latter strain only a 3-fold enrichment could be observed in the G_0/G_1 fraction. These results demonstrate that the majority of early hemopoietic progenitors are in the G_0/G_1 phase of the cell cycle.

ACKNOWLEDGMENTS

We thank Drs. J.-C. Cerottini and H. R. MacDonald for their constructive crit-icism, Dr. P. Zaech for operating the FACS, and Mrs. J. Duc for her invaluable assistance in the preparation of the manuscript.

REFERENCES

1. METCALF, D. 1977. Hemopoietic colonies. In vitro cloning of normal and leukemic cells. *In* Recent Results in Cancer Research. Vol. 61. Springer-Verlag. New York, N.Y.
2. QUESENBERRY, P. & L. LEVITT. 1979. Hemopoietic stem cells. N. Engl. J. Med. **301:** 755.
3. LAJTHA, L. 1979. Stem cell concepts. Differentiation **14:** 23.

4. POTTEN, C. S., R. SCHOFIELD & L. LAJTHA. 1979. A comparison of cell replacement in bone marrow, testis and three regions of surface epithelium. BBA Rev. Cancer **560**(6): 281.

5. CRONKITE, E. P. 1981. Leukemia revisited. Blood Cells **7:** 11-30.

6. TILL, J. E. & E. A. McCULLOCH. 1961. Direct measurement of the radiation sensitivity of normal mouse bone marrow cells. Radiat. Res. **14:** 213-222.

7. CURRY, J. L. & J. J. TRENTIN. 1967. Hemopoietic spleen colony studies. I. Growth and differentiation. Dev. Biol. **15:** 395-413.

8. TILL, J. E., E. A. McCULLOCH & L. SIMINOVITCH. 1964. A stochastic model of stem cell proliferation, based on the growth of spleen colony-forming cells. Proc. Natl. Acad. Sci. USA **51:** 29-36.

9. HUMPHRIES, R. K., A. C. EAVES & C. J. EAVES. 1981. Self-removal of hemopoietic stem cells during mixed colony formation *in-vitro*. Proc. Natl. Acad. Sci. USA **78:** 3629-3633.

10. GREGORY, C. J. & R. M. HENKELMAN. 1977. Relationships between early hemopoietic progenitor cells determined by correlation analysis of their numbers in individual spleen colonies. Exp. Hematol. Today **14:** 93-101.

11. MAGLI, M. C., N. N. ISCOVE & N. ODARTCHENKO. 1982. Transient nature of early haematopoietic spleen colonies. Nature **295:** 527-529.

12. LAJTHA, L. G., L. V. POZZI, R. SCHOFIELD & M. FOX. 1969. Kinetic properties of haemopoietic stem cells. Cell Tissue Kinet. **2:** 39.

13. ISCOVE, N. N., J. E. TILL & E. A. McCULLOCH. 1970. The proliferative status of mouse granulopoietic progenitor cells. Proc. Soc. Exp. Biol. Med. **134:** 33.

14. VASSORT, F., M. WINTERHALER, E. FRINDEL & M. TUBIANA. 1973. Kinetic parameters of bone marrow stem cells using in vivo suicide by tritiated thymidine or hydroxyurea. Blood **41:** 789.

15. HASKILL, J. S., T. A. McNEILL & M. A. S. MOORE. 1970. Density distribution analysis of *in vivo* and *in vitro* colony forming cells in bone marrow. J. Cell. Physiol. **75:** 167.

16. METCALF, D. & H. R. MacDONALD. 1975. Heterogeneity of *in vitro* colony- and cluster-forming cells in the mouse marrow: segregation by velocity sedimentation. J. Cell. Physiol. **85:** 643.

17. NICOLA, N. A., D. METCALF, H. VON MELCHNER & A. W. BURGESS. 1981. Isolation of murine fetal hemopoietic progenitor cells and selective fractionation of various erythroid precursors. Blood **58:** 376.

18. VISSER, J., G. VAN DEN ENGH & S. BOL. 1980. Characterization and isolation of murine haemopoietic stem cells by fluorescence activated cell sorting. Exp. Hematol. **9:** 644.

19. SEKALY, R. P., H. R. MacDONALD, P. ZAECH & M. NABHOLZ. 1982. Cell cycle regulation of cloned cytolytic T cells by T cell growth factor: analysis by flow microfluorometry. J. Immunol. **129:** 1407.

20. ISCOVE, N. N. 1977. The role of erythropoietin in regulation of population size and cell cycling of early and late erythroid precursors in mouse bone marrow. Cell Tissue Kinet. **10:** 323.

21. ISCOVE, N. N. 1978. Erythropoietin—independent stimulation of early erythropoiesis in adult marrow cultures by conditioned media from lectin-stimulated mouse spleen cells. *In* Hematopoietic Cell Differentiation. D. W. Golde, M. J. Cline, D. Metcalf & G. F. Fox, Eds.: 37. Academic Press, Inc. New York, N.Y.

22. RALPH, P. & I. NAKOINZ. 1977. Direct toxic effects of immunopotentiators on monocytic, myelomonocytic and histiocytic or macrophage tumor cells in culture. Cancer Res. **37:** 546.

23. SUZUKI, S. & A. A. AXELRAD. 1980. FV2 locus controls the proportion of erythropoietic progenitor cells (BFU-E) synthesizing DNA in normal mice. Cell **19:** 225.

24. METCALF, D., G. R. JOHNSON & J. WILSON. 1977. Radiation induced enlargement of granulocytic and macrophage progenitor cells in mouse bone marrow. Exp. Hematol. **5:** 299.

25. DICKE, K. A. & D. W. VAN BEKKUM. 1971. Evidence for the identity of CFUa and CFUs. *In* In Vitro Culture of Hemopoietic Cells. D. W. Bekkum & K. A. Dicke, Eds.: 136. Proceedings of a workshop/symposium held September/October 1971 at the Radiobiological Institute, TNO, Rijswijk, the Netherlands.

26. METCALF, D. 1972. Effect of thymidine suiciding on colony formation *in vitro* by mouse hematopoietic cells. Proc. Soc. Exp. Biol. Med. **139:** 511.
27. MILLARD, R. E., N. M. BLACKETT & S. F. OKELL. 1973. A comparison of the effect of cytotoxic agents on agar colony forming cells, spleen colony forming cells and the erythrocytic repopulating ability of mouse bone marrow. J. Cell Physiol. **82:** 309.
28. BERGERON, J. J. M. 1971. Different effects of thymidine and 5-fluorouracil 2-deoxyriboside on biosynthetic events in cultured P815 mast cells. Biochem. J. **123:** 385.
29. BAUESTAD, H. B. 1977. Hydroxyurea (HU) in experimental hematology. II. Similarities and dissimilarities between HU and ^{3}H-thymidine killing. Exp. Hematol. **5:** 415.
30. BLACKETT, N. M. 1975. Cell cycle characteristics of hemopoietic stem cells. *In* Stem Cells of Renewing Cell Populations. A. B. Cairnie, P. K. Lala & D. G. Osmond, Eds.: 157. Academic Press, Inc. New York, N.Y.
31. BLACKETT, N. M. 1974. Statistical accuracy to be expected from cell colony assays, with special reference to the spleen colony assay. Cell Tissue Kinet. **7:** 407.
32. QUESENBERRY, P. J. & R. STANLEY. 1980. A statistical analysis of murine stem cell suicide technique. Blood **56:** 1000.
33. MacDONALD, H. R. & R. G. MILLER. 1970. Synchronization of mouse L-cells by a velocity sedimentation technique. Biophys. J. **10:** 834.

Stem Cell Proliferation and ^{125}IdUrd Incorporation into Spleen and Whole Skeletal Tissue[a]

TOHRU INOUE,[b,c,d] JAMES E. BULLIS,[c]
EUGENE P. CRONKITE,[c,e] AND SACHIHO KUBO[b]

[b]Department of Pathology
Tokyo Metropolitan Institute of Gerontology
Itabashi, Tokyo-173, Japan

[c]Medical Research Center
Brookhaven National Laboratory
Upton, New York 11973

INTRODUCTION

The specific DNA precursor, 5-[^{125}I]-iodo-2′-deoxyuridine (^{125}IdUrd), has been reported by Siegers et al.[1,2] to be a useful tool to study proliferation and differentiation of the hemopoietic stem cell. Successive studies have shown that ^{125}IdUrd incorporation into spleen and bone marrow (BM) represents seeding, proliferation, and differentiation of the stem cell.[3,4]

In a previous report[5] on the development of spleen colonies using the Till and McCulloch method[6] and incorporation of ^{125}IdUrd, it was suggested that undefined factors suppressed stem cell seeding and/or proliferation in the spleen. To measure stem cell proliferation in the BM, ^{125}IdUrd incorporation[3] is advantageous because BM colonies are much more difficult to identify and evaluate than spleen colonies. In addition, ^{125}IdUrd incorporation into BM as a function of the number of BM cells injected is very different[5] from that into spleen.

^{125}IdUrd incorporation in the BM can be used to evaluate factors that may reduce the seeding of stem cells in the BM. Earlier studies had suggested that stem cells in DNA synthesis preferentially seed the BM.[5] Thus if one treats BM cells with a cytocidal dose of [^{3}H]thymidine prior to injection into irradiated recipient mice, one can determine the percentage of the population in S phase by measuring the reduction in the amount of ^{125}IdUrd incorporated in the BM of the recipients in the same manner as one does with the standard method for stem cells seeding the spleen.

In this paper we present new concepts of stem cell seeding and proliferation that

[a]Research supported by the Environmental Protection Agency under agreement No. EPA-79-D-X0533 and the U.S. Department of Energy under Contract DE-AC02-76CH00016.

[d]Present address: Department of Pathology, Yokohama City University School of Medicine, Minamiku, Yokohama-232, Japan.

[e]Author to whom correspondence should be addressed.

have been derived from the application of the technique of ^{125}IdUrd incorporation into the spleen and the femoral and other skeletal marrow.

MATERIALS AND METHODS

Mice

C57BL/6(BNL) male mice 8 to 12 weeks old, obtained from the Jackson Laboratory (Bar Harbor, Maine) and bred in the Animal Facilities of Brookhaven National Laboratory (Upton, N.Y.), were used. C57BL/6 mice obtained from the Charles River Japan (Atsugi, Japan) were also used at the Animal House at Tokyo Metropolitan Institute of Gerontology, Itabashi, Japan. Groups of 10 to 15 mice were used at each assay point unless otherwise stated.

Bone Marrow Cell Preparation

Either Medium 199 (Microbiological Associates, Inc., Washington, D.C.) or RPMI-1640 (Nissui Seiyaku, Co. Ltd., Tokyo, Japan) containing antibiotics was used with 10% fetal calf serum (GIBCO, N.Y.). Media for cell suspension were replaced by serum-free media when the cells were injected into irradiated mice. BM cells from two to three mice were harvested by flushing both femurs.[6,7] Briefly, a 27-gauge needle was inserted into the femoral bone cavity through the proximal and/or distal end of the bone shaft, and 3 ml of ice-cold media was injected under pressure. A single-cell suspension was prepared by aspirating two times through 26- and 27-gauge needles; it was then washed twice and resuspended in serum-free media for intravenous (i.v.) injection into fatally irradiated mice.

Irradiation

A fatal dose (750 rad) was given by a GE 250-kVp Maxitron X-ray machine at 250 kV, 30 mA, with 0.5 mm Cu plus 1.0 mm Al filtration at a dose rate of 110 rad/min. The mice were irradiated 2 to 3 hr before the BM cell transfusion. A biologically comparable dose of γ rays (915 rad) was given by ^{60}Co in the Therapeutic Gamma-Irradiator (RFG-2D, Shimazu, Inc., Tokyo, Japan) with a 0.2-cm Al filter. With the above doses of X rays and ^{60}Co γ rays endogenous colonies were not observed in over 300 spleens in the C57BL/6(BNL) or C57BL/6 mice that were injected with cell-free media.

Assay for Pluripotent Stem Cells (CFU-S)

The Till and McCulloch method[6] was used to assay for CFU-S. The recipient mice were injected with media or 10^1, 3.5×10^1, 10^2, 3.5×10^2, 10^3, 3.5×10^3, 6×10^3, 10^4, 2×10^4, 3.5×10^4, 10^5, 5×10^5, or 10^6 cells. In certain experiments groups were given up to 6×10^6 cells. The mice were killed 9 days after irradiation and BM transfusion. Spleens were fixed in Bouin's solution for 24 hr and then placed in 3.6% formaldehyde. Spleens were scored for colonies and prepared for routine histological sectioning.

$^{125}IdUrd$ Labeling and Measurement of ^{125}I Activity

The mice to be assayed were allowed water (0.1% NaI solution, pH 3) and food *ad libitum* after irradiation and injection of media or BM cells. Cells in S phase were labeled by 3 μCi of 5-[^{125}I]-iodo-2'-deoxyuridine (NEX 072; New England Nuclear, Boston, Mass.; specific activity over 2000 Ci/mmol; 1 Ci = 3.7×10^{10} Bq) diluted in 0.2 ml of phosphate-buffered saline. ^{125}IdUrd was injected on day 8, exactly 24 hr before the animals were killed. As described earlier by Commerford and Joel[8] and Burki *et al.*,[9] the nonincorporated precursor is degraded and excreted by 24 hr after labeling, so that over 90% of the remaining activity of the spleen or BM is ^{125}IdUrd incorporated into DNA.[3] Spleens and femoral bones were fixed with Bouin's solution. ^{125}I incorporation was measured in a well-type crystal scintillation counter with an efficiency of 60% prior to the colony counting. In three pilot studies in which 1-20 μCi of ^{125}IdUrd was injected into lethally irradiated mice, there was a linear correlation between the amount injected and the amount incorporated into spleen and BM between 1 and 10 μCi.[10] No cytotoxic effect of ^{125}IdUrd on CFU-S was observed at a dose less than 10 μCi.

Regenerating Bone Marrow

By injecting phenylhydrazine (PHZ) intraperitoneally (i.p.) (50 mg/kg)[11,12] on days 7, 6, and 4 prior to sacrifice, regenerating BM was produced. Most cells from regenerating BM are considered to be in cycle.

[³H]Thymidine Cytocide

To assay the fraction of CFU-S in S phase, BM cells were treated with a cytocidal dose of [³H]thymidine to kill CFU-S in S phase prior to injection. The method of Becker *et al.*[13] was used. Briefly, the technique involved 30 min incubation at 37°C of 1-ml aliquots of working cell suspension with 200 μCi [³H]thymidine (20 Ci/mmol, NEX-027X, New England Nuclear) or the equivalent amount of "cold" thymidine, followed by dilution 1:40, washing with ice-cold medium, and immediate i.v. injection of 0.2 ml of suspension into recipient mice.

Preparation of Clean Skeletons

To assay ^{125}IdUrd incorporated into total body BM, whole body skeletons were cleaned. Dermestid beetles, *Dermestes haemorrhoidalis* Kuster, both larva and adult, were kindly provided by Dr. Okugi, Department of Animal Service, Tokyo Metropolitan Institute of Gerontology, Tokyo, Japan. The beetles eat muscle, connective tissue, and intracranial and intraspinal nervous and connective tissue leaving skeletons devoid of other tissue; this allows the total ^{125}I activity in the whole skeleton to be measured. *Dermestes maculatus,* obtained from Carolina Biological Supply Company, Burlington, North Carolina, was used at Brookhaven National Laboratory.

Several thousand beetles, housed in a plastic container ($25 \times 35 \times 37$ cm^3) placed in a room in which the temperature and humidity were maintained at 25°C and 60% respectively, took 2 to 5 days to clean three to five mice whose skin and visceral organs had been removed in advance. Skeletons were separated into skull and jaw, forelegs, vertebrae, femurs, tibiae, and tail bones and the bone groups from individual animals were placed into gamma-counting tubes separately after being cleaned completely; then the ^{125}IdUrd incorporation was measured by an auto-gamma-counter. A background count was subtracted from the count of each skeleton. The background consisted of the skeletal counts of a group of mice that had been irradiated and given cell-free media and ^{125}IdUrd as above.

Splenectomy

Twelve-week-old mice were used in this experiment. Splenectomy was performed 2 weeks before the mice were irradiated and used as recipients of bone marrow. Control mice underwent a sham operation at the same time.

RESULTS AND DISCUSSION

Spleen Colony Formation and ^{125}IdUrd Uptake in Spleen and Bone Marrow

A comparison of the number of spleen colonies and the amount of ^{125}IdUrd incorporated into spleen as a function of the number of bone marrow cells injected suggests that there is a factor(s) suppressing the development of spleen colonies. This notion arises from observations on the relationship of the number of bone marrow cells injected to the number of spleen colonies observed.

The linearity of this relationship has been examined only within a limited range, usually between 1×10^4 and 1×10^5 BM cells injected.[14-16] One study reported by Till[17] shows the role of overlap error in counting spleen colonies starting with an injection of 2×10^4 cells. The linearity when fewer cells are injected has not been ascertained.

The amount of ^{125}IdUrd incorporated into spleen as a function of the number of BM cells injected is linear in a log-log plot when the number of BM cells injected is below that producing confluency of spleen colonies.[2-4] The possibility that spleen colony formation is controlled by factors other than those that determine ^{125}IdUrd incorporation must be considered. Therefore, both procedures were performed simultaneously over a wide range in number of injected BM cells from 0, 10, 2 × 10, up to 10^6. The mice (C57BL/6) chosen for this study produce no endogenous colonies with injection of cell-free media, and their day 9 colonies are quite discrete and equally developed. The results are presented in FIGURE 1. The spleen colony curve and ^{125}IdUrd curve are linear on the log-log plot between 2 × 10^3 and 1-2 × 10^5 cells injected and are essentially parallel (slopes, 0.755 and 0.788).

FIGURE 2 shows spleen colony formation as a function of number of BM cells injected from 0 to 10^5. Two regression lines are shown, one for up to 2 × 10^4 cells injected and one for 2 × 10^4-10^5 cells injected. Within these ranges there are very good fits, whereas it is not possible to get a good linear fit over the whole range.

Confluency of spleen colonies was considered improbable at the lower portion of the curve and the average number of CFU-S per unit number of BM cells injected that had been calculated based on the Poisson distribution (data not shown, see Reference 5) was not constant but showed a positive slope; therefore, the existence of a factor(s) suppressing the development of spleen colonies was suggested.[5] The suppressive cell that competes with stem cells for colony formation reported by Tange et al.[18] might be a factor. It is to be noted that if the regression line is straight and crosses the origin, then the same data plotted on the log-log scale should have a slope of 1.0. It is of interest that preliminary data in our recent studies in which BM cells are concentrated by centrifugal elutriation[7] show a steeper slope (0.965) for both ^{125}IdUrd and spleen colony curves (unpublished data).

^{125}IdUrd Incorporation into Femur—Ability of the Stem Cell to Penetrate into and Proliferate in BM

The amount of ^{125}IdUrd incorporated into femur as a function of number of BM cells injected is shown by solid triangles in FIGURES 1 and 3. Unless more than 3.5 × 10^4 BM cells are injected, no significant radioactivity is detected in the femoral BM after background is subtracted. In addition, no femoral colonies are seen upon microscopic examination, whereas colonies are easily found when more than 10^5 BM cells are injected. A possible explanation, described earlier,[5] is that only 1 per 10^5 BM cells are pluripotent stem cells with a proclivity for lodging in and proliferating in the femur. In addition, the ^{125}IdUrd curve for spleen (FIGURE 1) first starts to rise at 2 × 10^3 BM cells injected. Therefore, the relative ratio between stem cells seeding into spleen and into femur is about 50:1 to 80:1 or 1 per 50 stem cells is capable of seeding the femoral marrow. The morphologic identification of this subpopulation of stem cells has not been accomplished. The finding is, however, reasonably compatible with the fact that lethally irradiated mice are rescued from fatal irradiation only when they receive more than 10^6 BM cells.[19] Corresponding data by Vos[20] have shown that the BM was significantly repopulated with CFU-S only when more than 2 × 10^5 BM cells were injected.

A greater fraction of BM cells were in cycle when mice were treated with PHZ. This regenerating BM was more effective in repopulating BM at the lower number of bone marrow cells injected as shown in FIGURE 3 by open triangles with a broken line. The idea that "CFU-S in cycle are more effective in repopulating bone marrow than are CFU-S out of cycle" suggested by this study was directly supported by the thymidine cytocide study for BM-competent stem cells discussed next.

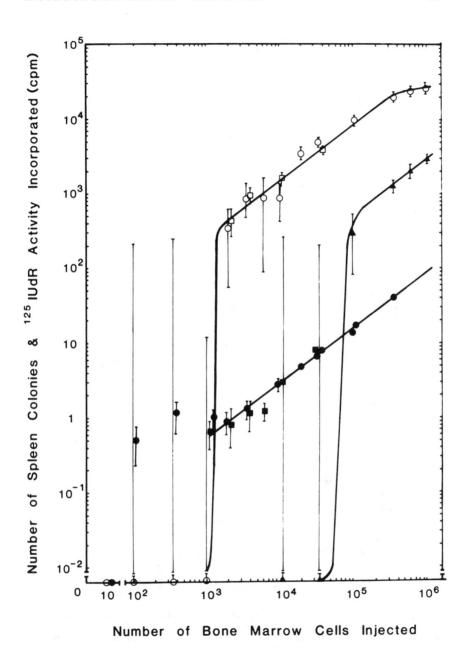

FIGURE 1. Relationship among number of BM cells injected, number of spleen colonies produced, and amount of ¹²⁵IdUrd (abbreviated ¹²⁵IUdR in figure) incorporated into the spleen and BM. Solid circles and squares, spleen colonies; open circles and squares, ¹²⁵IdUrd in spleens; solid triangles, ¹²⁵IdUrd uptake in the femur. (Reprinted with permission from Reference 5.)

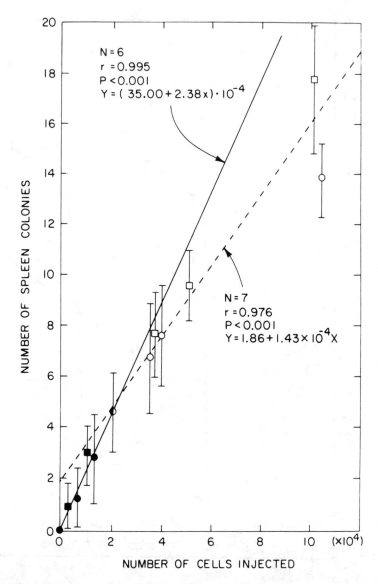

FIGURE 2. The number of day 9 spleen colonies as a function of number of bone marrow cells injected is shown on a linear scale. Note that the linearity of the relationship between the number of spleen colonies and the number of cells injected is seen only over a limited range. The solid regression line was obtained from six solid symbols within a range of 0 to 2×10^4 cells injected, whereas the broken line was obtained from seven open symbols in a range between 2×10^4 and 10^5 cells injected. Circles and squares represent separate experiments. Vertical bars indicate the standard error of the mean (SEM).

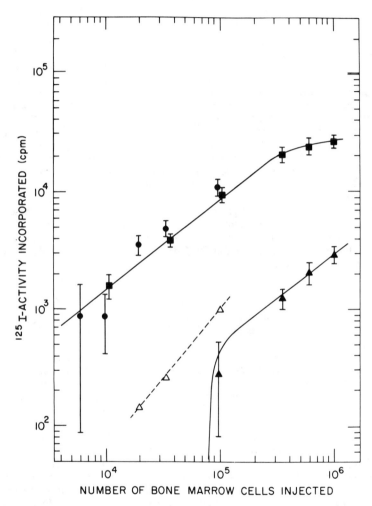

FIGURE 3. Magnified graph of the upper left part of FIGURE 1. The open triangles with the broken regression line indicate [125]IdUrd incorporated into femur when regenerating bone marrow was injected.

^{125}IdUrd Incorporation into Spleen and Femoral BM after Injection of BM Cells Treated with Cytocidal Doses of Tritiated Thymidine—Repopulation of Spleen and Femur

The number of cells in S phase is significantly reduced by [^{3}H]thymidine cytocide, and this provides the relative ratio in S phase. Changes in the number of spleen colonies after [^{3}H]thymidine cytocide of BM is an indication of whether S or non-S cells preferentially seed into the spleen and/or BM.[21,22] ^{125}IdUrd incorporation in the femur after injection of BM cells treated with cold thymidine or a cytocidal dose of [^{3}H]thymidine ([^{3}H]TdR) is shown in FIGURE 4. The incorporation of ^{125}IdUrd into spleen after treatment with cold thymidine or [^{3}H]TdR is also shown. Since spleen colonies become confluent when more than 2×10^5 cells are injected, the stem cell cytocidal test for spleen seeding must be performed with lower doses of BM cells (2×10^4-3.5×10^5), than in femur (3.5×10^5-6×10^6). Reduction of ^{125}IdUrd activity in BM was nearly 100% after injection of 3.5×10^5 cells, 90% after injection of 1×10^6 cells, and 87.5% after injection of 5×10^6 cells. The reduction in splenic ^{125}IdUrd was much smaller (21 to 8%). These observations are possibly inconsistent with those of Monette and DeMellow[22] whose studies suggested that a few CFU-S in S phase do seed the spleen. Our observations suggest that CFU-S in S phase do in part seed the spleen. Our data suggest that about 10-20% of CFU-S in S phase seed the spleen. Our data also show that CFU-S in S phase are primarily responsible for seeding and proliferating in the femoral BM. We cannot eliminate the possibility that CFU-S helper cells are being killed by [^{3}H]TdR cytocide and that CFU-S seeded in the BM are not proliferating.

^{125}IdUrd Incorporated into BM of the Whole Skeleton—Is There Any Difference between the Femur and Other Parts of the Skeleton?

To answer the above question the incorporation of ^{125}IdUrd into the whole skeleton was compared to incorporation into the femur. This was accomplished by removing viscera and skin and then allowing dermestid beetles to eat the muscle, connective tissue, and contents of the head and spinal canal. ^{125}IdUrd uptake in the whole skeletons of media-injected controls was compared to that in skeletons of mice that had received graded doses of BM cells. The results are shown in FIGURE 5.

All parts of the bone marrow begin to show ^{125}IdUrd incorporation only when more than 10^5 cells are injected as seen previously in the femur. In this experiment, ^{125}IdUrd incorporated into whole skeletal BM was not summed from the individual skeletal incorporations but by counting the complete skeleton. The ratio between the sum of the parts and the complete skeletons ranged from 0.91 to 1.10. In FIGURE 5, it should be noted that the amount of ^{125}IdUrd incorporated into whole skeletal BM was nearly the same as that incorporated into spleen when more than 10^5 cells were injected. Details of ^{125}IdUrd incorporation into various skeletal portions when mice were injected with 10^6 cells are given in TABLE 1. In this table, it should also be noted that the incorporation of ^{125}IdUrd is not only a function of the seeding of stem cells (and other progenitors) but also of their proliferation, differentiation, and exit from BM or spleen. Since the preceding may be different in spleen and BM, an estimation of the number of BM colonies cannot be obtained from the amount of incorporation of ^{125}IdUrd per spleen colony. Nevertheless, "amount of hemopoietic activity" in the

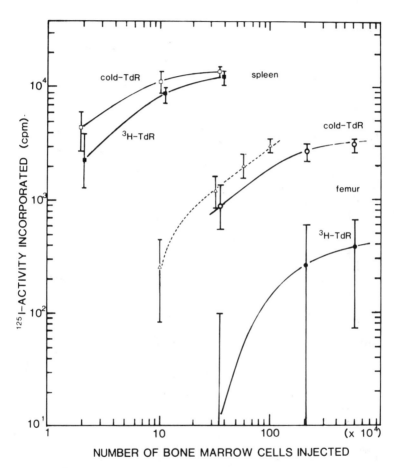

FIGURE 4. Relationship between number of BM cells injected and amount of ^{125}IdUrd incorporated into the spleen (squares) and BM (circles). Solid symbols indicate ^{125}IdUrd incorporation when the BM cells were treated with [^{3}H]thymidine, whereas open symbols indicate the control in which the BM cells were treated with the same amount of cold thymidine. Note a drastic reduction of ^{125}IdUrd uptake by thymidine cytocide is seen in the femur and a relatively small reduction is seen in the spleen. Open triangles refer to bone marrow obtained from anemic phenylhydrazine-treated mice.

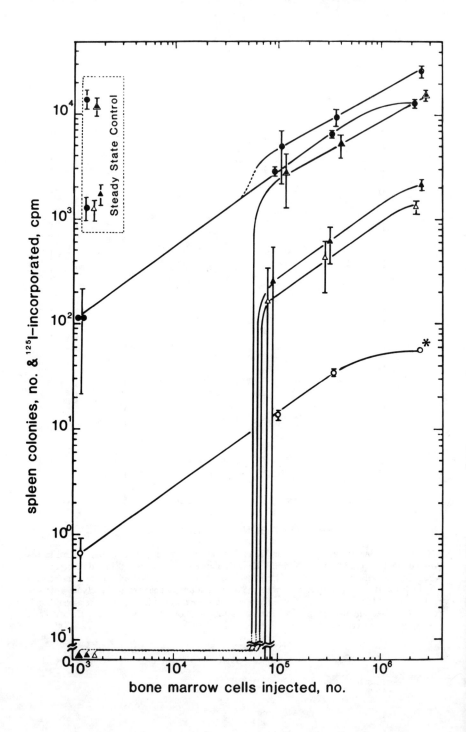

spleen suggested in this table is much larger than expected to date if one takes into account the "f" factor[23] in stem cell seeding.

When one compares these data to those of steady-state controls in which recipients were not irradiated, it is of interest that the incorporation of ^{125}IdUrd into whole skeletal BM is about the same ranging from 100.8 to 128.8% except for that in skull and jaw, whereas incorporation into spleen for the regenerating state is about 10 times higher than that for the steady-state control. These data show that in the steady state the ratio of spleen uptake to BM uptake is not the same as that seen in the regenerating state indicating that regeneration proceeds at different rates in the spleen and BM. In addition, these studies are relevant to the significance of the "f" factor. Published studies report f to be between 0.025 and 0.25.[23–25]

Our data suggest that when less than 10^5 BM cells are injected stem cells either do not seed the bone marrow or do not proliferate in the BM. Furthermore, our data suggest that the "f" factor may change as a function of BM cells injected.

Effect of Splenectomy on ^{125}IdUrd Incorporation into BM—Do Spleen-Competent Stem Cells Seed into BM when Spleen is Removed?

The data presented previously suggest that stem cells seeding into the spleen and bone marrow are in different phases of the cell cycle to a large extent. If stem cells that are trapped in the spleen can in part penetrate the bone marrow, splenectomized mice should have a greater uptake in BM than nonsplenectomized control sham-operated mice. To explore this further ^{125}IdUrd incorporation was studied in splenectomized mice and compared to that in sham-operated mice. In FIGURE 6 the results are expressed as a percentage of the uptake in the sham-operated controls. When 3.5 $\times$ 10^3 BM cells are injected there is essentially no incorporation of ^{125}IdUrd in splenectomized or sham-operated mice. When 2×10^4 BM cells are injected there is essentially no significant difference. When 1×10^5 BM cells are injected the uptake in BM of splenectomized mice is 29% of that in control sham-operated mice. There is equal uptake after injection of 3.5×10^6 BM cells. When 1.0×10^6 BM cells are injected the uptake in splenectomized mice is 200% of that in the sham-operated controls. Thus it appears that when a sufficient number of BM cells are injected the stem cells ordinarily seeding the spleen may penetrate into the BM. Details of the ^{125}IdUrd incorporation into each part of the skeleton when 10^6 cells were injected are given in TABLE 2. The average increase in incorporation (210%) is reasonable assuming that the stem cells ordinarily seeding the spleen are now entering the BM.

FIGURE 5. Relationship of the number of bone marrow cells injected to the amount of ^{125}IdUrd incorporated into various parts of the skeleton (femur (solid triangles), tibia (open triangles), whole skeletal marrow (double triangle, solid triangle within an open triangle)), into spleen (solid circle), into the spleen and whole skeletal BM (solid triangle within an open circle), and the number of spleen colonies (open circle). The amount of ^{125}IdUrd incorporated into bone marrow is obtained from cleaned skeletons followed by subtraction of skeletal uptake from control mice given irradiation and cell-free media. Asterisk shows confluency of spleen colonies. Vertical bars indicate standard error of the mean. Data from the steady-state control in which mice were not irradiated but given cell-free media on the same day as the experimental groups were irradiated and injected with media or BM cells are shown in the broken rectangle. Note, as seen in FIGURE 1, the amount of ^{125}IdUrd incorporated into any part of skeletal marrow was zero when 10^3 BM cells were injected.

TABLE 1. ¹²⁵IdUrd Incorporation (cpm) into Bone Marrow and Spleen

	Steady-State Control[a]			Regenerating State[b]			Percentage of Regenerating to Steady State
	cpm[c] ± SEM	% to (A)	% to (C)	cpm[c] ± SEM	% to (A)	% to (C)	
(A) Total (B) + (C)	14,004 ± 3,191	100.0	—	25,893 ± 2,322	100.0	—	184.9
(B) Spleen	1,288 ± 310	9.2	—	13,097 ± 899	50.5	—	1,015.5
(C) Whole skeletons	12,716 ± 2,881	90.8	100.0	12,814 ± 1,423	49.5	100.0	100.8
Skull & jaw	1,137 ± 238	8.1	8.9	363 ± 184	1.4	2.8	31.9
Forelegs	1,394 ± 250	10.0	11.0	1,585 ± 184	6.1	12.4	113.7
Vertebrae	7,244 ± 165	51.7	57.0	7,343 ± 602	25.4	57.3	101.4
Femurs	1,722 ± 352	12.3	13.5	2,218 ± 232	8.6	17.3	128.8
Tibiae	1,205 ± 274	8.6	9.5	1,305 ± 150	5.0	10.2	108.3
Tail	14 ± 114	0.1	0.1	0 ± 71	0.0	0.0	—

[a] Recipients were not irradiated but received media injection.

[b] Mice were given 915 rad whole-body irradiation and transfusion of 2.5×10^6 bone marrow cells. ¹²⁵IdUrd (3 μCi) was injected i.v., 24 hr prior to kill, 8 days after irradiation and transfusion of the bone marrow cells.

[c] Absolute gamma counts per minute determined by a crystal scintillation counter with a counting efficiency of 60%. All counts listed above have been corrected by subtracting the count from mice that had been irradiated and injected with media without cells. SEM: Standard error of the mean.

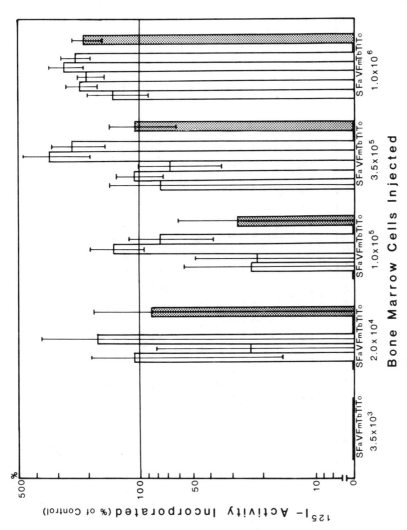

FIGURE 6. Effect of splenectomy on the amount of [125]IdUrd incorporated into various parts of skeletal bone marrow as a function of number of BM cells injected after lethal irradiation, shown as a percentage of the sham-operated control. Vertical bars indicate the standard error of the mean (SEM). S, skulls and jaw; Fa, forearms; V, vertebral bones; Fm, femurs; Tb, tibiae; Tl, tail bones; To, total skeletons.

TABLE 2. Effect of Splenectomy on ^{125}IdUrd Incorporation into Bone Marrow

	Mean ± SEM[a]		Mean Percentage of (A) to (B) ± SEM
	Splenectomized[b] (A)	Sham Operated[b] (B)	
Skull & jaw	2,816 ± 750 (6.6)	1,954 ± 557 (9.7)	144 ± 56
Forelegs	5,314 ± 706 (12.5)	2,398 ± 348 (11.9)	221 ± 43
Vertebrae	23,288 ± 2,310 (54.9)	11,554 ± 1,240 (57.2)	201 ± 29
Femurs	6,524 ± 402 (15.4)	2,376 ± 446 (11.8)	274 ± 64
Tibiae	4,510 ± 532 (10.6)	1,902 ± 300 (9.4)	237 ± 46
Tail	0 ± 93 (0.0)	0 ± 138 (0.0)	—
(a) Whole skeletons	42,452 ± 4,793 (100.0)	20,184 ± 3,029 (100.0)	210 ± 40
(b) Spleen	—	24,950 ± 2,296	
Total (a) + (b)	42,452 ± 4,793	45,134 ± 5,325	

[a] Each mean value represents 11 to 12 mice. SEM: Standard error of the mean. Numbers in parentheses are percentages of whole skeleton value.
[b] Mice underwent splenectomy or sham operation 3 weeks before use. Fatal, whole-body irradiation was given followed by transfusion of bone marrow, 1×10^6 cells. Eight days after irradiation, 3 μCi ^{125}IdUrd was injected i.v., and the mice were killed exactly 24 hr later.

ACKNOWLEDGMENTS

The authors appreciate the excellent technical assistance of B. Heldman, L. Honikel, E. Moriizumi, N. Pappas, L. Cook, and M. Utsuyma at Tokyo Metropolitan Institute of Gerontology and Brookhaven National Laboratory. Critical discussions with Drs. K.-H. v. Wangenheim and L. E. Feinendegen at Kernforschungsanlage (KFA), Federal Republic of Germany also are appreciated.

REFERENCES

1. SIEGERS, M. P., L. E. FEINENDEGEN, S. LAHIRI & E. P. CRONKITE. 1979. Proliferation kinetics of early hemopoietic precursor cells with self sustaining capacity in the mouse, studied with ^{125}I-labeled iododeoxyuridine. Exp. Hematol. **7:** 469-482.
2. SIEGERS, M. P., L. E. FEINENDEGEN, S. LAHIRI & E. P. CRONKITE. 1979. Relative number and proliferation kinetics of hemopoietic stem cells in the mouse. Blood Cells **5:** 211-236.
3. V. WANGENHEIM, K.-H., M. P. SIEGERS & L. E. FEINENDEGEN. 1980. Repopulation ability and proliferation stimulus in the hemopoietic system of mice following gamma-irradiation. Exp. Hematol. **6:** 694-701.
4. HUBNER, G. E., K.-H. V. WANGENHEIM & L. E. FEINENDEGEN. 1980. An assay for the measurement of residual damage of murine hematopoietic stem cells. Exp. Hematol. **9:** 111-117.
5. INOUE, T. & E. P. CRONKITE. 1983. Relationship between number of spleen colonies and ^{125}IdUrd incorporation into spleen and femur. Proc. Natl. Acad. Sci. USA **80:** 435-438.
6. TILL, J. E. & E. A. McCULLOCH. 1961. A direct measurement of the radiation sensitivity of normal bone marrow cells. Radiat. Res. **14:** 213-222.
7. INOUE, T., A. L. CARSTEN, E. P. CRONKITE & J. E. T. KELLEY. 1981. Separation and concentration of murine hematopoietic stem cells (CFUs) using a combination of density gradient sedimentation and counterflow centrifugal elutriation. Exp. Hematol. **9(6):** 563-572.
8. COMMERFORD, S. L. & D. D. JOEL. 1979. Iododeoxyuridine administered to mice is deiodinated and incorporated into DNA primarily as thymidylate. Biochem. Biophys. Res. Commun. **86:** 112-118.
9. BURKI, K., J. C. SCHAER, A. GRIEDER, R. SCHINDLER & H. COTTIER. 1971. Studies on liver regeneration. I. ^{131}Iododeoxyuridine as a precursor of DNA in normal and regenerating rat liver. Cell Tissue Kinet. **4:** 519-527.
10. INOUE, T. Unpublished data.
11. TOKSOZ, D., T. M. DEXTER, B. I. LORD, E. G. WRIGHT & L. G. LAJTHA. 1981. The regulation of hemopoiesis in long-term bone marrow cultures. II. Stimulation and inhibition of stem cell proliferation. Blood **55:** 931-936.
12. HARA, H. 1980. Kinetics of pluripotent hemopoietic precursors in vitro after erythropoietic stimulation or suppression. Exp. Hematol. **8:** 345-350.
13. BECKER, A. J., E. A. McCULLOCH, L. SIMINOVITCH & J. E. TILL. 1965. The effect of differing demands for blood cell production on DNA synthesis by hemopoietic colony forming cells of mice. Blood **26:** 296-308.
14. McCULLOCH, E. A., J. E. TILL & L. SIMINOVITCH. 1965. Genetic factors affecting the control of hemopoiesis. In Proceedings, Canadian Cancer Conference. Pp. 336-356. Pergamon Press. New York, N.Y.
15. McCULLOCH, E. A. & J. E. TILL. 1962. The sensitivity of cells from normal mouse bone marrow to gamma radiation in vitro and in vivo. Radiat. Res. **16(6):** 822-832.
16. WOLF, N. S. & J. J. TRENTIN. 1975. Linearity of counts of endogenous and exogenous colonies in mouse bone marrow. Exp. Hematol. **3:** 54-56.
17. TILL, J. E. 1972. Overlap error in counts of splenic colonies. Ser. Haematol. **2:** 5-14.

18. TANGE, T., S. KANAMORI, R. HABBERSETT, M. MUKAIDA, T. SHIMAMINE & H. TSE.1982. Suppression of pluripotent stem cell development by syngeneic non-T adherent cells. Exp. Hematol. **10**(Suppl. 12): 168-178.

19. BOND, V. P., T. M. FLIEDNER & J. ARCHAMBEAU. 1965. Mammalian Radiation Lethality. A Disturbance in Cellular Kinetics. P. 305. Academic Press, Inc. New York, N.Y.

20. VOS, O. 1972. Multiplication of hemopoietic forming units (CFU) in mice after X-irradiation and bone marrow transplantation. Cell Tissue Kinet. **5**: 341-350.

21. LAJTHA, L. G. & R. SCHOFIELD. 1971. Regulation of stem cell renewal and differentiation: possible significance in aging. *In* Advances in Gerontological Research. B. L. Strehler, Ed. **3**: 131-146. Academic Press, Inc. New York, N.Y.

22. MONETTE, F. C. & J. B. DeMELLOW. 1979. The relationship between stem cell seeding efficiency and position in cell cycle. Cell Tissue Kinet. **12**: 161-175.

23. TILL, J. E. & E. A. McCULLOCH. 1972. The 'f-factor' of the spleen-colony assay for hemopoietic stem cells. Ser. Haematol. **5**(2): 15-21.

24. REINCKE, U., H. BURLINGTON, A. L. CARSTEN, E. P. CRONKITE & J. A. LAISSUE. 1978. Hemopoietic effects in mice of a transplanted, granulocytosis-inducing tumor. Exp. Hematol. **6**: 421-430.

25. VAN BEKKUM, D. W., M. J. VAN NOORD, B. MAAT & K. A. DICKE. 1971. Attempts at identification of hemopoietic stem cell in mouse. Blood **38**: 547-558.

Modulation of Radiation-Induced Hemopoietic Suppression by Acute Thrombocytopenia[a]

SHIRLEY EBBE,[b,c,d] ELIZABETH PHALEN,[b]
GREGORY THREATTE,[b] AND HELEN LONDE[b]

[b]Donner Laboratory
Lawrence Berkeley Laboratory
University of California
Berkeley, California 94720

[c]Department of Laboratory Medicine
University of California
San Francisco, California 94143

INTRODUCTION

Previous studies have shown that the thrombocytopoietic suppression induced in mice by sublethal doses of radiation could be modified by production of acute thrombocytopenia with heterologous anti-mouse platelet serum (APS) at the time of exposure to radiation.[1, 2] For 4 days after irradiation, mice maintain normal platelet counts; during this interval, recovery to about normal platelet counts occurs from superimposed immunothrombocytopenia. Thereafter, platelet counts decline from the effects of the radiation. However, the radiation-induced thrombocytopenia is neither as severe nor as prolonged in mice that are initially treated with APS as it is in mice that are just irradiated. The present studies were done to further characterize the hemopoietic response to radiation and APS and to determine the effect of acutely reducing the platelet count with the nonimmunological agent neuraminidase (N'ase).

MATERIALS AND METHODS

Female mice of the CF_1 strain (Charles River) were used at the age of 12-14 weeks. Blood for cell counts was obtained by cardiac puncture under ether anesthesia

[a]Supported, in part, by Grants R01-AM21355 and T32-AM07349 from the National Institutes of Health and, in part, by the Office of Health and Environmental Research of the U.S. Department of Energy under Contract DE-AC03-76SF00098.

[d]Author to whom correspondence should be addressed: Shirley Ebbe, M.D., Building 74, Lawrence Berkeley Laboratory, University of California, Berkeley, Calif. 94720.

179

and anticoagulated with dry K_2EDTA. Platelets were counted by phase microscopy,[3] leukocytes by Coulter counter, and reticulocytes by the method of Brecher and Schneiderman[4]; microhematocrits were done with a Drummond centrifuge. Student's t test was used to determine significance of differences.

Mice were exposed to γ radiation from ^{60}Co in the doses indicated under Results. All doses were below the lethal dose (LD) 50/30 for this strain, and radiation-induced deaths did not occur during the course of the experiments.

Anti-mouse platelet serum was produced in guinea pigs; before use it was heat inactivated and absorbed three times with equal volumes of washed mouse red blood cells. It was injected intraperitoneally in 0.1-ml volumes after appropriate dilution with saline. Normal guinea pig serum (NGpS) was not absorbed before use, and it was used in the same amounts as APS. Neuraminidase (Sigma Chemical Co., St. Louis, Mo.) was dissolved in saline and injected i.v. in 0.25-ml volumes; controls received 0.25 ml saline or no injection. The dose of N'ase was 0.025 unit/mouse, one unit being defined as the amount that will liberate 1.0 μmol of N-acetylneuraminic acid per minute at pH 5.0 and 37°C from N-acetyl neuramin-lactose. There were 5.0-6.5 units/mg protein. Blood cell counts were done 4 hr after injections and at subsequent times as indicated under Results.

Incorporation of [^{75}Se]selenomethionine was measured as previously described.[5] A dose of 2 μCi of ^{75}Se was injected intraperitoneally 6 or 9 days after irradiation. One and 2 days later, cohorts of mice were bled by cardiac puncture under ether anesthesia. Blood was anticoagulated with dry K_2EDTA and, after determination of the platelet count, undiluted plasma and platelets were separated by differential centrifugation. Platelets were washed a total of three times with 1% ammonium oxalate and saline. Radioactivity of injected material, platelets, and plasma was measured. The results were expressed as the percentage of injected radioisotope incorporated into platelets; plasma radioactivity was the same in treated and control mice in each experiment.

RESULTS

FIGURE 1 shows blood cell counts of cohorts of mice examined serially after exposure to 650 R and either APS or NGpS injected immediately after irradiation. The findings of significantly higher platelet counts (days 8-12), hematocrits (days 8-15), and reticulocyte counts (days 8, 9, and 11) during the second week after irradiation in mice given APS than in those receiving NGpS showed that an increase in erythropoiesis accompanied the modification of radiation-induced thrombocytopenia. Leukocyte counts did not show consistent differences.

The data in FIGURE 2 confirm the conclusion that the higher platelet counts in mice treated with APS after exposure to irradiation than in irradiated controls were due to increased platelet production rather than some other mechanism. In the two experiments shown, platelet counts done 4 hr after APS were < 5% of normal, but hematocrits were not lower than in controls. Platelet counts and platelet incorporation of ^{75}Se were greater on days 10 and 11 after irradiation and APS than in irradiated controls. Platelet counts in all treated groups were still lower than those in untreated controls, but initiation of recovery of platelet production in the APS-treated mice was apparent from isotope incorporation values that were at or near normal values on days 10 and 11. Substitution of NGpS for APS did not produce acute thrombocytopenia, did not modify the radiation-induced thrombocytopenia, and did not increase ^{75}Se incorporation over that seen in mice exposed to radiation only.

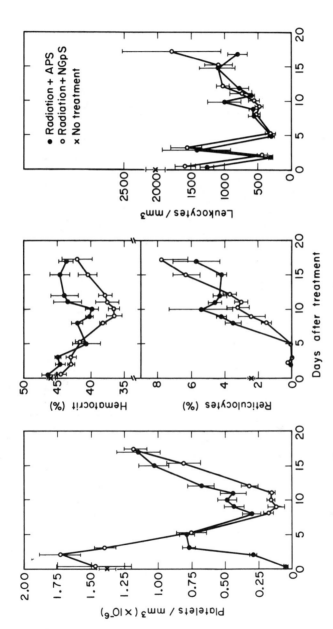

FIGURE 1. Platelet counts, hematocrits, reticulocytes, and leukocytes in mice treated with 650 R and APS or NGpS. Each point is the mean ± SEM for 9-10 mice from two experiments except for days 2, 3, and 17, when each point was derived from 5 mice from only one of the two experiments.

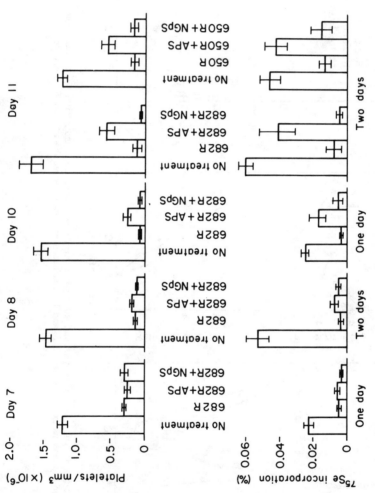

FIGURE 2. Platelet counts (top) and incorporation of ^{75}Se into platelets (bottom) on days 7, 8, 10, and 11 after no treatment, irradiation, irradiation plus APS, or irradiation plus NGpS. ^{75}Se incorporation was measured one day after injection of radioisotope on days 7 and 10 and two days after injection on days 8 and 11. Each bar is the mean ± SEM for 5-6 mice. The only significant differences among irradiated groups were on days 10 and 11 when platelet counts and isotope incorporation in mice receiving APS were significantly greater than irradiated controls (platelet counts: $p < 0.01$, < 0.01, < 0.01; isotope incorporation: $p < 0.05$, < 0.05, < 0.01).

The hematocrits listed in TABLE 1 are from the same groups of mice represented in FIGURE 2. The significance of differences between groups treated with APS or NGpS after irradiation is indicated. All APS-treated groups that showed increases in platelet production also showed elevations of hematocrits, and others did not.

Injection of N'ase into normal mice produced thrombocytopenia within 4 hr, and it increased in severity during the following day (FIGURE 3). Reactive thrombocytosis ensued before platelet counts returned to normal. Other blood cell counts did not show remarkable variances from normal after injection of N'ase.

When thrombocytopenia was produced by injection of N'ase immediately before exposure to 650 R, the course of the subsequent blood counts was similar to that described above for animals treated with APS plus radiation (FIGURE 4). Platelet counts were significantly greater than those in irradiated controls on days 9-12 and the same was true for reticulocytes on days 8-13 and hematocrits on days 10 and 11. Leukocyte counts were similar in both groups; apparent differences on days 17 and 18 were not significant.

TABLE 1. Hematocrits of Mice Depicted in FIGURE 2

Group	n	No Treatment	Radiation	Radiation + APS	Radiation + NGpS
Day 7	5	45.9 ± 0.8	42.1 ± 1.8	37.6 ± 0.2[a]	38.5 ± 0.7[a]
Day 8	5	46.2 ± 0.8	37.2 ± 1.0	38.4 ± 1.2[a]	35.9 ± 1.0[a]
Day 10	5	45.0 ± 1.0	34.9 ± 1.1	38.8 ± 1.0[b]	33.3 ± 0.3[b]
Day 11 (682 R)	5	46.2 ± 0.7	33.2 ± 2.2	42.4 ± 1.0[b]	32.9 ± 0.9[b]
Day 11 (650 R)	6	43.9 ± 1.0	31.5 ± 1.6	37.8 ± 1.4[c]	32.0 ± 1.2[c]

[a] Not significant.
[b] $p < 0.001$.
[c] $p < 0.05$.

DISCUSSION

The findings presented in this paper show that the combination of acute thrombocytopenia with sublethal irradiation in mice results in delayed stimulation of both thrombocytopoiesis and erythropoiesis relative to irradiated controls. This contrasts with the nonirradiated mice in which thrombocytopenia rapidly causes stimulation of platelet production without apparent stimulation of red cell production. The delay in the irradiated mice suggests either that the stimulation affected a compartment of precursor cells less mature than those responsible for the earlier burst of platelet production in response to thrombocytopenia in nonirradiated animals or that it was slowly generated by an interaction between the thrombocytopenic state and the radiation-induced marrow depletion. There is evidence to suggest that both thrombocytopoiesis[6] and erythropoiesis[7] may be dually regulated, with more mature marrow cells of each system responding to humoral regulators, i.e., thrombopoietin or eryth-

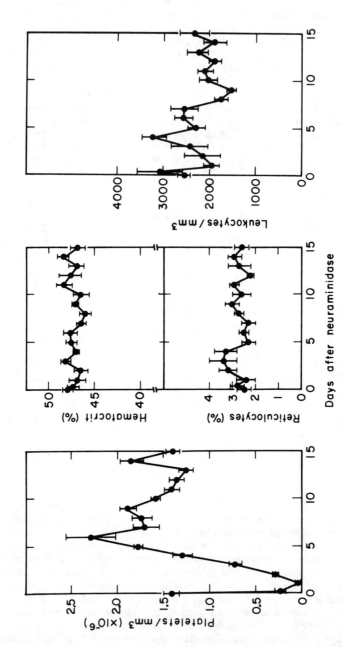

FIGURE 3. Platelet counts, hematocrits, reticulocytes, and- leukocytes in control mice (time zero) and mice injected with neuraminidase. Values are means ± SEM for 10 control mice or 6–8 treated mice at each time point.

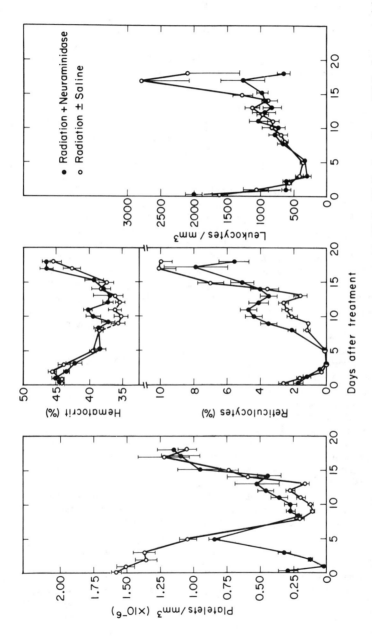

FIGURE 4. Platelet counts, hematocrits, reticulocytes, and leukocytes in mice treated with 650 R, 650 R plus saline, or 650 R plus neuraminidase. Each point is the mean ± SEM of 5-12 mice treated with radiation + N'ase or 7-17 mice treated with radiation ± saline.

ropoietin, that are controlled by the mass of circulating progeny, while less mature precursors are regulated by other mechanisms. In some marrow hypoplastic states, the numbers of circulating platelets[8] and red cells[9] are higher than would be expected from the low numbers of precursors in the marrow, and these observations support the notion that there may be a level of regulation that depends on marrow cellularity. In the experiments reported here, thrombocytopenia may have interacted with the hypoplastic marrow to induce a stimulus that eventuated in acceleration of production of both platelets and red cells. In the absence of differences in blood leukocyte counts, the findings imply that there was a selectivity to the stimulation of both thrombocytopoiesis and erythropoiesis.

There are a number of findings that suggest that there may be a particularly close linkage between thrombocytopoiesis and erythropoiesis which is manifested under special clinical or experimental conditions. Platelet production may be stimulated in the anemias of moderate iron deficiency,[10–13] pure red cell aplasia,[14, 15] and hemolysis in asplenic individuals.[16] However, this may not be a consistent finding in all patients or even a persistent one in a given patient. In experimental animals, stimulation of platelet production in anemia could be enhanced by administration of actinomycin D to block erythropoiesis,[17] and perturbations of erythropoiesis in irradiated mice have been reported to have either the same[18, 19] or the opposite[20] stimulatory or inhibitory effect on platelet production as they would on red cell production. The erythropoietic effect of hypoxia is well known; platelet production is also affected by hypoxia but in a less well defined manner. Human subjects whose erythropoiesis is chronically stimulated by environmental hypoxia generally do not have abnormal platelet counts,[21, 22] but acute, severe hypoxia in one person appeared to stimulate platelet production.[23] When animals are exposed to hypoxia, the results of most,[24–31] but not all,[32, 33] studies are consistent with platelet production showing a biphasic response: initially being higher than normal and, with continuation of hypoxia, declining to subnormal levels. These assorted observations provide additional examples of situations in which platelet and red cell production appear to be linked, but neither they nor the present results provide an explanation. Cross-reactivity of erythropoietin or thrombopoietin with cells of both systems might explain some of the findings but has not been demonstrable experimentally.[33] Thus the relationship in vivo remains enigmatic.

When hemopoietic cells are cultured in the presence of erythropoietin, megakaryocytes frequently appear in mixed colonies with erythroid cells,[34–37] and the chromosomal studies of such colonies by McLeod et al.[38] indicate that they originate from bipotential clonogenic cells. Paulus et al.[39] interpreted their analysis of ploidy and number of cells in pure megakaryocyte and mixed erythroid-megakaryocyte colonies to indicate that the process of commitment from a pluripotential to a unipotential megakaryocytic stem cell may proceed by way of bipotentiality for the two cell lines. It could thus be proposed that this bipotential progenitor cell may be the one that is expressed in the present experiments and in some of the other situations cited above. If so, it is clear that very special circumstances must exist for its demonstration in vivo.

The possibility that APS injections may induce hemopoietic stem cell changes by way of an immunological reaction rather than as a direct consequence of the thrombocytopenia has been introduced by Levin et al.[40] and Burstein et al.[41] The present findings that the effects of APS were duplicated by N'ase strongly suggested that the results with both were due to the common occurrence of thrombocytopenia or platelet lysis. If the effects of both were due to immunological reactions, then it would be necessary to postulate that identical reactions occurred to preformed heterologous antibodies and to the small amounts (4-5 μg) of foreign protein from Clostridium perfringens present in the N'ase preparation but not to the normal heterologous serum (~1 mg protein/injection).

The rapid onset of thrombocytopenia after injection of N'ase,[42, 43] the early development of reactive thrombocytosis,[43] the occurrence of ultrastructural abnormalities of platelets first in the circulation and later in the spleen,[43] and the damaging effect of N'ase on platelet survival[44] all support the conclusion that the major cause of thrombocytopenia is thrombocytolysis rather than damage to the bone marrow. However, any agent that reacts with circulating platelets might also react with mature megakaryocytes. Thus, modest damage to megakaryocytes by APS or N'ase, in addition to the thrombocytopenia itself, may have contributed to the apparent stimulation of early precursor cells that led to the delayed increase in production of platelets and red cells seen in these experiments. Other effects of N'ase were not apparent in the present studies. Hematocrits of irradiated mice treated with APS showed a sustained elevation over those of controls, whereas N'ase treatment resulted in only a transient rise in hematocrits on days 10 and 11 in spite of a more sustained reticulocytosis. This finding may have been related to the early senescence of red cells after N'ase treatment,[45] but delayed anemia did not occur in nonirradiated mice given N'ase. There was, likewise, no early reticulocytopenia which might have occurred in view of the known capability of N'ase to inactivate erythropoietin *in vivo*.[46] Therefore, N'ase may serve as a convenient alternative to APS to deplete experimental animals of circulating platelets.

In conclusion, a number of clinical and experimental situations suggest that severely disordered erythropoiesis may affect thrombocytopoiesis. The observations reported herein support the converse. These findings indicate that erythropoiesis may be stimulated by the thrombocytopenic state and that this stimulation will be manifested as increased red cell production under highly specific experimental conditions.

SUMMARY

Modifications of radiation-induced hemopoietic suppression by acute thrombocytopenia were evaluated. Immediately before or after exposure to sublethal irradiation, mice were given a single injection of anti-mouse platelet serum (APS), normal heterologous serum, neuraminidase (N'ase), or saline, or no further treatment was provided. Hemopoiesis was evaluated by blood cell counts, hematocrits, and incorporation of [75Se]selenomethionine into platelets. APS and N'ase induced an acute thrombocytopenia from which there was partial recovery before the platelet count started to fall from the radiation. During the second post-treatment week, both thrombocytopoiesis and erythropoiesis were greater in mice that received APS or N'ase in addition to radiation than in control irradiated mice. Differences in leukopoiesis were not apparent. Therefore, both thrombocytopoiesis and erythropoiesis appeared to be responsive to a stimulus generated by acute thrombocytopenia in sublethally irradiated mice.

REFERENCES

1. NAKAMURA, W., E. KOJIMA, H. MINAMISAWA, T. KANKURA, S. KOBAYASHI & H. ETO. 1968. Role of thrombocytopoietic system in radiation induced hematopoietic death. *In* Comparative Cellular and Species Radiosensitivity. V. P. Bond & T. Sugahara, Eds.: 202-210. Igaku Shoin Ltd. Tokyo, Japan.

2. EBBE, S. & F. STOHLMAN, JR. 1970. Stimulation of thrombocytopoiesis in irradiated mice. Blood **35**: 783-792.
3. BRECHER, G. & E. P. CRONKITE. 1950. Morphology and enumeration of human blood platelets. J. Appl. Physiol. **3**: 365-377.
4. BRECHER, G. & M. SCHNEIDERMAN. 1959. A time-saving device for the counting of reticulocytes. Am. J. Clin. Pathol. **20**: 1079-1083.
5. THREATTE, G. A., S. EBBE & E. PHALEN. 1981. Measurement of thrombocytopoiesis in W/W^v mice with evidence for an abnormality of sulfate metabolism. Proc. Soc. Exp. Biol. Med. **167**: 567-580.
6. BURSTEIN, S. A., J. W. ADAMSON, S. K. ERB & L. A. HARKER. 1981. Regulation of murine megakaryocytopoiesis. *In* Megakaryocyte Biology and Precursors: In Vitro Cloning and Cellular Properties. B. L. Evatt, R. F. Levine & N. T. Williams, Eds.: 127-138. Elsevier/North-Holland. New York, N.Y.
7. ISCOVE, N. N. 1977. The role of erythropoietin in regulation of population size and cell cycling of early and late erythroid precursors in mouse bone marrow. Cell Tissue Kinet. **10**: 323-334.
8. EBBE, S. & E. PHALEN. 1979. Does autoregulation of megakaryocytopoiesis occur? Blood Cells **5**: 123-138.
9. BAUM, S. J. & E. L. ALPEN. 1959. Residual injury induced in the erythropoietic system of the rat by periodic exposures to X-radiation. Radiat. Res. **11**: 844-860.
10. CHOI, S. I. & J. V. SIMONE. 1973. Platelet production in experimental iron deficiency anemia. Blood **42**: 219-228.
11. CHOI, S. I., J. V. SIMONE & C. W. JACKSON. 1974. Megakaryocytopoiesis in experimental iron deficiency anemia. Blood **43**: 111-120.
12. GROSS, S., V. KEEFER & A. J. NEWMAN. 1964. The platelets in iron-deficiency anemia. I. The response to oral and parenteral iron. Pediatrics **34**: 315-323.
13. SCHLOESSER, L. L., M. A. KIPP & F. J. WENZEL. 1965. Thrombocytosis in iron-deficiency anemia. J. Lab. Clin. Med. **66**: 107-114.
14. DIAMOND, L. K. 1978. Congenital hypoplastic anemia. Diamond-Blackfan syndrome. Historical and clinical aspects. Blood Cells **4**: 209-213.
15. ALTER, B. P. & D. G. NATHAN. 1979. Red cell aplasia in children. Arch. Dis. Child. **54**: 263-267.
16. HIRSH, J. & J. V. DACIE. 1966. Persistent post-splenectomy thrombocytosis and thromboembolism: a consequence of continuing anaemia. Br. J. Haematol. **12**: 44-53.
17. JACKSON, C. W., J. V. SIMONE & C. C. EDWARDS. 1974. The relationship of anemia and thrombocytosis. J. Lab. Clin. Med. **84**: 357-368.
18. GOODMAN, R., H. GRATE, E. HANNON & S. HELLMAN. 1977. Hematopoietic stem cells: effect of preirradiation, bleeding and erythropoietin on thrombopoietic differentiation. Blood **49**: 253-261.
19. BENTFELD-BARKER, M. E. & J. C. SCHOOLEY. 1981. Comparison of the effectiveness of bone marrow and spleen stem cells for platelet repopulation in lethally irradiated mice. Exp. Hematol. **9**: 379-390.
20. SMITH, P. J., C. W. JACKSON, M. A. WHIDDEN & C. C. EDWARDS. 1980. Effects of hypertransfusion on bone marrow regeneration in sublethally irradiated mice. II. Enhanced recovery of megakaryocytes and platelets. Blood **56**: 58-63.
21. MERINO, C. F. 1950. Studies on blood formation and destruction in the polycythemia of high altitude. Blood **5**: 1-30.
22. LAWRENCE, J. H., R. L. HUFF, W. SIRI, L. R. WASSERMAN & T. G. HENNESSY. 1952. A physiological study in the Peruvian Andes. Acta Med. Scand. **142**: 117-131.
23. SIRI, W. E., D. C. VAN DYKE, H. S. WINCHELL, M. POLLYCOVE, H. G. PARKER & A. S. CLEVELAND. 1966. Early erythropoietin, blood, and physiological responses to severe hypoxia in man. J. Appl. Physiol. **21**: 73-80.
24. BIRK, J. W., L. W. KLASSEN & C. W. GURNEY. 1975. Hypoxia-induced thrombocytopenia in mice. J. Lab. Clin. Med. **86**: 230-238.
25. SHREINER, D. P. & J. LEVIN. 1976. The effects of hemorrhage, hypoxia, and a preparation of erythropoietin on thrombopoiesis. J. Lab. Clin. Med. **88**: 930-940.
26. JACKSON, C. W. & C. C. EDWARDS. 1977. Biphasic thrombopoietic response to severe hypobaric hypoxia. Br. J. Haematol. **35**: 233-244.

27. LANGDON, J. R. & T. P. McDONALD. 1977. Effects of chronic hypoxia on platelet production in mice. Exp. Hematol. **5:** 191-198.
28. COOPER, G. W. & B. COOPER. 1977. Relationship between blood platelet and erythrocyte formation. Life Sci. **20:** 1571-1580.
29. McDONALD, T. P. 1978. Platelet production in hypoxic and rbc-transfused mice. Scand. J. Haematol. **20:** 213-220.
30. McDONALD, T. P. 1978. A comparison of platelet production in mice made thrombocytopenic by hypoxia and by platelet specific antisera. Br. J. Haematol. **40:** 299-309.
31. McDONALD, T. P., M. COTTRELL & R. CLIFT. 1978. Effects of short-term hypoxia on platelet counts of mice. Blood **51:** 165-175.
32. DEGABRIELE, G. & D. G. PENINGTON. 1967. Physiology of the regulation of platelet production. Br. J. Haematol. **13:** 202-209.
33. EVATT, B. L., J. L. SPIVAK & J. LEVIN. 1976. Relationships between thrombopoiesis and erythropoiesis: with studies of the effects of preparations of thrombopoietin and erythropoietin. Blood **48:** 547-558.
34. McLEOD, D. L., M. M. SHREEVE & A. A. AXELRAD. 1976. Induction of megakaryocyte colonies with platelet formation *in vitro.* Nature **261:** 492-494.
35. VAINCHENKER, W., J. BOUGUET, J. GUICHARD & J. BRETON-GORIUS. 1979. Megakaryocyte colony formation from human bone marrow precursors. Blood **54:** 940-945.
36. HUMPHRIES, R. K., A. C. EAVES & C. J. EAVES. 1979. Characterization of a primitive erythropoietic progenitor found in mouse marrow before and after several weeks in culture. Blood **53:** 746-763.
37. PAULUS, J. M., M. PRENANT, J. MAIGNE, M. HENRY-AMAR & J. F. DESCHAMPS. 1981. Ploidization of megakaryocyte progenitors *in vitro. In* Megakaryocyte Biology and Precursors: In Vitro Cloning and Cellular Properties. B. L. Evatt, R. F. Levine & N. T. Williams, Eds.: 171-177. Elsevier/North-Holland. New York, N.Y.
38. McLEOD, D. L., M. SHREEVE & A. A. AXELRAD. 1980. Chromosome marker evidence for the biopotentiality of BFU-E. Blood **56:** 318-322.
39. PAULUS, J., M. PRENANT, J. DESCHAMPS & M. HENRY-AMAR. 1982. Polyploid megakaryocytes develop randomly from a multicompartmental system of committed progenitors. Proc. Natl. Acad. Sci. USA **79:** 4410-4414.
40. LEVIN, J., F. C. LEVIN & D. METCALF. 1980. The effects of acute thrombocytopenia on megakaryocyte-CFC and granulocyte-macrophage-CFC in mice: studies of bone marrow and spleen. Blood **56:** 274-283.
41. BURSTEIN, S. A., S. K. ERB, J. W. ADAMSON & L. A. HARKER. 1982. Immunologic stimulation of early murine hematopoiesis and its abrogation by cyclosporin A. Blood **59:** 851-856.
42. GASIC, G. J., T. B. GASIC & C. C. STEWART. 1968. Antimetastatic effects associated with platelet reduction. Proc. Natl. Acad. Sci. USA **61:** 46-52.
43. CHOI, S., J. V. SIMONE & L. J. JOURNEY. 1972. Neuraminidase-induced thrombocytopenia in rats. Br. J. Haematol. **22:** 93-101.
44. GREENBERG, J. P., M. A. PACKHAM, M. A. GUCCIONE, M. L. RAND, H.-J. REIMERS & J. F. MUSTARD. 1979. Survival of rabbit platelets treated in vitro with chymotrypsin, plasmin, trypsin, or neuraminidase. Blood **53:** 916-927.
45. LANDAW, S. A., T. TENFORDE & J. C. SCHOOLEY. 1977. Decreased surface charge and accelerated senescence of red blood cells following neuraminidase treatment. J. Lab. Clin. Med. **89:** 581-591.
46. SCHOOLEY, J. C. & L. J. MAHLMANN. 1971. Inhibition of the biological activity of erythropoietin by neuraminidase in vivo. J. Lab. Clin. Med. **78:** 765-770.

The Question of Bone Marrow Stromal Fibroblast Traffic[a]

MARY A. MALONEY, ROSITO A. LAMELA, AND
HARVEY M. PATT[b]

Laboratory of Radiobiology and Environmental Health
University of California
San Francisco, California 94143

It is generally accepted that a radiation-induced deficiency of hemic cells in an irradiated site can be corrected by blood-borne stem cells from a shielded site.[1,2] It has been assumed that there is little, if any, similar migration of bone marrow stromal cell components. This assumption is based on the sequence of histologic events in the repopulation of a locally ablated marrow.[3] In general, the events leading to repopulation of a depleted marrow cavity in an unirradiated animal are the following: filling of the cavity with a blood coagulum, capillary invasion, appearance of primitive mesenchymal elements, osteoblastic proliferation, formation of trabecular bone, appearance of sinusoids, and hemic repopulation with the beginning of bone resorption. Disruption of the marrow without removal of the marrow leads to the same sequence of events. Recovery after ablation of a shielded depopulated femur in an otherwise whole-body-irradiated animal is similar to that in an unirradiated animal. Thus, restitution of the marrow stroma is thought to develop locally, preceding hematopoietic repopulation by migration of the blood-borne pluripotential stem cells.

Recently, however, Werts *et al.*[4] reported a study in which bone marrow stromal fibroblasts (CFU-F), components of bone marrow stroma known to transfer the microenvironment in heterotopic transplants,[5-7] migrated from unirradiated sites to irradiated sites via the blood after local X irradiation of a leg. This migration preceded hematopoietic repopulation, and it was concluded that migration of stromal cells facilitates this process.

The question of stromal fibroblast traffic is pertinent to interpretation of the secondary marrow aplasia that sometimes follows local irradiation. Therefore, we undertook a study to define stromal fibroblast traffic in male/female CBA/CaJ littermates in parabiotic equilibrium followed by X irradiation of one partner and separation of the partners 30 days later. Chromosome analysis by C-banding of the bone marrow fibroblasts in the parabiont pairs indicated that (1) bone marrow fibroblasts do not normally exchange sites, and (2) after X-ray damage to the bone marrow, repopulation of the CFU-F compartments of the bone marrow results primarily from recovery of the local CFU-F.

[a] This work was supported by the U.S. Department of Energy under Contract DE-AC03-76-SF01012.
[b] Deceased.

MATERIALS AND METHODS

Mice

CBA/CaJ mice (5 to 6 weeks old) were obtained from Jackson Laboratories, Bar Harbor, Maine.

Parabiosis

Male/female littermates were placed in parabiosis and maintained in parabiotic union for 3 weeks before irradiation, according to the method of Dorie *et al.*[8] Hematocrits of the parabiont partners at 3 weeks were 49.0 ± 0.4% in each partner, with a male:female ratio of 1.00 ± 0.01. This indicated that there was no parabiotic rejection, which would have caused extreme anemia in one animal and polycythemia in the other.[9]

X Irradiation

The radiation factors were 300 kVp, 20 mA, half-value layer (HVL) 1.65 mm Cu, target surface distance (TSD) 70 cm, and the dose rate was 0.59 Gy/min; the total dose of 10 Gy was determined by lithium fluoride dosimetry. In 15 parabiont pairs, one partner was X-irradiated with 10 Gy and the other was shielded with 2 mm lead. The remaining 7 pairs were not irradiated so that we could determine if normally there is an exchange of bone marrow fibroblasts from one site to another.

Spleen Colony Assay (CFU-S)

The spleens of the irradiated partners of the parabiont pairs were surgically excised at 7 days and fixed. The surface colonies were then counted.

Bone Marrow Transplantation

Seven CBA/CaJ male mice were whole-body-irradiated with 10 Gy and received 1×10^7 female CBA/CaJ bone marrow cells by intravenous injection 2 hr later.

Chromosome Analysis of Stromal Fibroblasts

The parabiont partners were separated at 30 days after irradiation, and bone marrow from both femurs of each parabiont was collected 24 hr later. The plug of bone marrow was flushed with 0.2 ml Hanks' balanced salt solution (Grand Island Biological Co., Grand Island, N.Y.) into a 50-ml centrifuge tube. The marrow was cut into four or five segments, incubated in 20 ml of 0.25% trypsin solution containing 0.02% EDTA for 20 min, and the samples were stirred every 5 min.[6] The trypsin-EDTA solution was decanted and replaced with Dulbecco's modified Eagle's medium containing 20% fetal calf serum (Grand Island Biological Co.). The suspension was centrifuged at 1000 rpm for 10 min, the medium was decanted, and the cells were resuspended in Hanks' balanced salt solution. A total nucleated-cell count was carried out on a hemocytometer. Cells were returned to the medium, and cultures containing 5×10^6 bone marrow cells per milliliter from the unirradiated parabionts or the shielded partner and 1×10^7 bone marrow cells per milliliter from the irradiated partner were incubated in a 60-mm cell culture dish at 37°C in an atmosphere of 90-100% relative humidity and 10% CO_2. At 4 hr, the unattached cells were removed and fresh medium was added to the culture. At 7 days, the medium was changed. At 10 days, the cultures were trypsinized and replated 1:3 for the shielded marrow and 1:1 for the irradiated marrow. At 12 days, 10^{-5} M Colcemid was added to the cultures. After 2 hr, the cells were harvested by trypsinization, resuspended in Dulbecco's medium containing 20% fetal calf serum, and centrifuged at 800 rpm for 4 min. The medium was decanted and 0.075 M KCl was added for 7 min. The KCl was decanted and the cells were fixed with 2:1 methanol:glacial acetic acid. The cells were dispersed on a warm slide held at a 30° angle. Slide preparations were aged for 3 days at room temperature and stained according to the modification by Dorie et al.[8] of an earlier protocol demonstrating centromeric heterochromatin.[10] The male or female origin of each metaphase figure in a 40-chromosome spread was identified by the absence or presence of the male Y chromosome. C-banding readily distinguishes the Y chromosome because it stains uniformly, whereas in the other chromosomes the centromere is more deeply stained.

Bone Marrow Stromal Fibroblast Colony Assay (CFU-F)

Bone marrow for total nucleated-cell counts and the clonogenic fibroblast colony assay was flushed from the femur with 1.0 ml Hanks' balanced salt solution. A single-cell suspension was made by passage through a 25-gauge needle; cells were counted on a hemocytometer. Cultures containing 2×10^6 bone marrow cells per milliliter of medium were grown as described for chromosome analysis. The medium was changed at 7 days, and at 14 days the medium was removed and the cells were fixed with methanol and stained with 1% crystal violet. Colonies containing 50 or more cells were scored for CFU-F.

RESULTS

At 7 days after X irradiation, the spleen colony count (CFU-S) in the surgically excised spleen of the irradiated partner was 39.4 ± 5.5. This demonstrates that there was good blood exchange between the partners.

At 30 days after irradiation, the number of bone marrow fibroblasts in the irradiated parabiont partner was only 8% of that in the unirradiated controls (TABLE 1). Chromosome analysis by C-banding revealed that 94% of these fibroblasts were of host origin, which amounts to only about one clonogenic fibroblast of donor origin per femur. In the unirradiated parabiont partner all of the fibroblasts were of host origin (TABLE 1). In parabiont pairs in which neither partner was irradiated all the fibroblasts were of host origin. Therefore, there is no indication that bone marrow fibroblasts normally exchange sites.

The recovery of the CFU-F population in X-irradiated mice that were injected with bone marrow cells was also studied. At 30 days, chromosome analysis revealed that 44% of the CFU-F were derived from the injected bone marrow (TABLE 1). However, the CFU-F assay revealed that the bone marrow contained only about 1% of the CFU-F observed in unirradiated mice. As in the irradiated parabiont mice, this represents only about one fibroblast of donor origin per femur.

Since recovery of the bone marrow fibroblasts was so low and did not seem to

TABLE 1. Number of Donor and Host CFU-F in Parabiont or Bone Marrow-Injected Mice at 30 Days after X Irradiation

Treatment	CFU-F per Femur[a] (% of Control)	Chromosome Analysis		CFU-F per Femur	
		Number Scored	% Host	Donor	Host
Parabiont partner irradiated (10 Gy)	7.98 ± 1.5 (6)[b]	182	94	0.7	10.3
Parabiont partner shielded	30.6 ± 7.2 (6)	1385	100	0	42
Whole-body irradiated (10 Gy) plus 1 × 10^7 bone marrow cells injected	0.76 ± 0.24(7)	69	56	0.5	0.5

[a] CFU-F per femur in unirradiated mice = 138 ± 26 (n = 24).
[b] Mean ± standard error; number of experiments in parentheses.

result from migration, we evaluated the time course for the recovery of total nucleated cells and bone marrow fibroblasts to determine if there was a correlation between marrow cellularity and CFU-F content. The recovery patterns were assayed in parabionts with one partner X irradiated, individual mice with one leg irradiated, and individual mice that were whole-body irradiated. The X-radiation dose in all instances was 10 Gy. In all irradiated sites there was a precipitous drop in the total nucleated-cell count (FIGURE 1). With whole-body irradiation there was no recovery and the mice died at about 10 days. In the shielded sites of the irradiated parabiont mice and the leg-irradiated mice there was a lesser decrease in cellularity. By 30 days, a normal value for bone marrow cellularity in both the irradiated and shielded sites in these mice was attained.

The whole-body-irradiated mice had no demonstrable CFU-F at 7 days (FIGURE 2). At 30 days, complete recovery had not occurred in the shielded or irradiated sites of the irradiated parabiont mice or the leg-irradiated mice.

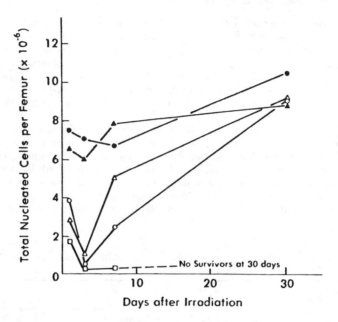

FIGURE 1. Recovery of bone marrow cellularity in the femurs of mice receiving 10 Gy X radiation. ○, Parabiont partner irradiated; ●, parabiont partner shielded; △, leg irradiated; ▲, leg shielded; □, whole-body irradiated. The control value is 8.5 ($\pm$ 0.4) $\times$ 10^6 (n = 24). Data are from six replicate experiments.

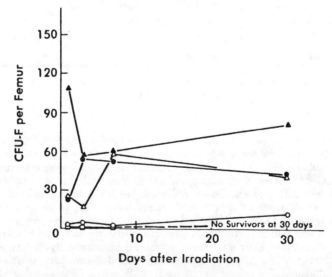

FIGURE 2. Recovery of bone marrow CFU-F in the femurs of mice receiving 10 Gy X radiation. ○, Parabiont partner irradiated; ●, parabiont partner shielded; △, leg irradiated; ▲, leg shielded; □, whole-body irradiated. The control value is 138 $\pm$ 26 (n = 24). Data are from six replicate experiments.

DISCUSSION

Bone marrow fibroblasts have been shown to transfer the hematopoietic microenvironment in heterotopic implants.[5-7] Therefore, it is important to determine if marrow stromal fibroblasts, either by migration from a shielded site or by transplantation, can colonize X-irradiated marrow and whether or not these fibroblasts enhance hematopoietic repopulation. Normally, bone marrow fibroblasts are considered to be in a quiescent state *in vivo*; there is little or no turnover of these cells in the adult.[11]

The assay for determining the number of bone marrow fibroblasts requires plating of bone marrow cells in single-cell suspension in medium that promotes their growth *in vitro*. The CFU-F assay tests the ability of the bone marrow fibroblasts to form colonies rather than directly enumerating the number of fibroblasts in the marrow or assaying the ability of fibroblasts to provide the proper microenvironment for hematopoiesis. In essence, the CFU-F assay measures the residual damage to the proliferative capacity of the stromal fibroblasts. We propose that the recovery of bone marrow CFU-F (FIGURE 2) reflects recovery from potentially lethal damage, which is a phenomenon extensively studied in plateau-phase cultures. When plateau-phase cells are X-irradiated and kept in a plateau phase before subculturing, there is repair of radiation damage that usually would be lethal in proliferating cells.[12] The bone marrow fibroblast population is akin to plateau-phase cultures. Since cell death is usually considered to be due to reproductive failure, and recovery from potentially lethal damage occurs primarily in quiescent cells, it appears that the recovery of the bone marrow fibroblasts after X irradiation is a reflection of repair of the potentially lethal damage.

In assaying the residual damage to this population, the total number of CFU-F is a more important criterion than the relative distribution of donor and host cells. Recently, Piersma *et al.*[13] reported an experiment in which they injected 2.5×10^7 bone marrow cells into mice that had received 9 Gy whole-body radiation. At 4 weeks, the CFU-F content was about 10% of control values and no further recovery was demonstrated up to 8 weeks. In chromosome analysis of the CFU-F, about one half of the metaphase figures scored were derived from donor cells. Thus, it appears that the injected bone marrow replaced only 5% of the CFU-F population. These results are similar to those we obtained after bone marrow transplantation. Therefore, assaying the relative distribution of donor and host cells among stromal cells of the *in vivo* population by chromosome analysis in bone marrow transplants is valid only if both the donor and host populations have the same potential to form colonies. If the bone marrow stromal fibroblasts have residual damage that is expressed only when they are forced into a cell cycle, relative distribution of the two populations probably does not reflect the stromal distribution *in vivo*.

This could explain the diverse results reported in bone marrow transplants in patients. Wilson *et al.*[14] and Golde *et al.*[15] reported that stroma in transplant patients was of host origin, whereas Keating *et al.*[16] reported that the stroma was primarily from the donor. In humans it is not possible to establish whether the number of CFU-F is normal. From our data, it would appear that if a large percentage of the stromal fibroblasts are of donor origin, it is probably a reflection of the residual damage to bone marrow stroma from treatment before implantation rather than repopulation of the CFU-F from the bone marrow transplant.

Our data demonstrate that it is not essential for bone marrow fibroblasts (assayed as CFU-F) to return to normal numbers for hematopoietic recovery to take place, as judged by total nucleated-cell counts of the bone marrow. In the X-irradiated parabiont partner, the CFU-F recovery was only about 8% of the control value but the total nucleated-cell count was normal. It is possible that bone marrow fibroblasts with residual damage that cannot be expressed in the CFU-F assay can support *in vivo* hematopoiesis. It has recently been demonstrated that bone marrow fibroblasts *in vitro* produce a large amount of procollagen III (R. Stern, D. F. Bainton, M. A. Maloney, and H. M. Patt, unpublished data), which is presumed to be the precursor of bone marrow reticulum. Since normal cellularity is obtained in marrow with a few CFU-F, the reticulum, which is the matrix for hemic cell repopulation, must still be intact. Collagens are known to have a relatively long biologic life.[17] It is not possible to assess from our data whether the bone marrow fibroblasts with residual X-radiation damage continue to produce the reticulum, but this could be tested *in vitro*.

The final consideration is whether bone marrow stromal fibroblasts can migrate. It is apparent from our work, the work of Piersma *et al.,*[13] and experience with bone marrow transplant patients[16] that bone marrow stromal fibroblasts can be demonstrated to have the karyotype of the injected bone marrow. Thus, it appears that if bone marrow fibroblasts are introduced into the circulating blood, a few of these cells may lodge in the marrow. However, there is limited restitution of this population *in vivo*. Bone marrow fibroblasts with residual X-ray damage probably are present in the marrow and are lost only in reproductive death.

Whether or not bone marrow fibroblasts can migrate from a shielded site to an irradiated site is an open question. Certainly, migration can at most play a minor role. Our data show that on the average less than one migratory fibroblast was found in the marrow of the X-irradiated parabionts.

SUMMARY

Bone marrow stromal fibroblasts (CFU-F) normally do not exchange bone marrow sites *in vivo*. Restitution of the CFU-F after radiation damage is primarily recovery by the local fibroblasts from potentially lethal damage. Migration of stromal fibroblasts from shielded sites to an irradiated site makes a minimal contribution, if any, to CFU-F recovery.

Determination of the relative contribution of donor stromal cells in bone marrow transplants by karyotyping the proliferating bone marrow stromal cells *in vitro* may not reflect the relative distribution of fibroblasts in the marrow. If there is residual damage to the host stromal fibroblasts from treatment before transplantation, these cells may not be able to proliferate *in vitro*. Therefore, an occasional transplanted fibroblast may contribute most of the metaphase figures scored for karyotype.

ACKNOWLEDGMENTS

We thank Dorothy F. Bainton and James E. Cleaver for valuable discussion, Mary McKenney for editorial assistance, and Susan Brekhus for secretarial assistance.

REFERENCES

1. DE VRIES, F. A. J. & O. VOS. 1966. Prevention of the bone-marrow syndrome in irradiated mice. A comparison of the results after bone-marrow shielding and bone-marrow inoculation. Int. J. Radiat. Biol. **11:** 235-243.
2. MALONEY, M. A. & H. M. PATT. 1972. Migration of cells from shielded to irradiated marrow. Blood **39:** 804-808.
3. PATT, H. M. & M. A. MALONEY. 1975. Bone marrow regeneration after local injury: a review. Exp. Hematol. **3:** 135-148.
4. WERTS, E. D., D. P. GIBSON, S. A. KNAPP & R. L. DEGOWIN. 1980. Stromal cell migration precedes hemopoietic repopulation of the bone marrow after irradiation. Radiat. Res. **81:** 20-30.
5. FRIEDENSTEIN, A. J., R. K. CHAILAKHYAN, N. V. LATSINIK, A. F. PANASYUK & I. V. KEILISS-BOROK. 1974. Stromal cells responsible for transferring the microenvironment of the hemopoietic tissues. Transplantation **17:** 331-340.
6. FRIEDENSTEIN, A. J., N. W. LATZINIK, A. G. GROSHEVA & U. F. GORSKAYA. 1982. Marrow microenvironment transfer by heterotopic transplantation of freshly isolated and cultured cells in porous sponges. Exp. Hematol. **10:** 217-227.
7. PATT, H. M., M. A. MALONEY & M. L. FLANNERY. 1982. Hematopoietic microenvironment transfer by stromal fibroblasts derived from bone marrow varying in cellularity. Exp. Hematol. **10:** 738-742.
8. DORIE, M. J., M. A. MALONEY & H. M. PATT. 1979. Turnover of circulating hematopoietic stem cells. Exp. Hematol. **7:** 483-489.
9. NISBET, N. W. 1973. Parabiosis in immunobiology. Transplant. Rev. **15:** 123-161.
10. SUMNER, A. T. 1972. A simple technique for demonstrating centromeric heterochromatin. Exp. Cell Res. **75:** 304-306.
11. HAAS, R. J., F. BOHNE & T. M. FLIEDNER. 1969. On the development of slowly-turning-over cell types in neonatal rat bone marrow (studies utilizing the complete tritiated thymidine labeling method complemented by C-14 thymidine administration). Blood **34:** 791-805.
12. LITTLE, J. B. 1969. Repair of sub-lethal and potential lethal radiation damage in plateau phase cultures of human cells. Nature **224:** 804-806.
13. PIERSMA, A. H., R. E. PLOEMACHER & K. G. M. BROCKBANK. 1983. Transplantation of bone marrow fibroblastoid stromal cells in mice via the intravenous route. Br. J. Haematol. **54:** 285-290.
14. WILSON, F. D., B. R. GREENBERG, P. N. KONRAD, A. K. KLEIN & P. A. WALLING. 1978. Cytogenetic studies on bone marrow fibroblasts from a male-female hematopoietic chimera. Evidence that stromal elements in human transplantation recipients are of host type. Transplantation **25:** 87-88.
15. GOLDE, D. W., W. G. HOCKING, S. G. QUAN, R. S. SPARKES & R. P. GALE. 1980. Origin of human bone marrow fibroblasts. Br. J. Haematol. **44:** 183-187.
16. KEATING, A., J. W. SINGER, P. D. KILLEN, G. E. STRIKER, A. C. SALO, J. SANDERS, E. D. THOMAS, D. THORNING & P. J. FIALKOW. 1982. Donor origin of the *in vitro* haematopoietic microenvironment after marrow transplantation in man. Nature **298:** 280-283.
17. NISSEN, R., G. J. CARDINALE & S. UDENFRIEND. 1978. Increased turnover of arterial collagen in hypertensive rats. Proc. Natl. Acad. Sci. USA **75:** 451-453.

Inhibition of Fibroblast Proliferation by Myelotoxic Drugs

ANTHONY V. PISCIOTTA,[a,b,c] RICHARD C. MILLER,[a]
SADAYUKI BAN,[a] AND CHRISTINA CRONKITE[b]

[a]Department of Experimental Pathology
Radiation Effects Research Foundation
Hiroshima 730, Japan

[b]Blood Research Laboratory
Medical College of Wisconsin
Milwaukee, Wisconsin 53226

Clinical treatment with certain drugs in dosages not harmful to the general population may result in an unexpected sudden loss of circulating leukocytes in highly sensitive individuals.[1] With most drugs, this reaction is mediated by immune destruction of circulating leukocytes. However, a class of drugs exists that exerts its effect by suppressing hematopoietic committed stem cells in the bone marrow. Such drugs kill living cells in higher concentrations and thereby prevent cellular proliferation. Individuals sensitive to these drugs are believed to have a cellular proliferative defect that prevents adequate compensatory response to drug-induced myelotoxicity.

Drugs known to affect marrow cells in this way are the phenothiazine derivatives of which chlorpromazine (CPZ) is a prototype.[2] A cluster of agranulocytosis was observed by Idänpään-Heikkilä et al.[3] in Finland in 1976 during treatment with clozapine (CZP) for mental illness. The mechanism of this type of agranulocytosis has not been established to date, but a number of features in common with CPZ have been suggested.

The mechanisms and predictability of agranulocytosis attributed to CPZ have been extensively studied. When randomly selected normal marrow cells were incubated with tritiated thymidine ([³H]TdR), for 5 hr, the labeling index more than doubled. When CPZ (8×10^{-5} M) was included the labeling index kept pace with, but lagged behind that of the preparation in which the drug was omitted. Similar observations on individuals who had had agranulocytosis induced by CPZ showed that the labeling index at each point over a 5-hr period was less than that of a normal subject; when CPZ is included in the same concentration as that used in normal subjects (8×10^{-5} M) any increment in labeling index is prevented. These data suggest that CPZ exerts its primary effect by suppressing cell division in an individual with limited proliferative potential.[4]

Similar results have been found using a 14-day culture of human marrow cells cultured over a feeder layer system as recommended by Robinson and Pike.[5] In randomly selected humans, CPZ suppressed accumulation of colony forming units

[c]Author to whom correspondence should be addressed: Anthony V. Pisciotta, Blood Research Laboratory, Medical College of Wisconsin, 8700 W. Wisconsin Ave., Milwaukee, Wis. 53226.

(CFU-GM) in direct relation to its concentration.[1] At 5×10^{-5} M, a few such colonies survived. Those who had had agranulocytosis had fewer colonies to begin with, in preparations that contained no drug. In all of these the number of colonies decreased in proportion to normals as the concentration of CPZ was increased. At 5×10^{-5} M, all colonies disappeared. Patients who developed benign leukopenia during the course of treatment with CPZ developed an intermediate number of CFU-GM. These were also diminished in number proportionate to normals as the concentration of CPZ was increased and disappeared entirely at 5×10^{-5} M. Similar suppression was observed

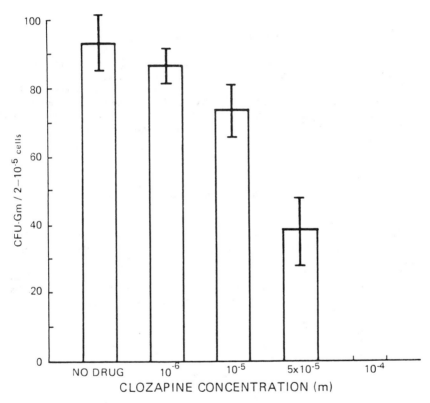

FIGURE 1. Effect of clozapine on accumulation of bone marrow colony forming units in a human culture system.

using clozapine (FIGURE 1), though a higher concentration (10^{-4} M) was required for complete suppression of CFU-GM in randomly selected young individuals.

Procedures to determine the effect of drugs on hematopoiesis, while direct in their approach, nevertheless require bone marrow samples which are often difficult to obtain. For this reason, alternate methodology was developed using more readily available cell lines. These studies were conducted not to predict individual susceptibility to toxic drugs, but to identify the suppressive potential of drugs such as CPZ and CZP.

Thus at a concentration of 10^{-4} M, CPZ suppressed proliferation of *Escherichia coli* and its DNA polymerase-deficient mutant P3478[6] and furthermore completely prevented repair in the ultraviolet-treated mutant strain. Similar concentrations inhibited the growth in a cell line of trophoblastic cells as well as phytohemagglutinin (PHA)-treated lymphocytes.

MATERIALS AND METHODS

The present studies were conducted on test cells such as human diploid fibroblasts (LU-235), hamster lung fibroblasts (V-79), and HeLa S$_3$ cells. They were grown suspended in Eagle's minimum essential medium (Eagle's MEM) supplemented by a batch of 10% fetal calf serum, previously found to support optimal growth by pretesting 50 μg/ml penicillin and 50 μg streptomycin. Confluent cells were subcultured into fresh medium and harvested with 0.125% trypsin. For estimation of colony growth, 6-cm plastic petri dishes were seeded with cells and were provided with fresh medium every 3 or 4 days. After 2 weeks the plates were stained with crystal violet and colonies were counted by macroscopic observation.

Treatment with Test Drug and X Irradiation

The cells in suspension were exposed to CPZ or CZP in concentrations of 10^{-3} to 10^{-7} M, for 2, 4, or 6 hr. Following this, the cells were washed and plated in the petri dishes.

In some experiments cells were treated with various doses of X rays in suspensions which consisted of 5×10^{-5} cells/ml. Some of these cells were treated with CZP at concentrations of 2 and 1×10^{-4} M in order to determine the effect of this drug on recovery from radiation injury.

RESULTS

Similar results were observed with each cell line for the two drugs and were reproducible with repeated experiments. FIGURE 2 illustrates cell survival following *in vitro* exposure to CPZ. With increasing drug concentration, the number of colonies decreased rapidly.

As shown in FIGURES 2 and 3, incubation for 4 hr with a CPZ concentration greater than 10^{-6} M resulted in increased killing of V-79 cells. Complete cell killing of V-79 was evident at 24 hr of incubation with a CPZ concentration of 10^{-4} M and was irreversible. Suppression was dissipated between 10^{-5} and 10^{-6} M, and at lower concentrations no further evidence of cell killing was observed. FIGURE 4 shows a similar relationship using human fibroblasts which failed to survive concentrations of CPZ greater than 10^{-5} M.

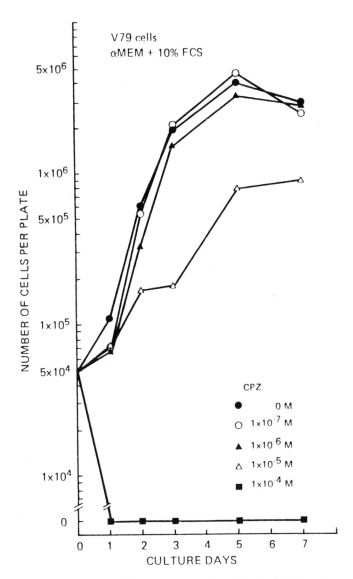

FIGURE 2. Effect of CPZ on accumulation of fibroblast V-79 units.

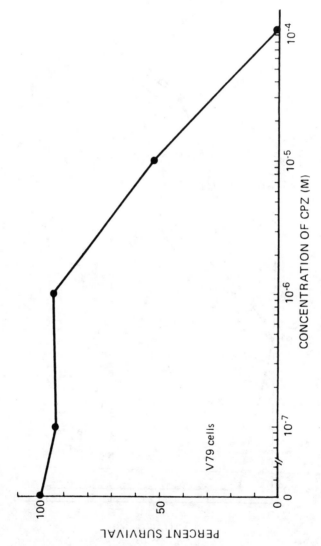

FIGURE 3. Suppression of V-79 colony forming units by CPZ in concentrations exceeding 10^{-6} M.

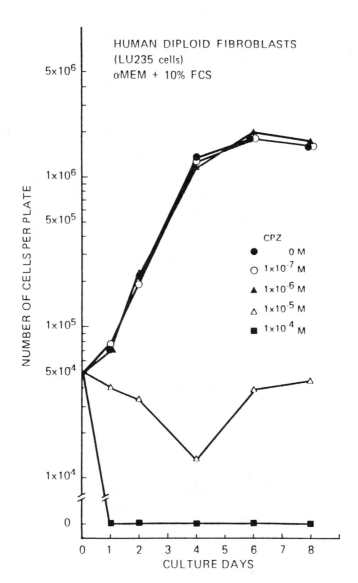

FIGURE 4. Effect of CPZ on accumulation of human diploid fibroblasts (LU-235 cells).

The effects of incubating fibroblasts in CPZ for various time periods are illustrated in FIGURE 5. The cells were exposed to CPZ for 2, 4, or 6 hr. Those preincubated with the drug for 6 hr were far more sensitive to lesser concentrations of the drug than those preincubated for 2 hr. Thus, length of time exposed, as well as concentration, played a role in suppressing cell growth.

When HeLa cells were incubated with CPZ (FIGURE 6), complete cell killing was observed at 10^{-4} M and partial killing at 10^{-5} M. In this system, cell killing was similarly completely dissipated at 10^{-6} M. Treating HeLa cells in continuous culture for an entire week with CPZ concentrations between 10^{-6} and 10^{-5} M resulted in cell death (FIGURE 7). On the other hand, incubation for 2 hr before plating killed HeLa cells only at 10^{-4} M.

CZP also killed human fibroblasts but at concentrations that exceeded 1.2×10^{-4} M. FIGURE 8 shows that CPZ was 10 times more toxic to cell survival than CZP during a 4-hr exposure period.

FIGURE 9 shows that V-79 cells were not exposure time dependent to CZP. Incubation for 2, 4, or 6 hr did not alter cell killing which remained constant at concentrations of 2×10^{-5} M. The simultaneous incubation of cells with both CPZ and CZP in nontoxic concentrations failed to show simple additivity of toxicity (FIGURE 9). In fact, the resulting cell killing was no greater than that when both drugs were used separately. The failure to demonstrate synergistic effects with drug combinations in tissue culture suggests that both drugs used together do not potentiate each other's toxicity.

The potentiating effect of CZP (2×10^{-4} M for 4 hr) on recovery of surviving cells from X irradiation was investigated (FIGURE 10). When V-79 cells were exposed to concentrations of 2×10^{-4} M and irradiated, the initial plateau in the curve depicting attempts at recovery was removed. Furthermore, at the highest concentration the slope of the curve depicting cell killing was steeper than that at a lesser concentration or no drug at all.

DISCUSSION

The aim of the present studies was to test the potential use of several tissue culture models as a means of testing drug toxicity. They confirm that CPZ is toxic to living cells in concentrations that exceed 10^{-5} M and CZP is toxic in concentrations greater than 10^{-4} M. The mechanisms whereby drug-induced cell killing is induced are better known for CPZ than for CZP.

CPZ potentiates membrane permeability and thereby results in a loss of macromolecules by passive diffusion to the outside of the cell. A similar effect on mitochondrial membranes is associated with the uncoupling of oxidative phosphorylation. Furthermore, CPZ combines with complex macromolecules leading to coprecipitation and denaturation. Such properties remove substances of biochemical importance from participation in intracellular biochemical reactions. Thus, the precipitation of soluble protein complexes which constitute intracellular enzymes would deprive the cell of its enzymatic machinery. Furthermore, coprecipitation with complex polynucleotides would deprive cells of compounds required for nucleic acid synthesis.

The concentrations of drugs used in these experiments far exceed those employed therapeutically. However, CPZ is rapidly cleared from the circulation and accumulates by attaching to tissue cellular proteins. In this way, a toxic blood level is never built up and an accurate definition of tissue cellular concentration is not yet available.

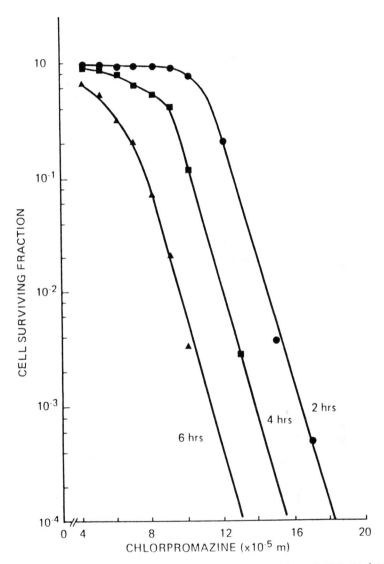

FIGURE 5. Effect of length of time exposed to toxic concentrations of CPZ (10^{-5} M) on accumulation of fibroblast colony forming units.

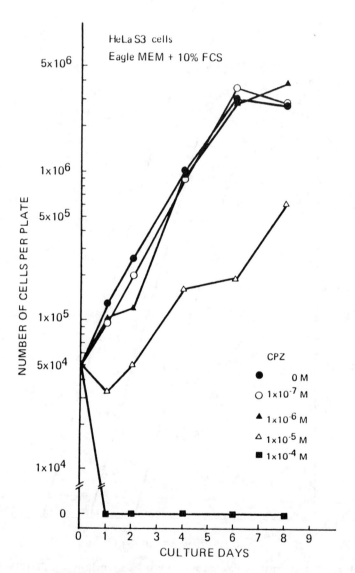

FIGURE 6. Effect of CPZ on proliferation of HeLa cells.

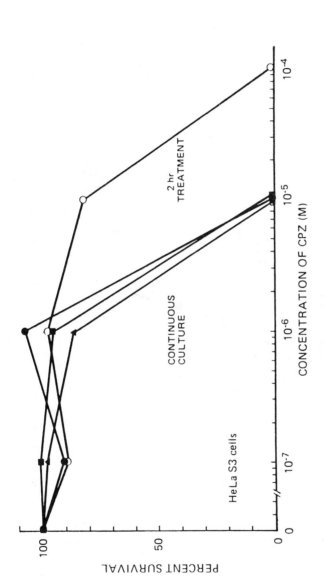

FIGURE 7. Effect of CPZ on proliferation of HeLa cells. Comparison between 2 hr exposure and continuous treatment for entire culture period.

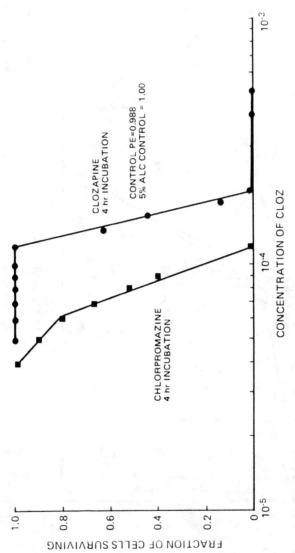

FIGURE 8. Comparison of the effects of toxic concentrations of chlorpromazine and clozapine in fibroblast cultures.

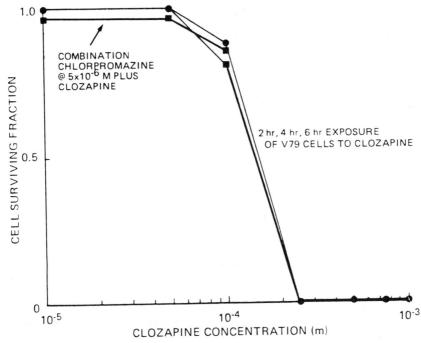

FIGURE 9. The lack of cumulative toxicity when nontoxic concentrations of chlorpromazine and clozapine are combined is shown.

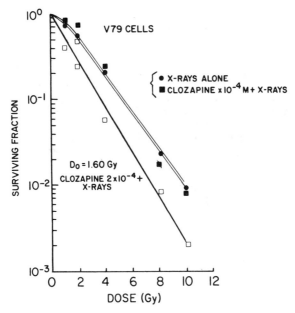

FIGURE 10. Suppression of recovery from irradiation by clozapine (2×10^{-4} M).

CONCLUSIONS

Enumeration of fibroblast colony forming units is affected by substances usually used therapeutically. Both chlorpromazine and clozapine are capable of suppressing colony formation, but at differing concentrations, and clozapine has a demonstrable effect on repair of X-ray-induced cellular damage. Such procedures may be useful in identifying potential drug toxicity.

REFERENCES

1. PISCIOTTA, A. V. 1973. Immune and toxic mechanisms in drug-induced agranulocytosis. Semin. Hematol. **10:** 279.
2. PISCIOTTA, A. V. 1962. Agranulocytosis induced by certain phenothiazine derivatives. J. Am. Med. Assoc. **208:** 1862.
3. IDÄNPÄÄN-HEIKKILÄ, J., A. ALAAVA, M. OLKINUORA & I. P. PALVA. 1977. Agranulocytosis during treatment with clozapine. Eur. J. Clin. Pharmacol. **11:** 193.
4. PISCIOTTA, A. V. 1971. Studies on agranulocytosis. IX. A biochemical defect in chlorpromazine sensitive marrow cells. J. Lab. Clin. Med. **78:** 435.
5. ROBINSON, W. A. & B. L. PIKE. 1970. Colony growth of human bone marrow cells *in vitro*. *In* Hematopoietic Cellular Proliferation. F. Stohlman, Jr., Ed. Grune & Stratton. New York, N.Y.
6. PISCIOTTA, A. V., L. PETERSON, K. WALZ & S. FARMER. 1978. Effect of chlorpromazine (CPZ) on proliferation of DNA polymerase deficient E. coli. Fed. Proc. **32**(No. 3).

DISCUSSION OF THE PAPER

J. W. BYRON (*Meharry Medical College, Nashville, Tenn.*): Concentrations of clozapine and chlorpromazine of 10^{-4} and 10^{-5} M are extremely high. How do they compare with the concentrations of both compounds *in vivo*?

A. V. PISCIOTTA: Indeed, the concentrations were very high. However, the purpose of the present experiments was to establish the toxicity of chlorpromazine and clozapine *in vitro*. Moreover, chlorpromazine sulfoxide, a major metabolic end product, promethazine, and Phenergan all failed to demonstrate a similar suppression in concentrations as high as 10^{-3} M.

BYRON: Can you test fibroblasts from a patient?

PISCIOTTA: I think we could. In fact, it is on the agenda, if we can get our human experimentation committee to approve such a protocol.

The Critical Cell Concept and Its Application in the Assessment of Effects from Different Dose Rates and Different Radiation Qualities

L. E. FEINENDEGEN, V. P. BOND,[a] AND
C. A. SONDHAUS[b]

Institute of Medicine
Nuclear Research Center Jülich GMBH
D-5170 Jülich, Federal Republic of Germany

Nowhere else has hematology and radiobiology been brought together so well and so creatively as around E. P. Cronkite at Brookhaven National Laboratory. Beginning with the measurement of radiation-induced changes in the structure and cellular composition of the hemopoietic system, he was the first to proceed to unravel the kinetic parameters of hemopoiesis by employing [³H]thymidine ([³H]TdR) and autoradiography.[1] His studies over many years on the control of hemopoiesis, and especially on granulopoiesis and lymphopoiesis, were stimulated by constant and intimate contact with clinical medicine. Of course, the question of radiation effects from ³H and other radionuclides incorporated into the genetic material inevitably arose. Under the chairmanship of Eugene Cronkite, Committee 24 of the National Council on Radiation Protection (NCRP), on which the senior author has served, was set up to work out guidelines for the use of radiation protection dosimetry in the incorporation of [³H]TdR.[2] How was one to proceed with the problem of detriment generated by radionuclides that were heterogeneously distributed within a fraction of proliferating cells, or were eventually distributed among resting cells? After long deliberation, the question was finally addressed in NCRP Report 63; in the process, this effort helped to advance a new concept of absorbed dose and its consequences with respect to late effects.[3] It was becoming increasingly clear at this time, from microdosimetric and other considerations, that the conventional concept of dose was inapplicable in the case of low-dose exposure.

In discussing this problem, we will briefly deal with the following three questions:

(a) In the case of low-dose exposures, what and how big is the apparent critical volume of the individual cell "target" which gives rise to late effects such as cancer?

(b) What is the fate of this critical volume in the low-dose-exposure case?

(c) How does this critical volume react to being hit by different-sized energy packages, or "hit sizes"?

---

[a] Von Humboldt Fellow; on leave from Brookhaven National Laboratory, Upton, N.Y.

[b] Guest Scientist; on leave from the University of California, Irvine, Calif.

LOW-DOSE EXPOSURE

The solution to the problem of predicting the damage from heterogeneously distributed radionuclides was found by assuming that the critical target for DNA-bound tritium and other radionuclides was the nucleus of the stem cell. This followed from a paper published in 1961 by Cronkite et al.[4] on the diminution of tracer labeling intensity in a cell nucleus through cell division, and a paper by Bond and Feinendegen[5] in 1966 on the dosimetric, radiobiological, and radioprotection aspects of intranuclear tritium.

NCRP Report 63 developed this approach by specifying the hemopoietic and spermatogonial stem cells to be the critical cells, and the nuclei within these cells to be the critical volumes. The calculations took into account the estimated degree of stem cell labeling per unit of labeled precursor administered, and derived the proliferation kinetics of these cells. By obtaining the relationship between the amount of administered [3H]TdR and the dose, it was possible to calculate the amount of injected isotope that would deliver 5 rad to the stem cells. This resulted in the recommendation of a maximum permissible single intake, by injection, of 1.4 mCi [3H]TdR per total body, i.e., 1/50th of the recommended limit for tritiated water.[3]

In terms of microdosimetry,[c] the critical volume concept had earlier been extended to the case of external exposure.[6] Here again the "critical volume" within a relevant cell was taken to be spherical and was assumed to be the apparent volume within which certain specific targets are considered to be responsible for cell killing as well as the sublethal changes responsible for late effects such as cancer. This brings us to the second question above: What is the fate of this critical volume in the case of low-dose exposure?

THE FATE OF CRITICAL VOLUME IN LOW-DOSE EXPOSURE

Having defined an apparent critical volume, the concepts of low dose and low dose rate need to be considered. This is particularly necessary now that the concept of dose in terms of energy absorbed per unit mass averaged over a given tissue is increasingly seen to be inapplicable to the low-dose and low-dose-rate situation. Let us briefly explain this. To begin with, it is essential to understand that the primary radiation flux, i.e., the photon flux, determines the spatial density of electron tracks produced by photon collisions with atomic orbital electrons in the target material. The electrons are of course a consequence of the collisions of photons with the orbital electrons of the target atoms. In the case of 100-kV X rays, these electrons have an average energy of ~ 10 keV and an average range of ~ 1 μm.

FIGURE 1 is a schematic representation of a tissue and its individual cells.[6,7] For 100-kV X rays a dose of 1 rad results, on the average, in three electron tracks in each cell nucleus, whereas a dose of 0.03 rad produces an electron track in only one out of 10 nuclei. In other words, a low enough dose produces what is essentially a partial-body irradiation.

[c]The absorbed dose to a cell nucleus calculated from tritium-containing DNA or RNA precursors is not to be equated to the dosimetrically determined "hit size" to a like volume. The absorbed dose usually includes the total energy from a number of tritium disintegrations. The "hit size" includes all or part of the energy from a single disintegration only.

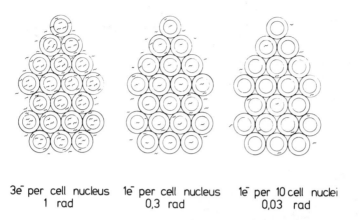

3e⁻ per cell nucleus   1e⁻ per cell nucleus   1e⁻ per 10 cell nuclei
1 rad   0,3 rad   0,03 rad

FIGURE 1. Distribution of Compton electrons in tissues from 100-kV X irradiation (diameter of cells 10 μm and of cell nuclei 8 μm). Reprinted with permission from Reference 7.

Hence *two parameters* need to be considered in describing an exposure:

(a) the average specific energy deposited, or "hit size," and

(b) the number (or fractional number) of cellular critical volumes that are hit.

These have been calculated for a number of different radiation qualities. FIG-URE 2, for example, depicts the two parameters for a range of ^{60}Co γ-ray doses.[8] The figure illustrates several important features of low and high doses of ^{60}Co γ rays in critical volumes of 8 μm diameter, and deserves further comment:

(a) *Thick vertical lines:* subdivision of absorbed dose range into low-dose, medium-dose, and high-dose regions.

(b) *Thick solid curves:* mean specific energy in affected critical volumes as a function of absorbed dose. Low dose: a constant mean specific energy per critical volume, since no more than one hit occurs in any affected critical volume. High dose: the mean specific energy is proportional to absorbed dose, since most critical volumes are now hit more than once.

(c) *Shaded area:* the fluctuation or distribution of deposited specific energy, or "hit size," within one standard deviation. Low dose: large fluctuation, independent of absorbed dose; high dose: small fluctuation, decreasing with absorbed dose.

(d) *Thick broken curves:* the fraction F of affected volumes as a function of absorbed dose. Low dose: F increasing with absorbed dose; high dose: $F = 1.0$, i.e., 100% of volumes affected (at least once).

One may thus propose to define a "low dose" as one producing no more than one hit in less than, say, 20% of the cellular critical volumes, and a "low dose rate" as a level of exposure per unit time which is low enough that any two consecutive hits in the same critical volume are separated by a length of time sufficient to allow for (maximum) repair. This approach to the specification of a low-dose exposure in terms of the average number of hits and their average size (in the critical volume) and by the fraction of critical volumes affected is useful for radiation protection. But for investigating late effects, additional information is needed, namely, a relation between the response of the critical volume and the amount of specific energy deposited in it when it is hit. We shall therefore turn now to the third question above.

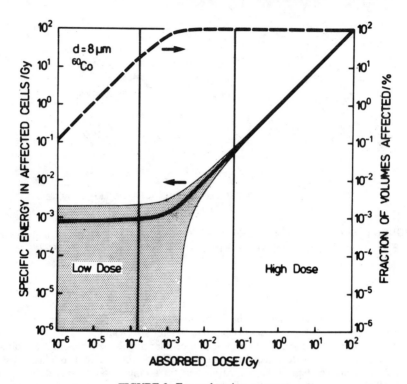

FIGURE 2. For explanation, see text.

RESPONSE OF CRITICAL VOLUME TO BEING HIT

We must begin by pointing out that there is a spectrum of hit sizes in a given-sized critical volume per unit dose, and in the low-dose ranges this distribution is constant, as is illustrated in FIGURE 2. In FIGURE 3, taken from Reference 9, a hit size spectrum is depicted in panel a. In panel b, the curve represents the probability that each hit size will cause a definite reaction. This relationship, developed by Bond and Varma,[9] has been called the "hit size effect function." If the frequency of each hit size (panel a) is multiplied by its probability of causing a defined effect (panel b), the observed incidence of effect in the exposed population of cells is obtained (panel c); and conversely. In the low-dose region, the dose-effect curve will be linear and will be determined by the number of critical volumes actually hit.

Now what are the responses of the critical volume to the individual hits? We will discuss two cases:

    (a) *sparsely ionizing radiation, and*

    (b) *densely ionizing radiation.*

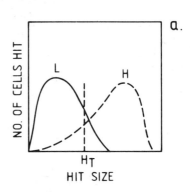

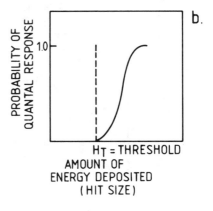

FIGURE 3. For explanation, see text.

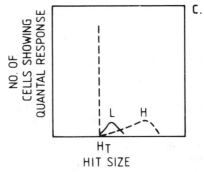

Sparsely Ionizing Radiation

For sparsely ionizing radiation, we know from the work of Veatch and Okada that on the average, each rad produces three to five single-strand breaks and about 0.15 double-strand breaks in the DNA of a cell nucleus,[10] and that nearly all of the damage is repaired. But some low-dose experiments done by us are of interest in this regard, since at the radiation level we used, strand breaks are unlikely and few cells are even affected.[11]

Briefly, it was found that whole-body irradiation of mice with 0.01 Gy or less caused a reduction in uptake of [³H]thymidine and ¹²⁵I-deoxyuridine (¹²⁵I-UdR) into

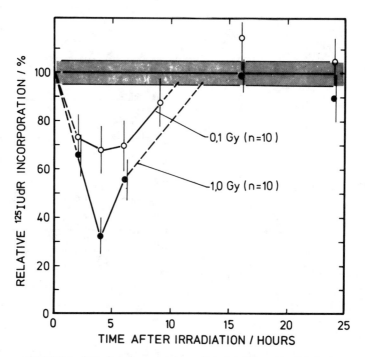

FIGURE 4. Data from bone marrow cells isolated from irradiated mice.

isolated bone marrow cells, and an elevation of thymidine in the blood serum. The effects were maximal at 4 hr and subsided about 10 hr after exposure (FIGURE 4). To further elucidate this phenomenon, bone marrow cells were obtained at various times after whole-body exposure and incubated *in vitro* using different media, buffers, and pH ranges. Thymidine kinase, the enzyme catalyzing the phosphorylation of thymidine and IUdR into DNA precursors, was assayed in the high-speed supernatant of cell homogenates, again with different buffers and pH ranges. Tracer intake into bone marrow cells *in vitro*, following irradiation *in vivo*, was depressed when the cells were buffered to pH 7.2-7.4 with NaHCO₃. Outside this pH range and without NaHCO₃, tracer uptake was not depressed. Along with depression of tracer uptake, thymidine kinase was found to be inhibited, but beyond a dose of 0.01 Gy the effect was dose independent and 65% of the thymidine kinase remained uninhibited. There was no inhibition when intact cells were collected outside the optimal pH range and in the absence of $NaHCO_3$, and addition of $NaHCO_3$ failed to restore enzyme inhibition. Procaine chloride given to the mice 1 hr before to 1 hr after irradiation fully abolished the effect on cells *in vitro*.

Enzyme inhibition, depression of [^{3}H]TdR or ^{125}I-UdR incorporation, and increase of TdR concentration in blood serum are all maximum at about 4 hr after exposure and recover to control levels about 6 hr later. This suggests that all three effects are related to each other and that inhibition of tracer uptake by cells after low-dose exposure leads to an increase of TdR in the reutilization pathway. It is noteworthy that the inhibition of both tracer incorporation and kinase activity takes 4 hr to reach maximum effect and that within the first hour after exposure no clear effect is seen. Thus, after the radiation energy absorption events, a cascade of reactions must be set in motion within the cell before the enzyme responds with inhibition.

Extracellular influences must also be taken into consideration. In fact, side experiments have shown that the effect also develops in cells placed in suspension within minutes after whole-body exposure and kept *in vitro* under optimal conditions; in this system also, there was no inhibition of tracer uptake 1 hr after exposure.

Three questions arise: (1) What is the signal that is created by radiation absorption events and that, with a delay of at least 1 hr, leads to enzyme inhibition? (2) How is the signal transferred from the site of radiation absorption to the site of the enzyme, i.e., what is the chain of events from signal initiation until final expression of effect? (3) How does the signal or chain of events finally interact with the structural complex that transduces enzyme inhibition?

Densely Ionizing Radiation

The second example of individual critical response to single hits is the *Auger Effect* from the decay of ^{125}I when it is attached to DNA.

FIGURE 5a gives the decay scheme for ^{125}I. The first step in the decay is electron capture in which an inner-shell electron is absorbed into the nucleus producing an inner-shell vacancy. The atom will be in an excited state and this energy is rapidly released by stepwise photon and electron emission. The portion of this energy carried by electrons is governed by the probabilities of K- and L-X-ray characteristic emissions and X-ray escape, and varies greatly. In some cases all of the energy released (67.2 keV) is carried by the electrons.

The filling of vacancies in the atom by these orbital transitions produces what has been called an electron cascade and, depending upon which transitions occur during the de-excitation, a very large number of electrons may be emitted by a single decay; FIGURE 5b shows typical spectra.[12] Here the data are plotted as histograms of the number of electrons with energy E emitted per disintegration. Line 3 in the figure is the average electron energy spectrum for the condensed phase in matter.

The electron cascade described above leads to high ionization densities in the immediate neighborhood of the decaying nucleus. As a result, the biological effects of ^{125}I if incorporated in DNA considerably exceed those which could be expected from the same energy deposited in the nucleus as a whole. In several experiments, these effects were demonstrated by measurement of DNA strand breaks; experiments with ^{60}Co γ rays were made for comparison.[13]

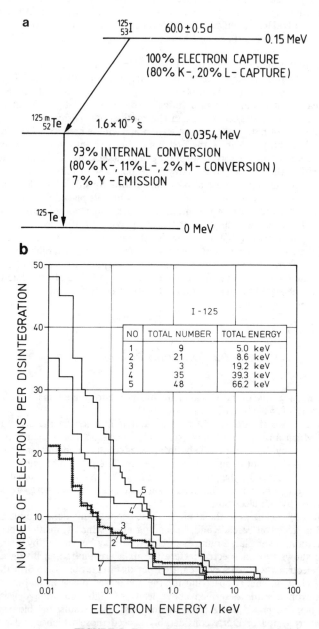

FIGURE 5. For explanation, see text.

[125]I was incorporated by unifilar labeling of the DNA of an asynchronous population of human kidney cells, using iododeoxyuridine as a carrier. Radiation doses were accumulated at −196°C. Single-strand breaks (SSBs) were measured in sucrose gradients of pH 12.0. Double-strand breaks (DSBs) were measured in a gradient of pH 9.4. The number of SSBs after exposure to ^{60}Co was 3.8 per 100 eV absorbed energy. The number of DSBs per 100 eV was 0.16 to 0.20. For ^{125}I, 4.1 SSBs per decay were found in intact cells. After exposure of the DNA in an isolated state, 2.0 SSBs per decay were measured. The number of DSBs per decay in intact cells was 1.5 to 1.9.

Repair of both SSBs and DSBs was measured by incubation of the cells at 37°C before strand break determination. For SSBs, repair was indicated by a corresponding shift of the molecular weight distribution. No repair of DSBs was detectable.

The following brief evaluation relates to the probability that more than one DSB is produced per ^{125}I decay. (For this purpose, the DNA was taken to be geometrically arranged in the cell nucleus in straight, parallel, and equidistant rods which reach across the cell nucleus from one side of the membrane to the other.) Assuming a diameter of the double helix proper of 2 nm, the mean distance between the DNA strands—including the DNA diameter—is very close to 10 nm in this pile configuration. According to calculations by Charlton and co-workers[11] the mean energy deposited per ^{125}I decay in a spherical volume of 10 nm radius is 1.6 keV. Since this dimension is only a very crude approximation of the effective sensitive volume of ^{125}I decay in DNA, it is not possible to express precisely the numbers of induced DSBs in terms of required electron volts. Nevertheless, 1.6 keV, the amount of energy leading to more than one DSB, may be used as an orientation value and compared with 600 eV per DSB, the amount obtained on an average from experiments with external γ irradiation.

CONCLUSION

Clearly, many aspects of radiation energy transfer on the cellular and molecular levels remain to be explored. Nevertheless, in further attempts to understand the processes and their consequences for radiation protection, low dose should be specified by (1) defining the critical volume to be the *cell nucleus,* and quantified by (2) the fraction of *critical volumes* being hit, (3) the *frequency of hits* per unit time, and (4) the distribution of *hit sizes.* If the frequency of each hit size (for a given exposure) is multiplied by its probability of causing an effect, then the biological response is predictable for any quality of radiation. This approach, moreover, offers the opportunity to compare effects of external exposure with those produced by heterogeneous microdistributions of incorporated particle emitters.

REFERENCES

1. BOND, V. P., T. M. FLIEDNER & J. O. ARCHAMBEAU. 1965. Mammalian Radiation Lethality. Chapter 2. Academic Press, Inc. New York, N.Y.

2. FEINENDEGEN, L. E. & E. P. CRONKITE. 1977. Effect of microdistribution of radionuclides on recommended limits in radiation protection: a model. Curr. Top. Radiat. Res. Q. **12:** 83-99.
3. NATIONAL COUNCIL ON RADIATION PROTECTION. 1979. Handbook 63: Tritium and Other Radionuclide Labelled Organic Compounds Incorporated in Genetic Material. NCRP. Washington, D.C.
4. CRONKITE, E., S. GREENHOUSE, G. BRECHER & V. BOND. 1961. Implications of chromosome structure and replication on hazards of tritiated thymidine and the interpretation of data on cell proliferation. Nature **189:** 153-154.
5. BOND, V. P. & L. E. FEINENDEGEN. 1966. Intranuclear ^{3}H thymidine: dosimetric, radiobiological and radiation protection aspects. Health Phys. **12:** 1007-1020.
6. ROSSI, H. H. 1968. Microscopic energy distribution in irradiated matter. *In* Radiation Dosimetry. F. H. Attix & W. C. Roesch, Eds.: 43-92. Academic Press, Inc. New York, N.Y.
7. FEINENDEGEN, L. E. 1977. Das Strahlenrisiko bei Kernreaktoren und Radioaktiven Müll. Das Öffentliche Gesundheitswesen **39:** 584-598.
8. INTERNATIONAL COMMISSION ON RADIOLOGICAL UNITS AND MEASUREMENTS. 1983. Report 36: Microdosimetry. Pp. 44 and 55. ICRU. Washington, D.C.
9. BOND, V. P. & M. VARMA. 1983. A stochastic, weighted hit size theory of cellular radiobiological action. *In* Proceedings, Eighth Symposium on Microdosimetry. J. Booz & H. Ebert, Eds.: 424-437. Commission of the European Communities. Luxembourg.
10. VEATCH, W. & S. OKADA. 1969. Biological damage from the Auger effect: radiation induced breaks in DNA. Biophys. J. **9:** 330-346.
11. FEINENDEGEN, L. E., H. MÜHLENSIEPEN, C. LINDBERG, J. MARX, W. PORSCHEN & J. BOOZ. 1983. Acute effects of very low dose in mouse bone marrow cells: a physiological response to background radiation? *In* Biological Effects of Low-Level Radiation. Pp. 459-471. International Atomic Energy Agency. Vienna, Austria.
12. CHARLTON, D. E., J. BOOZ, J. FIDORRA, TH. SMIT & L. E. FEINENDEGEN. 1978. Microdosimetry of radioactive nuclei incorporated into the DNA of mammalian cells. *In* Proceedings, Sixth Symposium on Microdosimetry. J. Booz & H. Ebert, Eds.: 91-110. Commission of the European Communities. Luxembourg.
13. TISLJAR-LENTULIS, G., P. HENNEBERG, M. MIELKE & L. E. FEINENDEGEN. 1978. DNA strand breaks induced by ^{125}I in cultured human kidney cells and their repair. *In* Proceedings, Sixth Symposium on Microdosimetry. J. Booz & H. Ebert, Eds.: 111-120. Commission of the European Communities. Luxembourg.

DISCUSSION OF THE PAPER

D. PRICE (*University of California Hospitals, San Francisco, Calif.*): I would like to congratulate Dr. Feinendegen on a very interesting presentation and I would like to point out a practical problem in dosimetry. What is the critical volume? Is it the cell nucleus? My question particularly concerns blood cells labeled with indium-111.

L. E. FEINENDEGEN: I would support the concept of choosing the cell nucleus to be the critical volume.

D. W. VAN BEKKUM (*Radiobiological Institute TNO, Rijswijk, the Netherlands*): A number of years ago we measured the repair of breaks induced by iodine-125. We found that there were both single-strand and double-strand breaks, which makes the repair process extremely complicated.

FEINENDEGEN: I think you are right. I did not get a chance to cover this subject. We have to take into consideration that there are two major mechanisms of double-strand breaks in the cell. One is by decay of iodine directly on DNA and the other is radiogenic.

Long-term Residual Radiation Effect in the Murine Hematopoietic Stem Cell Compartment[a]

K.-H. V. WANGENHEIM, H.-P. PETERSON,
G. E. HÜBNER,[b] AND L. E. FEINENDEGEN

Institute of Medicine
Nuclear Research Center Jülich GmbH
D-5170 Jülich, Federal Republic of Germany

INTRODUCTION

Long-term radiation effect in the hematopoietic system is well known.[1,2] Labeling repopulating bone marrow with the thymidine analogue [^{125}I]iododeoxyuridine (^{125}IUdR)[3,4] indicated that, at least in part, reduction in stem cell quality is involved.[5,6] Therefore, an assay was developed which measures long-term residual effect that is expressed in the hematopoietic system as reduction in proliferation ability of progeny of spleen repopulating cells following transfusion of marrow cell suspensions into lethally irradiated recipient mice. Since cell proliferation is measured by incremental increase in ^{125}IUdR uptake, the assay appears to be largely independent of donor stroma, number of spleen colony forming units (CFU-S) transfused, and changes in seeding efficiency.[7-9]

Residual radiation effect was observed in the hematopoietic system for at least 1 year after 500 rad γ irradiation. Various studies on number and size of spleen colonies from irradiated marrow complemented the data from tracer experiments and suggested that sublethal damage persists in surviving stem cells, is passed on to their progeny, and causes changes in cellular proliferation kinetics.

[a] The investigations were supported by the Bundesamt für Zivilschutz of the Federal Republic of Germany.

[b] Present address: Institute for Immunology and Oncology, Bayer A. G., D-5600 Wuppertal 1, Federal Republic of Germany.

MATERIALS AND METHODS

Animals

As described previously,[9] 10- to 14-week-old C57BL6 mice were used. With the exception of a few early experiments, control and irradiated donors were always taken from the same batches of female mice. Recipients were from uniform batches, preferentially of male mice, and received 0.1% NaI in drinking water after cell transfusion. Irradiations were performed with a ^{137}Cs source.

The Test System

General Procedures

The original test system[7,8] was modified to include the additional measurement of cell loss from the regenerating spleens.[9] This is shown in FIGURE 1. Donor mice either remained unirradiated in order to serve as controls or received 500 rad whole-body irradiation. Bone marrow was harvested after various times of recovery up to 1 year. In each experiment three dilutions were prepared from each cell suspension, usually 1.0, 1.5, and 2.25 × 10^6 nucleated cells in 0.2 ml Hanks' solution; 8 and 21 days after 500 rad, higher cell numbers were used to compensate for the reduced CFU-S content. The cell dilutions were transfused into groups of 800-rad-irradiated recipients who were then divided into subgroups of six to seven recipients. Two subgroups were needed for the measurement of proliferation ability and a third permitted the observation of cell loss needed for calculating the doubling time of proliferating cells. Thus subgroup I was injected with ^{125}IUdR^c at day 3 after cell transfusion, subgroup II at day 5. Two hours after tracer injection the spleens were fixed and washed for 48 hr in 4% formaldehyde in order to remove nonincorporated tracer. Subgroup III received ^{125}IUdR at day 3 and was sacrificed at day 5 for collecting and fixing the spleens. All spleens were measured in a scintillation well counter.

Proliferation Factor (PF)

FIGURE 2 shows, as an example, the results of a complete assay for nonirradiated control marrow cells on the left and for donors with a recovery period of 1 year after 500 rad on the right. The data given by the open triangles refer to subgroup I, that is, the activity incorporated in the spleens at day 3 after transfusion of the three cell suspensions. The solid triangles give the corresponding values at day 5 from subgroup II. The open circles refer to subgroup III, which was labeled at day 3 but measured 2 days later.

^{c} 5-[^{125}I]Iodo-2'-deoxyuridine: New England Nuclear, Boston, Mass., NEX 072, sp act > 2000 Ci/mmol, 5 μCi per recipient, i.p.

It can be seen in each subgroup that incorporated activity increases with increasing cell numbers transfused. This indicates proportionality between [125]IUdR uptake and number of proliferating cells that are progeny of spleen repopulating cells. The increase in tracer uptake from day 3 to day 5, thus indicates an increase in number of cells in cycle over that period of time. This increase is expressed by the proliferation factor (PF) which is the average ratio of tracer uptake at day 5 to that at day 3. In the example (FIGURE 2) it amounts to 18.1 ± 1.6 for the controls and 14.6 ± 1.2 for the progeny of irradiated bone marrow. Thus, in spite of the long recovery period, PF is still reduced to 81% of control.

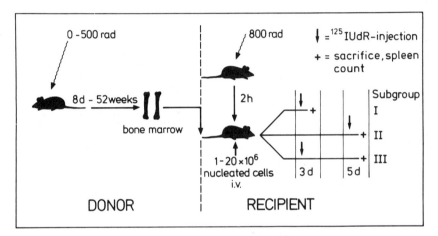

FIGURE 1. Experimental scheme.

Cell Loss

The difference between subgroups I and III, that is, the reduction in incorporated activity over 48 hr following labeling at day 3, indicates a loss of labeled cells from the spleens which averages 51% for the controls and 57% for the irradiated bone marrow. This loss was previously shown to be mainly due to maturation and migration of labeled cells from the spleen.[9]

Quotient (Q) and Cell Doubling Time (t_d)

The doubling time of proliferating cells (t_d) is calculated by use of the quotient (Q) of label from subgroup II to that of subgroup III:

$$t_d \text{ (hours)} = 48 \, \frac{\ln 2}{\ln Q}$$

With this calculation of t_d cell loss is excluded.[9] In the controls t_d averaged 8.75 hr and is, thus, close to normal average mitotic cycle time of 8.5 hr in the normal bone marrow.[10] In the example shown in FIGURE 2, t_d amounts to 8.5 hr for the controls and 8.9 hr 1 year after 500 rad.

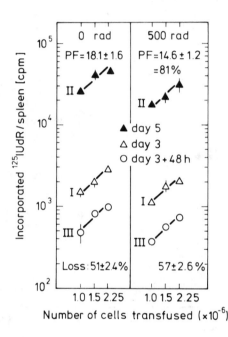

FIGURE 2. Example of an assay of proliferation ability of progeny of spleen repopulating cells including measurement of cell loss carried out 1 year after irradiation with 500 rad. Controls were not irradiated. Vertical bars indicate ± SE when larger than the symbols drawn.

Spleen Colonies

The numbers of CFU-S were determined by the spleen colony assay.[11] Colonies > 0.25 mm in diameter were counted with a stereomicroscope. For the assay at day 7 usually 4×10^4 nucleated cells were transfused; for comparisons of colony number and size at days 7 and 12 the number was 2×10^4. The average diameter of the colonies was measured with a stereomicroscope by use of an eyepiece micrometer under $20 \times$ magnification. For noncircular colonies the largest diameter was measured.

RESULTS AND DISCUSSION

Recovery of Proliferation Factor

In FIGURE 3 open circles represent average proliferation factors in percentage of control from 4 to 10 experiments per point at various times of recovery up to 1 year.

The solid triangles show the number of CFU-S per femur in the irradiated donors; these data are from separate experiments with 3-7 assays per point except for day 8 with one experiment. It can be seen that PF improves up to 6 months but then remains at about 80% of control. In 10 experiments 1 year after 500 rad, PF and CFU-S varied from 58% of control for PF and 48% of control for CFU-S to control level. Thus, recovery varies perhaps due to changes in factors that influence the ability of the organism to replace injured stem cells by less injured or normal stem cells.

Recovery of Increased Cell Loss and Doubling Time

FIGURE 4 summarizes the results of experiments simultaneously measuring PF, cell loss between days 3 and 5 after cell transfusion, and t_d from two to five experiments per point at the various times of recovery after 500 rad γ irradiation. The open circles and the heavy line represent PF in percentage of control. The solid squares and the broken line show the loss of labeled cells in percentage of controls between days 3 and 5 of the assay. The solid circles and the light line refer to the deviation of the doubling time from control(Δt). It can be seen that normalization of cell loss and doubling time is closely related to improvement of PF. Yet, even 1 year after exposure the average PF is still significantly reduced and also cell loss rate and Δt_d still appear to be elevated.

Possible Reasons for Radiogenic Reduction of Proliferation Factor

Changes in Age Structure of CFU-S Compartment

An increased loss of mature cells from spleens between days 3 and 5 of the assay would be sufficient to explain a reduction in PF. This could be brought about by a change in age structure of the stem cell compartment.[12] Thus, if younger CFU-S or "true" stem cells were more radiosensitive than the more advanced stages, the proportion of these committed CFU-S would increase after irradiation. Consequently, a larger proportion of cells would cease proliferation, mature, and disappear between 3 and 5 days after cell transfusion than seen in controls.

Magli *et al.*[13] demonstrated that the spleen colonies at day 7 after cell transfusion are partially transient, being derived from committed CFU-S. The proportion of transient colonies, thus, would increase if radiation preferentially eliminated the younger CFU-S. Since these transient colonies disappear by day 12, the number of spleen colonies at that time should be smaller than in controls.

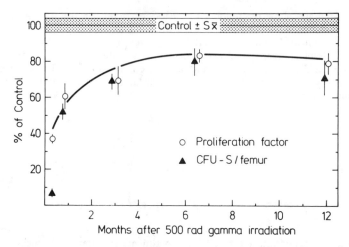

FIGURE 3. Recovery of proliferation factor (PF) and number of CFU-S per femur in percentage of controls at various times of recovery after 500 rad. The CFU-S were assayed at day 7 after cell transfusion. The shaded area refers to the controls of PF ± average SE. Vertical bars indicate ± SE.

We determined therefore the number of spleen colonies at day 7 and at day 12 after transfusion of marrow cells from normal donors and donors 1 year after 500 rad. FIGURE 5 shows results from four different experiments. In each experiment, the number of CFU-S per 10^6 nucleated cells of controls is given by white columns and that of irradiated donors by hatched columns. It is obvious that the number of colonies of controls tends to increase from day 7 to day 12, the average increase being 19%.

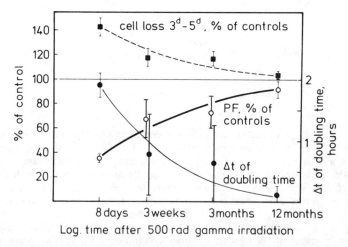

FIGURE 4. Summary of experiments showing recovery of proliferation factor (PF) and cell loss in percentage of controls and increased doubling time of proliferating progeny of spleen repopulating cells.

For irradiated cells the average increase is 45% which surpasses the control value. Thus there was no reduction in number of 12-day spleen colonies and a preferential killing of younger CFU-S with concomitant change in age structure appears to be excluded from being the reason for reduction in PF after irradiation.

Slow Growth of Progeny of Irradiated CFU-S and Cell Loss

It was obvious, however, that the 12-day colonies from irradiated marrow were smaller than those from the controls. Indeed, as shown in FIGURE 6, the mean colony size increased from day 7 to day 12; however, the 12-day colonies from irradiated

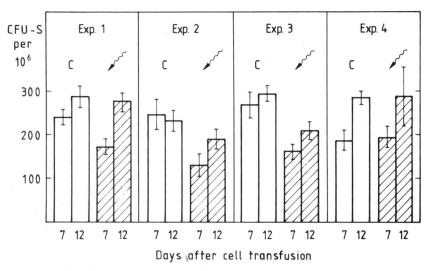

FIGURE 5. Numbers of CFU-S per 10^6 nucleated bone marrow cells in controls (C) and 500-rad-irradiated donors (⬅〰) following 1 year of recovery, assayed at days 7 and 12 after cell transfusion.

bone marrow, represented by hatched columns, were always distinctly smaller, and had an average size of 80% of the controls.

A significant correlation between radiogenic reduction in PF and reduction in size of 4-day and 6-day spleen colonies was also found from measurements of midsagittal spleen sections.[14] Three months after the last fraction of 3000 rad γ irradiation given in daily doses of 50 rad, PF was reduced to 56% of control; immediately after 50 rad acute exposure PF was 39% of control. In both cases the reduction of spleen colony size was between 40 and 60%.

It appears therefore that, on the average, colonies from CFU-S that survive radiation grow more slowly. Slow-growing colonies can be produced by radiation-induced loss of acentric chromosome fragments.[15,16] Slow growth, i.e., prolonged mitotic cycle time of progeny of spleen repopulating cells alone, however, is not sufficient to explain

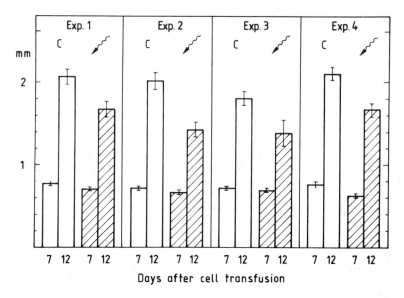

FIGURE 6. Average diameters of 7-day and 12-day spleen colonies from controls (C) and 500-rad-irradiated donors (➤⌁) following 1 year of recovery. The colonies are from the same spleens used for FIGURE 5.

the reduction of PF after irradiation. Q, that is, the quotient of incorporated activity at day 5 to that at day 3 minus activity lost up to day 5, is a function of cell doubling time t_d, which is, in this case, close to the mitotic cycle time. Q from irradiated donors, expressed in percentage of controls, was always larger than PF, expressed in percentage of controls (TABLE 1), the difference being in the order of the radiogenic increase in cell loss above the control level (FIGURE 4). Two effects, therefore, appear to be involved in causing a decrease in PF after irradiation: increase in mitotic cycle time and increase in the proportion of cells that mature and migrate from the spleen. Both effects may be caused by chromosomal lesions, for example, acentric chromosome fragments or point mutations. Prolonged mitotic cycle times, due to such lesions, are a probable cause of enhancement of differentiation and maturation through interference with endocellular control of cell differentiation and proliferation.[17] At any rate, sublethal lesions appear to persist in irradiated hematopoietic stem cells, as suggested earlier.[18]

Slow Recovery of CFU-S following Irradiation

Enhanced cell differentiation may lead to a reduction of the self-renewal capacity of CFU-S, as is seen in the slow recovery in the number of CFU-S after irradiation or other mutagenic treatment (FIGURE 3).[12,19,20] Sublethal chromosomal lesions must have similar consequences for all mitotically active cells, including cells with helper function in the hematopoietic system. The present data indicate that recovery following radiation exposure depends on the ability of the organism to replace sublethally injured stem cells by less injured or normal stem cells.

Conclusion

We conclude that long-term residual radiation effect in the hematopoietic system can be measured by a proliferation factor (PF) that describes the net gain in the number of proliferating progeny of spleen repopulating cells over 48 hr. Radiation reduces PF and residual effects are seen even 1 year after recovery from acute exposure. Residual injury resides in a certain proportion of stem cells leading, apparently, to an increase of mitotic cycle time in stem cell progeny and an enhanced loss of cells from the site of proliferation, probably via precocious differentiation and maturation.

SUMMARY

For the measurement of long-term residual radiation effect in the murine hematopoietic system a test system was developed that quantifies the proliferation ability of progeny of spleen repopulating cells by the proliferation factor (PF). The PF expresses the ratios of ^{125}IUdR incorporation in the recipient spleens at days 3 and 5 following cell transfusion, thus measuring the relative increase in number of proliferating cells. Following 500 rad whole-body γ irradiation, PF recovered up to 6 months and remained thereafter, on the average, at 80% of control. Recovery of the number of 7-day CFU-S was similar to recovery of PF.

Various studies were aimed at elucidating the reasons for reduction in PF. Loss of incorporated ^{125}IUdR activity from spleens between days 3 and 5 after cell transfusion indicates loss of mature labeled cells. When the doubling time of proliferating cells of CFU-S progeny (t_d) is corrected for cell loss, t_d for control bone marrow approaches mitotic cycle time in normal bone marrow as was found elsewhere.[10] Following 500 rad, both cell loss and t_d were initially increased and recovered in parallel with PF and number of CFU-S.

Reduction of PF could be brought about by radiation-induced increase in transient CFU-S with the consequence of increased loss of mature cells between days 3 and 5. This possibility was excluded by the observation that 1 year after 500 rad the number of colonies per spleen did not decrease from day 7 to day 12 after cell transfusion,

TABLE 1. Average Proliferation Factor (PF) and Quotient (Q) in Percentage of Controls at Various Times after 500 rad, $\overline{x} \pm$ SE

Time after 500 rad	PF (% of Control)	Q (% of Control)
8 days	35.2 ± 3.3	52.5 ± 5.9
3 weeks	67.6 ± 15.3	76.7 ± 18.2
3 months	72.8 ± 12.7	81.7 ± 9.8
12 months	92.0 ± 6.5	96.0 ± 4.1

as was expected from a higher proportion of transient CFU-S, but increased more than in the controls. Measurement of these 12-day colonies showed a significantly reduced size. Average progeny from irradiated CFU-S, apparently, grow more slowly.

It is concluded that sublethal injury resides in stem cells, increases mitotic cycle time, and causes precocious loss of cells from spleens probably by enhanced differentiation and maturation due to interference with endocellular control of cell proliferation and differentiation. Probably the observed recovery proceeds via replacement of injured stem cells by less injured or normal stem cells.

ACKNOWLEDGMENTS

The authors are indebted to Mrs. S. Fassbender and Miss M. Bröckling for excellent technical assistance.

REFERENCES

1. BAUM, S. J. & E. L. ALPEN. 1959. Residual injury induced in the erythropoietic system of the rat by periodic exposures to X-irradiation. Radiat. Res. **11:** 844-860.
2. BOND, V. P., T. M. FLIEDNER & J. O. ARCHAMBEAU. 1965. Mammalian Radiation Lethality. Academic Press, Inc. New York, N.Y.
3. SIEGERS, M. P., L. E. FEINENDEGEN, S. K. LAHIRI & E. P. CRONKITE. 1979. Relative number and proliferation kinetics of hemopoietic stem cells in the mouse. Blood Cells **5:** 211-236.
4. SIEGERS, M. P., L. E. FEINENDEGEN, S. K. LAHIRI & E. P. CRONKITE. 1979. Proliferation kinetics of early hemopoietic precursor cells with self sustaining capacity in the mouse, studied with 125-I-labeled iodo-deoxyuridine. Exp. Hematol. **7:** 469-482.
5. V. WANGENHEIM, K.-H., M. P. SIEGERS & L. E. FEINENDEGEN. 1980. Repopulation ability and proliferation stimulus in the hematopoietic system of mice following gamma-irradiation. Exp. Hematol. **8:** 694-701.
6. SIEGERS, M. P., K.-H. V. WANGENHEIM, G. E. HÜBNER & L. E. FEINENDEGEN. 1981. Residual damage and discontinuity of recovery in the hematopoietic system of mice following gamma-irradiation. Exp. Hematol. **9:** 346-354.
7. HÜBNER, G. E., K.-H. V. WANGENHEIM & L. E. FEINENDEGEN. 1981. An assay for the measurement of residual damage of murine hematopoietic stem cells. Exp. Hematol. **9:** 111-117.
8. HÜBNER, G. E. & E. P. CRONKITE. 1982. Drug-induced residual damage of murine hematopoietic stem cells measured by a new assay. Leuk. Res. **6:** 815-818.
9. V. WANGENHEIM, K.-H., E. P. CRONKITE, H.-P. PETERSON, G. E. HÜBNER & L. E. FEINENDEGEN. Persisting radiation effect in the hematopoietic stem cell compartment of mice. In preparation.
10. FRINDEL, E., M. TUBIANA & F. VASSORT. 1967. Generation cycle of mouse bone marrow. Nature **214:** 1017-1018.
11. TILL, J. E. & E. A. McCULLOCH. 1961. A direct measurement of the radiation sensitivity of normal mouse bone marrow cells. Radiat. Res. **14:** 213-222.
12. ROSENDAAL, M., G. S. HODGSON & T. R. BRADLEY. 1979. Organization of haemopoietic stem cells: the generation-age hypothesis. Cell Tissue Kinet. **12:** 17-29.
13. MAGLI, M. C., N. N. ISCOVE & N. ODARTCHENKO. 1982. Transient nature of early hematopoietic spleen colonies. Nature **295:** 527-529.

14. INOUE, T., E. P. CRONKITE, G. E. HÜBNER, K.-H. V. WANGENHEIM & L. E. FEINEN-DEGEN. 1984. Stem cell quality following irradiation: comparison of 125-IUdR uptake in the spleen and number and size of splenic colonies in bone marrow transfused, fatally irradiated mice. J. Radiat. Res. **25**: 261-273.

15. GROTE, S. J. & S. H. REVELL. 1972. Correlation of chromosome damage and colony-forming ability in Syrian hamster cells in culture irradiated in G_1. Curr. Top. Radiat. Res. Q. **7**: 303-309.

16. JOSHI, G. P., W. J. NELSON, S. H. REVELL & C. A. SHAW. 1982. Discrimination of slow growth from non-survival among small colonies of diploid Syrian hamster cells after chromosome damage induced by a range of X-ray doses. Int. J. Radiat. Biol. **42**: 283-296.

17. V. WANGENHEIM, K.-H. & A. HOWARD. 1978. Different modes of cell sterilization: cell killing and early differentiation. Radiat. Res.**73**: 288-302.

18. BAUM, S. J., M. I. VARON & D. E. WYANT. 1970. Radiation induced anemia in rats exposed repeatedly to mixed gamma-neutron radiation. Radiat. Res. **41**: 492-499.

19. SCHOFIELD, R. 1978. The relationship between the spleen colony-forming cell and he-mopoietic stem cell. A hypothesis. Blood Cells **4**: 7-25.

20. CRONKITE, E. P., A. L. CARSTEN & G. BRECHER. 1979. Hemopoietic stem cell niches, recovery from radiation and bone marrow transfusion. *In* Radiation Research, Proceedings of the Sixth International Congress on Radiation Research. S. Okada, M. Imamura, T. Terashima & H. Yamaguchi, Eds.: 648-656. Japanese Association for Radiation Research. Tokyo, Japan.

Enhanced Proliferation of Transfused Marrow and Reversal of Normal Growth Inhibition of Female Marrow in Male Hosts 2 Months after Sublethal Irradiation[a]

G. BRECHER AND K. MULCAHY

Donner Laboratory
Lawrence Berkeley Laboratory
University of California
Berkeley, California 94720

J.-H. TJIO AND E. RAVECHÉ

Section on Cytogenetics
National Institute of Arthritis, Metabolism, and Digestive Diseases
National Institutes of Health
Bethesda, Maryland 20205

It is well established that 0.5 to 1 million marrow cells suffice to rescue (though not necessarily fully restore) lethally irradiated mice, while even 40 million cells result only in minimal seeding in isogeneic, nonirradiated mice.[1-3] It was originally suggested that the results imply the existence of special proliferative sites which are filled in the nonirradiated animal, but are emptied by high doses of irradiation.

In 1982 we demonstrated the feasibility of establishing substantial numbers of donor cells in normal, nonirradiated hosts[4] as suggested by Saxe *et al.*[5] After four daily transfusions of 50 million marrow cells, 20-40% of the host's marrow consisted of cells of donor origin. The present paper reports the marked enhancement of the proliferation of transfused marrow cells in mice exposed to sublethal doses of irradiation of 300-900 R. Two months later, when the peripheral blood counts of the irradiated animals had returned to normal, transfusion of 100 million cells resulted in donor cell percentages of 55-100% in the peripheral blood and marrow.

We have previously found that male donor cells proliferated as readily in female as in male hosts, while female donor cells proliferated to a comparable degree only

[a]Supported by National Institutes of Health Grant AM 27454. Research was conducted at Lawrence Berkeley Laboratory which is supported by the U.S. Department of Energy under Contract DE-AC03-7600098.

in female hosts.[6] In the present study, male animals that had been exposed to 600-900 R 2 months earlier sustained proliferation of male and female donor cells equally well.

MATERIALS AND METHODS

The mice used were CBA/CA(PGK-1,AB) characterized by two X-linked alloenzymes, A and B of phosphoglycerate kinase (PGK), which can be distinguished electrophoretically. Hence, donor cells can be readily traced in the isogeneic recipients by using animals with the A variant as donor and those with B as recipient or vice versa. The mice were raised at the University of California, Berkeley, from a breeding stock kindly provided by Dr. H. S. Micklem of the Department of Zoology, University of Edinburgh, Edinburgh, Scotland, who had developed the strain by backcrossing the original C3H(PGK-1A) variant onto the CBA/CA(PGK-1B) genetic background. It had gone through 12 generations by the time we obtained it.[4] The males carrying only the A or B genes are designated YA or YB, respectively; the females AA or BB, respectively.

Peripheral blood was hemolyzed in distilled water, the red cell ghosts were removed by centrifugation, and the supernatant was used for analysis. Marrow samples were exposed to distilled water for 10 sec. Electrophoretic separation of the PGK alloenzymes A and B was slightly modified from the method of Buecher *et al.*[7] Samples were applied to a cellulose acetate membrane and run in a Sartorius cell, at a constant voltage of 400 V for 45 min in the buffer system specified by Buecher,[7] except that the anodal buffer was also used on the cathodal side. On completion of the electrophoresis, the cellulose acetate membrane was inverted on a 1.5% agarose plate which was flooded with the staining solution. That solution contained the enzyme mixture which generates 1,3-diphosphoglycerate as substrate for PGK, which converts it to 3-phosphoglycerate and ATP. Glucose, hexokinase, glucose-6-phosphate dehydrogenase (G-6-PD), and NADP were added. The conversion of NADP to NADPH as glucose is converted to 6-phosphogluconate parallels the production of ATP. NADPH was assayed by thiazolyl blue, a tetrazolium dye, and meldola blue. The intensity of the blue color on the electrophoresis membrane was read in a densitometer, the curves traced manually in an integrator which automatically computed the areas under the peaks. The A peak was then computed as a percentage of A+B. The results were checked by preparing a wide range of mixtures of A and B from blood or marrows of AA and BB animals.

Irradiation was from a ^{60}Co source at 1.22 m at a dose rate of 22 R/min measured with a Victoreen condenser R-meter. Mice carrying only the A gene were irradiated and later transfused with B cells from mice of the same or opposite sex as indicated under Results and in FIGURE 1, or B cells were transfused into A hosts. No differences were noted in the outcome between transfusion of B cells into A hosts and the reverse procedure. Mice were exposed to 300, 600, or 900 R which did not induce mortality. Two to 4 months after irradiation the hematocrit, white cell and platelet counts of each animal were checked to make sure that the peripheral blood values had returned to normal. In the few animals in which any of the counts were low, they returned to normal within another 2 weeks. At that time the irradiated animals and controls were

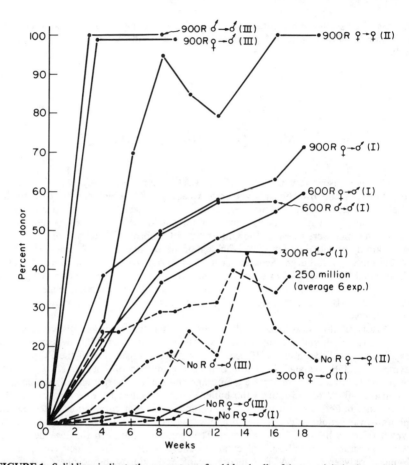

FIGURE 1. Solid lines indicate the percentage of red blood cells of donor origin in the peripheral blood following transfusion in animals that had been exposed to 300, 600, or 900 R 2 months earlier; broken lines indicate that in the unirradiated controls. All animals received 100 million marrow cells, the same suspensions being used to transfuse irradiated and control mice in a given experiment. The dose of irradiation, the sex of the donor and the recipient, and the number of the experiment (roman numerals) are indicated at the end of each line. For comparison the average values of six experiments in which unirradiated animals received 250 million marrow cells from sex-matched donors are also shown.

given 100 million marrow cells intravenously from donors whose alloenzyme differed from that of host.

RESULTS

The results of the three experiments which form the basis of this report are shown in FIGURE 1. In Experiment I, groups of six male (B) animals were exposed to 300,

600, or 900 R or no irradiation. Two months later all animals received 100 million marrow cells from either female or male (A) donors in groups of 3, except for the nonirradiated controls. The 100 million cells were given in two divided doses on successive days. In the animals irradiated with 900 or 600 R, the 100 million donor cells resulted in percentages of cells of donor origin of more than 50% in the peripheral blood in all groups by 16 weeks post-transfusion. When the animals were killed at 18 weeks their marrows contained 55 to 70% donor cells. Four male (B) animals in the 600- and 900-R groups that had been given female (A) cells 2 months after irradiation were also examined cytogenetically for the presence or absence of the Y chromosome. They were found consistently to have female donor cell percentages compatible with the electrophoretic results.

In contrast to the 600- and 900-R groups in which transfused marrow from male and female donors had a comparable rate of proliferation, there was a marked difference in the 300-R group in which male donor cells rose to 45% by 16 weeks, while female cells remained undetectable in two of three animals and in a third rose to 40% giving an average of 14%.

Six unirradiated male controls had received female donor marrow. Five of them had no detectable donor enzyme in their blood, while one had a maximum of 8%. There was thus no significant difference between male controls and male animals that had received 300 R. Both groups had minimal or no proliferation of donor cells when transfused with 100 million female donor cells. Due to an oversight, no unirradiated males were given 100 million male donor cells as a further control. However, results of six other experiments with four to nine animals each are available in which 200-300 million cells were given to unirradiated animals of the same sex. In each of these six experiments donor cells averaged 43% or less in the peripheral blood on repeated examination over 16 to 19 weeks, except for a single instance in one experiment in which the average rose to 48%. There was no difference in the results when male hosts were given male cells and female hosts were given female cells. The mean of all six experiments is shown in FIGURE 1 for comparison with the various groups given 100 million cells. It may be noted that the average percentage of donor cells in all previously irradiated groups given 100 million cells exceeded that in unirradiated hosts given 250 million marrow cells, with the exception of the male recipients of female cells in the 300-R group.

At the end of the experiment, when the peripheral blood as well as the bone marrow could be examined, the percentages of donor cells were similar. This was also the case in all other experiments (TABLE 1).

In Experiment II, six female (A) animals were exposed to 900 R and transfused with 100 million cells from female (B) donors 2 months later. Seven unirradiated controls received 100 million (B) cells from the same suspension. In the previously irradiated group, percentages of cells of donor origin averaged 95, 85, 79, and 100% at 8, 10, 12, and 16 weeks after transfusion and all marrows had 100% cells of donor origin when killed at 19 weeks. The control animals averaged 24% from 8 to 16 weeks, with a single rise to 44% at 14 weeks.

In Experiment III, groups of five male (A) recipients were exposed to 900 R and transfused with 100 million male or female (B) marrow cells 2 months later. Nonirradiated controls of A type received the same suspensions of male or female donor cells. All irradiated recipients had 100% cells of donor origin in the peripheral blood 3 weeks after transfusion, whether they had received male or female cells. When reexamined at 9 weeks, they had maintained the 100% replacement by donor cells. The unirradiated controls given male cells reached 28%, with a range of 25-32% 7 weeks after transfusion. At the same time four of five recipients of female marrow had no evidence of B cells; the fifth had 28% B cells, an average of 6% for the group.

DISCUSSION

The PGK alloenzymes A and B make it possible to follow the cells of donor origin in the peripheral blood, as well as in the marrow, by using donors having only one of these alloenzymes and recipients having only the other. The peripheral blood values reflect the enzyme content of red cells. Since their life span is 52 days,[8] it may be expected to take 7-8 weeks for their complete replacement. Multiple experiments in which marrow was transfused into normal recipients confirmed that the rise in peripheral blood cells of donor origin is indeed quite slow as a rule. The delay in the rise of donor cells in the peripheral blood in the present experiments is in keeping with that experience except for the unexpectedly rapid rise in Experiment III.

TABLE 1. Comparison of the Percentages of Cells of Donor Origin in the Bone Marrow and Peripheral Blood in 10 Experiments[a]

Peripheral Blood		Bone Marrow		No. in Group
Mean	SE	Mean	SE	
43	2.8	40	6.3	6
19	3.5	12	4.9	6
31	3.5	33	2.2	4
26	6.0	28	5.2	4
30	5.0	15	5.2	8
55	1.6	61	7.2	5
37	2.2	41	12.5	5
29	3.0	5	1.0	5
35	2.5	36	7.9	3
41	5.8	20	3.6	3

[a] The figures represent average percentages of three to eight animals and standard errors (SE). Both peripheral blood and bone marrow values were determined on the day the animals were killed at the end of each experiment. At that time, 14-18 weeks after transfusion, the peripheral blood was expected to reflect the marrow values. The expectation was generally fulfilled with the three instances in which the marrow value was significantly lower being ascribed to greater technical problems in marrow examinations than in peripheral blood examinations.

The observation that donor cells can replace 100% of host cells in animals that had been irradiated sublethally 2 months earlier and whose peripheral blood values had returned to normal appears incongruous at first. Even if every pluripotential stem cell in the transfused 100 million cells were to seed and proliferate successfully, they could not replace 100% of the host cells which number at least 240 million in the normal mouse.[9] Therefore, it must be assumed that the host cells, though capable of maintaining a normal peripheral blood picture, nevertheless suffered permanent damage resulting in a reduced capacity for self-renewal. The donor cells could thus outgrow and replace the host cells to varying degrees, providing 60-100% of host marrow. The replacement of cells with reduced self-renewal rates by more normal cells has been well established. It was first utilized by Micklem et al.[10] in their competitive repopulation assay and subsequently used extensively by Harrison.[11]

In experiments reported earlier,[6] we explored the response of animals exposed to a uniformly lethal dose of radiation and given a transfusion of marrow within hours to assure their survival. These animals were given a second transfusion of 40 million marrow cells 2 months later, when their peripheral blood values had returned to normal. The cells derived from these second donors subsequently averaged 10% of the host's marrow, while unirradiated controls given the same suspensions of marrow cells never contained more than 2% donor cells. The difference was highly significant, though not as striking as in the present experiment. This must have been due at least in part to the small inoculum of 40 million cells used.

The increased proliferation of marrow cells given 2 months after sublethal irradiation was ascribed to radiation damage of the host stem cells. This explanation cannot be applied to lethally irradiated mice since their marrow was entirely replaced by the progeny of the donor cells given immediately after irradiation. These cells, though not subject to direct radiation, may nevertheless have been damaged indirectly by their sojourn in the recently irradiated environment. Such indirect radiation damage was documented by a markedly shortened life span of normal red cells transfused into dogs 2-5 days after irradiation with 475 R.[12] Further studies are, therefore, indicated to verify the postulated indirect damage of donor cells in the recently irradiated environment.

The inhibition of growth of female cells in the male can be abolished not only by sublethal irradiation of the host as shown here, but also by anti-Thy-1 serum and complement added to the female donor cells as recently observed.[13] The indication that the inhibition is immunologic in nature should aid in identifying the specific mechanism responsible.

SUMMARY

We have previously shown that bone marrow will seed and proliferate in normal recipients. Transfusion of 50 million cells on each of 4 or 5 consecutive days, a total of 200-250 million cells, resulted in the recipient's marrow being 20-40% of donor origin. The present paper reported on the marked enhancement of proliferation of donor cells in animals that were exposed to sublethal doses of irradiation of 300-900 R. Two months later, when their peripheral blood values had returned to normal, they were transfused with 100 million cells. The number of donor cells in the recipients exposed to 600-900 R reached 55-100% at various intervals after transfusion, with controls averaging 24% and never exceeding 40%. Since the transfused cells numbered less than 40% of the host's own complement of marrow cells, they could not replace 100% of them unless they proliferated more rapidly than the host cells. The implied competitive advantage of the donor cells was ascribed to a reduced capacity for self-renewal of the host's irradiated cells.

In recipients exposed to 300 R and in nonirradiated controls, female cells failed to grow in male recipients, while male cells grew as well in female as in male hosts. The inibition of growth of female cells in the male host was abolished by irradiation with 600 or 900 R, or by the exposure of the female donor cells to anti-Thy-1 serum and complement prior to transfusion. Experiments are under way to test the suggested immunologic nature of the inhibition phenomenon.

REFERENCES

1. MICKLEM, H. S., C. M. CLARKE, E. P. EVANS & C. E. FORD. 1968. Fate of chromosome-marked mouse bone marrow cells transfused into normal syngeneic recipients. Transplantation 6: 299-301.
2. TAKADA, A., Y. TAKADA & J. L. AMBRUS. 1971. Proliferation of donor spleen and bone marrow cells in the spleens and marrow. Proc. Soc. Exp. Biol. Med. 136: 222-226.
3. BRECHER, G., J.-H. TJIO, J. E. HALEY, J. NARLA & S. L. BEAL. 1979. Transplantation of murine bone marrow without prior host irradiation. Blood Cells 5: 237-246.
4. BRECHER, G., J. D. ANSELL, H. S. MICKLEM, J.-H. TJIO & E. P. CRONKITE. 1982. Special proliferative sites not needed for seeding and proliferation of transfused bone marrow cells in normal syngeneic mice. Proc. Natl. Acad. Sci. USA 79: 5085-5087.
5. SAXE, D. F., S. S. BOGGS & D. R. BOGGS. 1981. Transplantation of syngeneic marrow into nontreated recipients. Exp. Hematol. 9(Suppl. 9): 173. (Abstract.)
6. BRECHER, G., H. LAWCE & J.-H. TJIO. 1981. Bone marrow transfusions in previously irradiated, hematologically normal syngeneic mice. Proc. Soc. Exp. Biol. Med. 166: 389-393.
7. BUECHER, T., R. BENDER, R. FUNDELE, H. HOFNER & I. LINKE. 1980. Quantitative evaluation of electrophoretic allo- and isozyme patterns. FEBS Lett. 115: 319-324.
8. LANDAW, S. A., T. TENFORDE & J. C. SCHOOLEY. 1977. Decreased surface charge and accelerated senescence of red blood cells following neuraminidase treatment. J. Lab. Clin. Med. 89: 581-591.
9. CHERVENIK, P. A., D. R. BOGGS, J. C. MARSH, G. E. CARTWRIGHT & M. H. WINTROBE. 1968. Quantitative studies of blood and bone marrow neutrophils in normal mice. Am. J. Physiol. 215: 353-360.
10. MICKLEM, H. S., C. E. FORD, E. P. EVANS, D. A. OGDEN & D. S. PAPWORTH. 1972. Competitive in vivo proliferation of foetal and adult haemopoietic cells in lethally irradiated mice. J. Cell. Physiol. 79: 293-299.
11. HARRISON, D. E. 1980. Competitive repopulation: a new assay for long-term stem cell functional capacity. Blood 55: 77-81.
12. STOHLMAN, F., JR., G. BRECHER, M. SCHNEIDERMAN & E. P. CRONKITE. 1957. The hemolytic effect of ionizing radiations and its relationship to the hemorrhagic phase of radiation injury. Blood 12: 1061-1085.
13. RAVECHÉ, E., T. SANTORO, G. BRECHER & J. TJIO. 1985. Role of T cells in sex differences in syngeneic transfer of bone marrow. Exp. Hematol. 13: 975.

Neon-20 Ion- and X-Ray-Induced Mammary Carcinogenesis in Female Rats

CLAIRE J. SHELLABARGER,[a] JOHN W. BAUM,[b]
SEYMOUR HOLTZMAN,[a] AND J. PATRICK STONE[a]

[a]Medical Department
and
[b]Safety and Environmental Protection Division
Brookhaven National Laboratory[c]
Upton, New York 11973

INTRODUCTION

The acceleration of heavy ions ($^{12}_6$C, $^{20}_{10}$Ne, $^{40}_{18}$Ar) to energies of 400-500 MeV/amu has been achieved at the BEVALAC of the University of California in Berkeley.[1] In addition to radiation therapy, one of the proposed uses of heavy-ion irradiation is to image lesions of the human female breast.[2] It is now generally accepted that radiation exposure of the human female breast will increase the risk of breast cancer development.[3-5] It is known that radiation-induced mammary carcinogenesis in the female rat occurs by a scopal mechanism[6] that is similar to the scopal mechanism of radiation-induced breast cancer in the human female.[7] Thus, the rat model system was chosen to assess the carcinogenic potential of heavy-ion irradiation in the belief that data obtained from rat studies would have a qualitatively predictive value for the human female. Accordingly, female rats were exposed to ^{20}Ne ions at the BEVALAC and studied for the development of mammary neoplasia for 312 ± 2 days at Brookhaven National Laboratory along with rats exposed concurrently to X irradiation or to no irradiation.

MATERIALS AND METHODS

Female Sprague-Dawley rats were purchased from Taconic Farms, Germantown, New York and shipped by air to California. They were irradiated two days after their arrival at 43 ± 1 days of age, and two days later all were returned to Brookhaven via air shipment where they were studied for some 312 days.

[c]Brookhaven National Laboratory is operated by Associated Universities, Inc., under contract to the U.S. Department of Energy (Contract DE-AC02-CH00016).

A 7.36-GeV ^{20}Ne ion beam from the BEVALAC facility was passed through a 0.2-cm-thick lead scatterer to provide a uniform field approximately 5 cm in diameter at the rat position. The resulting beam energy at the sample position was estimated at 6.6 GeV. ^{20}Ne ions of this energy have a linear energy transfer (LET) and a range in water of 33 keV/μm and 20 cm, respectively. ^{20}Ne ion irradiation and dosimetry were done as follows. Nominal doses of 2, 6, 18, or 54 rad (100 rad = 1 Gy) were given in 1-3 min. Each rat was exposed individually, facing the beam, in a Plexiglas cylinder 5 cm in diameter and 14 cm long. The cylinder was placed concentric with the beam. Dose was measured upstream, dowstream, and radially, using ionization chambers normally employed at the BEVALAC facility supplemented by TLD and film dosimeters placed anteriorly and posteriorly to the rat position. Each rat was placed in the plateau region of the depth-dose pattern immediately before the Bragg peak, as evidenced by the slightly higher dose measured at the posterior dosimeters than at the anterior dosimeters. On the basis of these measurements, and available information on the ^{20}Ne ion depth-dose pattern,[8] it was concluded that dose increased by 50% from the anterior end of the rat to the posterior end, and dose decreased from the central longitudinal axis of the beam out to the wall of the rat holder by approximately 15%. The increased dose and LET near the posterior end contributed an estimated 14% greater mean dose and mean LET to the posterior half of the rat than to the anterior half of the rat. As a positive control, and as reference radiation, either 60 or 180 R (1 R = 0.95 rad) of total-body 230-kVp X irradiation was given at an exposure rate of approximately 14 R/min by operating a Phillips X-ray machine at 15 mA with 0.5 mm Cu and 1.0 mm Al filtration. Fifteen rats at a time were exposed, from the top, at a target-to-sample distance of 95 cm. The exposure was measured in air, under maximum backscatter conditions, with a Victoreen ionization chamber. The calculated nominal doses given were 57 and 171 rad.

After their return to Brookhaven National Laboratory, all rats were kept five per cage on corncob bedding in rooms maintained at 21-23°C under conditions of 7 A.M.-7 P.M. fluorescent light, and given commercial rat chow and water *ad libitum*. Each rat was identified by a numbered ear tag. The anatomical location of each mammary tumor, discovered by once a week palpation, was recorded using the nipples as reference points. All mammary tumors were removed under ether anesthesia at a size of about 2 cm. All suspected mammary tumors were studied microscopically, and were classified as either mammary adenocarcinomas or mammary fibroadenomas using criteria consistent with those published by Young and Hallowes.[9] In the case of a mammary neoplasm appearing at the site of a previous neoplasm, if the second neoplasm was of a different pathological type, or if more than 90 days had elapsed and the neoplasm was of the same pathological type, it was considered a separate neoplasm. The time of appearance of mammary tumors was taken as the date of the initial palpation of a tumor that proved to be a mammary tumor upon subsequent histological study. The time of tumor appearance, and death, was reckoned as days after the date of the exposure to radiation. The experiment was ended 312 ± 2 days after the day of irradiation when all rats were killed and examined for pathology.

RESULTS AND DISCUSSION

In the ^{20}Ne ion-irradiated rats, 41 mammary neoplasms were found in the posterior half of the rats and 17 were found in the anterior half. In contrast, the anterior-posterior distribution was approximately equal, 31 and 33 respectively, in the X-ray-irradiated rats. The right-left distribution was approximately the same in both the [20]Ne ion-irradiated rats, 28 and 30, and in the X-ray-irradiated rats, 29 and 35. The finding, in the [20]Ne ion-irradiated rats, of more neoplasms in the posterior half than in the anterior half is in agreement with the calculation of a larger [20]Ne ion dose in the posterior half than in the anterior half. This result, more mammary neoplasia in the volume with the larger [20]Ne ion dose, is in agreement also with a dose-related mammary neoplastic response as well as the concept that the mode of action of radiation-induced mammary neoplasia is scopal in nature.

There are some uncertainties about whether or not the development of a mammary adenocarcinoma and a mammary fibroadenoma within the same rat is an interdependent process.[10] In the current experiment, using 301 rats, 13 developed only an adenocarcinoma, 46 developed only a fibroadenoma, and 12 rats developed both types. A χ^2 analysis of these data indicates ($p < 0.001$) a dependence between the occurrences of the two types of tumor. Even so, we have chosen to analyze the percentage of rats

TABLE 1. The Type and Dose of Radiation, the Number of Rats Irradiated at 43 ± 1 Days of Age and Alive 312 ± 2 Days Later, and the Number and Percentage of Rats with Mammary Adenocarcinomas (AC) or with Mammary Fibroadenomas (FA)

| Radiation | | | | Rats with: | | | |
| Type | Dose (rad) | Number of Rats at: | | AC | | FA | |
		Start	End	N	%	N	%
None	None	76	75	0	0	6	8
Neon-20	2	58	57	2	3	6	10
Neon-20	6	49	49	1	2	6	12
Neon-20	18	21	20	3[a]	14	3	14
Neon-20	54	22	19	9[b]	41	8[a]	36
X ray	57	45	45	1	2	11[b]	24
X ray	171	30	29	9[b]	30	18[b]	60

[a] Significantly different (χ^2) from control, nonirradiated value; $p < 0.01$.
[b] Significantly different (χ^2) from control, nonirradiated value; $p < 0.001$.

with at least one adenocarcinoma (with or without a fibroadenoma), or at least one fibroadenoma (with or without an adenocarcinoma). We accept as proven that the irradiated female rat and the irradiated human female are at risk for the development of both benign and malignant mammary neoplasia.[4]

We have chosen not to "correct" or modify the final incidence of rats with either an adenocarcinoma or a fibroadenoma for intercurrent mortality. Some 98% of the rats survived the 312-day study period (TABLE 1). Only 7 of the 301 rats died and these deaths did not appear to be related to the type of radiation.

Similarly, we have chosen not to study the time-to-tumor data, in part, because the experiment was severely truncated and no account was taken of possible late-appearing mammary neoplasia. Also, some statisticians[11] argue that no meaningful distinction can be made between earlier onset (acceleration) and extra onset (higher incidence).

Data on the mean number of mammary neoplasms per rat were not analyzed. It has been reported[12,13] that the distribution of the number of rats with a specified number of mammary neoplasms (rats with no mammary neoplasms, rats with one mammary neoplasm, rats with two mammary neoplasms, etc.) departs from a Poisson distribution. Thus, even though the mean number of mammary adenocarcinomas and mammary fibroadenomas tended to increase with dose (data not shown), there were too few rats with multiple tumors to allow a meaningful analysis of these data.

The percentage of rats with one or more mammary adenocarcinomas, and the percentage of rats with one or more mammary fibroadenomas, tended to increase as the dose of ^{20}Ne ion irradiation, or X irradiation, was increased (TABLE 1). The two highest doses of ^{20}Ne ion irradiation, 18 and 54 rad, and the higher dose of X irradiation, 180 R, increased the incidence of rats with mammary adenocarcinomas, as compared to the nonirradiated controls, using the χ^2 test. The highest ^{20}Ne ion

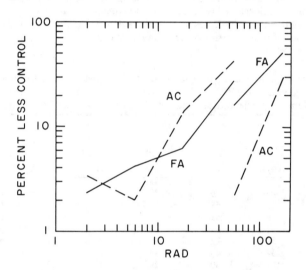

FIGURE 1. AC = mammary adenocarcinomas; FA = mammary fibroadenomas. Lines on right represent X-ray results; lines on left represent neon ion results.

dose, 54 rad, and both doses of X rays, 60 and 180 R, increased the incidence of rats with mammary fibroadenomas above the control value.

To compare the dose-response relationships for the two types of radiation, the percentage of irradiated rats with one or more mammary adenocarcinomas, or with one or more mammary fibroadenomas, after subtracting the appropriate nonirradiated control value, was plotted in a log-log fashion with the points joined by straight lines (FIGURE 1). At a prevalence of 20%, a response that is bracketed by all groups, the RBE (relative biological effectiveness) for rats with mammary fibroadenomas appears to be less than 2, and for those with adenocarcinomas, more than 5. No attempts to derive confidence limits of the RBE values has been made because we believe the data are not adequate for this purpose. Also, it is not possible using these data to determine if the RBE values vary inversely with dose.

SUMMARY AND CONCLUSIONS

Female Sprague-Dawley rats were given 2, 6, 18, or 54 rad of 6.6-GeV neon-20 ions at 43 ± 1 days of age. Concurrently, additional rats were either exposed to 60 or 180 R of 230-kVp X rays or were not irradiated. Mammary neoplasms were removed as they occurred and all rats were killed after 312 $\pm$ 2 days of study. As the dose of either type of radiation was increased the percentage of rats with mammary adenocarcinomas, and the percentage of rats with mammary fibroadenomas, tended to increase. At a prevalence of 20%, the RBE for neon-20 ions for mammary adenocarcinomas was estimated to be larger than 5 and for mammary fibroadenomas the RBE was estimated to be less than 2. No conclusion was reached concerning whether or not the RBE might vary with dose. We suggest that neon-20 ions do have a carcinogenic potential for rat mammary tissue and that this carcinogenic potential is likely to be greater than that for X irradiation. This finding is in accord with reports indicating that neutron radiation has a high RBE for mammary carcinogenesis in several strains of rats.[13-18] Thus, although we conclude that neon-20 ions are likely to be carcinogenic for the human breast, the question of what the precise RBE might be remains unanswered.

EPILOGUE

When Dr. Eugene Cronkite moved to Brookhaven National Laboratory in 1954, he was interested in the study of the hematopoietic aspects of the acute radiation syndrome and in developing a model system to simulate the radiation conditions of the Marshallese in regard to the possible interaction of β burns and total-body γ radiation. In regard to the study of hematopoietic cellular proliferation—the rest is history—witness the scientific content of this conference.

In regard to the possible interaction of β burns and total-body irradiation on the risk for the development of skin cancer in the Marshallese, Dr. Cronkite along with Drs. Victor Bond and Claire Shellabarger, started an experiment where female Sprague-Dawley rats received total-body irradiation and/or β irradiation of the skin. It turned out that the β sources were calibrated incorrectly and only a trivial amount of β dose was delivered to the skin. However, the rats that received total-body irradiation, either 200 or 400 R, began to develop subcutaneous tumors on the ventral surface some 60-90 days after exposure. With the help of Dr. Stuart Lippincott, it was soon shown that these tumors were of mammary gland origin. The incidence of rats with mammary neoplasms increased to approximately 60% at 11 months after starting the experiment, while no mammary neoplasms developed in nonirradiated rats. It was soon recognized that this experimental system could be used to study radiation-induced mammary carcinogenesis[19] and, indeed, many investigators did and still do use this rat model system.

The above account shows another example of serendipity at work.

REFERENCES

1. ALPEN, E. 1977. National Biomedical Heavy-Ion Research Program at the BEVALAC. *In* Biological and Medical Research with Accelerated Heavy Ions at the BEVALAC 1974-1977. Pp. 13-25. Lawrence Berkeley Laboratory Report LBL-5610. University of California. Berkeley, Calif. (Available from National Technical Information Service, Springfield, Va. 22161.)
2. TOBIAS, C. A., E. V. BENTON & M. P. CAPP. 1977. Heavy-ion radiography. *In* Biological and Medical Research with Accelerated Heavy Ions at the BEVALAC 1974-1977. Pp.

164-186. Lawrence Berkeley Laboratory Report LBL-5610. University of California. Berkeley, Calif. (Available from National Technical Information Service, Springfield, Va. 22161.)

3. McGREGOR, D. H., C. E. LAND, K. CHOI, S. TOKUOKA, P. I. LIU, T. WAKABAYASHI & G. W. BEEBE. 1977. Breast cancer incidence among atomic bomb survivors, Hiroshima and Nagasaki. J. Natl. Cancer Inst. **59:** 799-811.

4. SHORE, R. E., L. H. HEMPLMANN, E. KOWALUK, P. S. MANSUR, B. S. PASTERNAC, R. E. ALBERT & G. E. HAUGIE. 1977. Breast neoplasms in women treated with X-rays for acute postpartum mastitis. J. Natl. Cancer Inst. **59:** 813-822.

5. BOICE, J. D., JR. & R. R. MONSON. 1977. Breast cancer in women after repeated fluorescopic examinations of the chest. J. Natl. Cancer Inst. **59:** 823-832.

6. BOND, V. P., C. J. SHELLABARGER, E. P. CRONKITE & T. FLIEDNER. 1960. Studies on radiation-induced mammary gland neoplasia in the rat. V. Induction by localized radiation. Radiat. Res. **13:** 318-328.

7. MACKENZIE, I. 1965. Breast cancer following multiple fluoroscopies. Br. J. Cancer **19:** 1-8.

8. LYMAN, J. T. & J. HOWARD. 1977. Biomedical research facilities and dosimetry. *In* Biological and Medical Research with Accelerated Heavy Ions at the BEVALAC 1974-1977. Pp. 26-35. Lawrence Berkeley Laboratory Report LBL-5610. Univesity of California. Berkeley, Calif. (Available from National Technical Information Service, Springfield, Va. (22161.)

9. YOUNG, S. & R. C. HALLOWES. 1973. Tumors of the mammary gland. *In* Pathology of Tumors in Laboratory Animals. Vol. 1, Tumors of the Rat. V. S. Tursov, Ed. IACR Scientific Publication No. 5. International Agency for Cancer Research. Lyons, France.

10. HOLTZMAN, S., J. P. STONE & C. J. SHELLABARGER. 1979. Synergism of diethylstilbestrol and radiation in mammary carcinogenesis in female F344 rats. J. Natl. Cancer Inst. **63:** 1071-1074.

11. PETO, R., M. C. PIKE, N. E. DAY, R. G. GRAY, P. N. LEE, S. PARISH, J. PETO, S. RICHARDS & J. WAHRENDORF. 1980. Guidelines for simple, sensitive significance tests for carcinogenic effects in long-term animal experiments. *In* International Agency for Cancer Research. Supplement 2: 311-426. Lyons, France.

12. CLIFTON, K. H. & J. CROWLEY. 1978. Effects of radiation type and dose and the role of glucocorticoids, gonadectomy, and thyroidectomy in mammary tumor induction in mammotropin-secreting pituitary tumor-grafted rats. Cancer Res. **38:** 1507-1513.

13. SHELLABARGER, C. J., D. CHMELEVSKY & A. M. KELLERER. 1980. Induction of mammary neoplasms in the Sprague-Dawley rat by 430 keV neutrons and X-rays. J. Natl. Cancer Inst. **64:** 821-833.

14. VOGEL, H. H., JR. 1969. Mammary gland neutron irradiation. Nature **222:** 1279-1289.

15. CLIFTON, K. H., E. B. DOUPLE & B. N. SRIDHARAN. 1976. Effects of grafts of single anterior pituitary glands on the incidence and type of mammary neoplasms in neutron- or gamma-irradiated Fischer female rats. Cancer Res. **36:** 3732-3735.

16. MONTOUR, J. L., R. C. HARD & R. E. FLORA. 1977. Mammary neoplasia in the rat following high-energy neutron irradiation. Cancer Res. **37:** 2619-2623.

17. BROERSE, J. J., S. KNAAN, D. W. VAN BEKKUM, A. L. NOOTEBOOM & C. F. HOLLANDER. 1977. Incidence of mammary tumors in rats of different strains after fast neutron irradiation. Int. J. Radiat. Biol. **31:** 378-379.

18. YOKORO, K., M. NAKANO, A. ITO, K. NAGO, Y. KADAMA & K. HAMADA. 1977. Role of prolactin in rat mammary carcinogenesis: detection of carcinogenicity of low-dose carcinogens and persisting dormant cancer cells. J. Natl. Cancer Inst. **58:** 1777-1783.

19. SHELLABARGER, C. J., E. P. CRONKITE, V. P. BOND & S. W. LIPPINCOTT. 1957. The occurrence of mammary tumors in the rat after sublethal whole-body irradiation. Radiat. Res. **6:** 501-512.

Role of DNA Polymerase α in Chromosomal Aberration Production by Ionizing Radiation[a]

MICHAEL A BENDER

Medical Department
Brookhaven National Laboratory
Upton, New York 11973

INTRODUCTION

Aphidicolin is a tetracyclic diterpenoid fungal antibiotic which inhibits DNA synthesis in eucaryotic cells by interfering specifically with DNA polymerase α, but not polymerases β or γ.[1] It appears that aphidicolin inhibits by binding to and inactivating the DNA-polymerase α complex.[2] We have shown that aphidicolin, like other inhibitors of DNA synthesis, both induces chromosomal aberrations in human peripheral lymphocytes and, as a post-treatment, interacts synergistically with X rays to produce greatly enhanced aberration yields.[3] Because DNA polymerase α is the only DNA-synthetic or repair enzyme known to be affected by aphidicolin, we infer that this enzyme is directly involved in the repair of DNA lesions which, if unrepaired, can result in visible chromosomal aberrations.

The present experiments were undertaken to further explore the effects of aphidicolin in human lymphocytes in the post-DNA-synthetic G_2 phase of the cell cycle. Earlier experiments in which cells were simply fixed at times after treatment when the frequency of metaphases in the DNA-synthetic S phase of the cell cycle is zero in typical percentage labeled mitoses curves for human lymphocytes did not completely rule out the possibility that the aberrations induced by aphidicolin actually arose in a small subpopulation of cells actually in the S phase, and not in G_2 cells. Furthermore, the yield of X-ray-induced aberrations in G_2 cells falls rapidly as a function of increasing irradiation-fixation interval,[4] so comparisons of yields at particular fixation times can be misleading if the cells in each group do not progress through G_2 at the same rate. The experiments reported here utilized labeling with tritiated thymidine to positively identify cells in the S phase at the time of treatment and serial Colcemid collections and fixations to determine aberration yields over as much of the G_2 phase as feasible.

[a] Work supported by Contract DE-AC02-76CH00016 with the U.S. Department of Energy. Accordingly, the U.S. Government retains a nonexclusive, royalty-free license to publish or reproduce the published form of this contribution, or allow others to do so, for U.S. Government purposes.

MATERIALS AND METHODS

Lymphocyte Culture

Sterile, heparinized blood samples were obtained from normal, healthy, adult volunteers. Whole blood was inoculated into 10 ml of RPMI 1640 (GIBCO) containing 15% fetal calf serum in a quantity sufficient to give 5×10^6 leukocytes per culture, based upon prior cell counts. Cultures were incubated at 37°C in 15-ml screw-capped conical plastic centrifuge tubes following addition of 0.25 ml of phytohemagglutinin (GIBCO). They were incubated for 72 hr prior to treatment. Colcemid was added, $1\frac{1}{2}$ hr prior to fixation, to a level of 0.1 μg/ml.

Aphidicolin

The drug was the generous gift of Dr. A. H. Todd of Imperial Chemical Industries, Ltd., Macclesfield, Cheshire, England. It was dissolved in dimethyl sulfoxide (DMSO) to give a 5×10^{-2} M stock solution which was stored at -20°C. It was added to treated cultures to give a final concentration of 5×10^{-5} M. The dimethyl sulfoxide concentration in cultures was thus 0.1%, and all controls also had solvent added to this level. The drug or solvent was added immediately after the X-ray treatments and allowed to remain while the culture was reincubated for the indicated treatment times (see Experiments section). If the drug or solvent was removed, this was done by aspiration of the supernate from centrifuged cultures, followed by two washes with prewarmed medium. All procedures were carried out in a warmroom at 37°C to avoid temperature-induced effects on progression through the cell cycle.

Labeling

Immediately before treatment tritiated thymidine ([*methyl*-³H]thymidine; 2 Ci/ mM; Amersham) was added to the cultures to a level of 1 μCi/ml in order to tag S-phase cells. The label was allowed to remain until the drug or solvent was washed out (or until fixation).

X Irradiation

Cultures were irradiated with a General Electric Maxitron operated at 250 kVp with 1.0 mm Al and 0.5 mm Cu added filtration. The exposure rate was approximately 100 R/min. Irradiations were done at room temperature, though the cultures were removed from incubation immediately before irradiation and returned immediately after, and so probably did not cool very much during irradiation.

Experiments

Two types of experiment were done. In the first, an X-ray exposure of 100 R was used and the aphidicolin or solvent remained until the time of fixation. Colcemid was added either immediately after irradiation and/or drug addition, or after 1.5, 3, 4.5, or 6 hr, and the cultures were fixed 1.5 hr later at 1.5, 3, 4.5, 6, and 7.5 hr, respectively. Thus mitoses were collected through successive 1.5-hr "windows" yielding samples of cells treated at successively earlier stages, with successively longer and longer aphidicolin post-treatment times.

The second type of experiment was carried out according to the same general plan, except that the aphidicolin or solvent was washed out of the cultures fixed at 3 hr and later after 1.5 hr of post-treatment time (e.g., immediately prior to addition of Colcemid to the cultures to be fixed at 3 hr). Thus successive 1.5-hr "windows" were again sampled, but this time following a constant 1.5-hr post-treatment immediately following X irradiation.

Fixation and Slide Preparation

Cultures were treated for 15 min in 75 mM KCl, fixed in 3:1 methanol:acetic acid, washed twice with fresh fixative, spread on the surfaces of clean wet slides, and air dried. They were then dipped in Kodak NTB emulsion diluted 1:1 with distilled water, dried, and stored for approximately 2 weeks exposure time in lightproof boxes at 4°C. Autoradiographs were developed in D-19 developer (Kodak), fixed, and subsequently stained with 5% Giemsa in phosphate citrate buffer at pH 5.75 for 20-30 min. Metaphases were scored for presence or absence of label, and unlabeled mitoses with 44-46 chromosomes were scored for chromosomal aberrations according to conventional criteria.

RESULTS

Continuous Post-treatment

Two separate experiments involving a total of three subjects were done. As no significant differences were seen between them, all results have been pooled over all three donors. The X-ray dose was 100 R. Percentages of labeled mitoses were ascertained on 200 metaphase samples for each treatment at each time point. No labeled mitoses were seen at 1.5 hr. For the solvent control the 50%-labeled point was at 3.0 hr, while the X-ray-plus-solvent-treated cells reached the 50% point somewhat later at about 4.5 hr. Naturally, neither of the aphidicolin-treated cultures showed any labeled metaphases at any fixation time. Unexpectedly, however, though metaphases were plentiful in cultures treated with aphidicolin alone or with X rays alone, the 3-hr cultures given both X rays and aphidicolin from all three donors contained very few mitoses, and by 4.5 hr none of the cultures from any donor contained more than an odd mitosis here and there with the later fixations containing none at all.

The pooled results for aberrations at 1.5 hr scored in 150 metaphases per donor per point are shown in TABLE 1, and are typical of our earlier results.[3] Only chromatid aberrations, mainly achromatic lesions and chromatid deletions, were seen. Their frequency was significantly, if not dramatically, increased by aphidicolin alone. The yield for the combined treatment was greater than the sum of the yields for X rays alone and aphidicolin alone; 2.5 times in the case of achromatic lesions and over 4 times in the case of chromatid deletions. Just as in our earlier experiments, though X rays alone induced some chromatid exchanges, none at all were seen in aphidicolin-treated cultures.

Because of the paucity of mitoses in the 3-hr X-ray-plus-aphidicolin cultures, it was possible to score only a total of 170 mitoses on the slides from all three donors. Scoring of mitoses from samples treated with aphidicolin alone and X rays alone was accordingly limited to an arbitrary total of 250 cells distributed among donors in approximately the same way as the metaphases from the combined treatment. Despite the smaller samples, the pooled data for the 3-hr fixation still show a dramatic effect. As expected, the frequencies of aberrations in the 3-hr cultures treated with X rays alone are substantially lower than those for the first collection interval, while those in the cultures treated with aphidicolin alone are significantly increased. The excesses over additivity for the combined treatment are fivefold for achromatic lesions and ninefold for deletions, or about twice as much as in the 1.5-hr samples.

Limited Post-treatment

Only one experiment involving blood samples from two different donors has been done. This time, to try to minimize induced delay, an X-ray dose of 50 R was used. Again, because there were no significant differences in the results for the two donors they have been pooled for presentation here. FIGURE 1 shows the percentages of labeled mitoses in graphic form. As expected, removal of the aphidicolin did allow labeled mitoses to appear eventually, though it will be seen that the 50%-labeled-mitoses point is still reached at successively later sampling intervals according to treatment (in the solvent control cultures again by about 3 hr, in the X-irradiated cultures perhaps an hour later at about 4 hr, and in the aphidicolin-treated cultures by about 6 hr), while the cultures receiving the combined treatment never achieved more than 30% labeling of their mitoses.

The pooled results for chromosomal aberrations are shown in TABLE 2. An attempt was made to score 100 metaphases per donor per point, but as may be seen this was not always achieved, particularly for the later times. This was caused by a paucity of mitoses in general and particularly of the required unlabeled mitoses for the less drastic treatments in later collection intervals. Despite the lower X-ray exposure, the combined treatment still resulted in a substantial increase in chromatid deletions over additivity at 1.5 hr, though not much effect is still apparent for achromatic lesions.

Aberration frequencies as a function of sampling time are shown graphically in FIGURE 2. As is commonly seen, the samples treated with X rays alone show a rapid decrease with time in aberration frequencies, a decrease approximating an exponential decay curve. Clearly, however, the situation is more complex with the combined treatment. It is immediately apparent that the synergistic effect for chromatid deletions has completely disappeared after the first 1.5-hr collection interval; indeed, it appears significantly reversed in the 3.0- and 4.5-hr samples. In a somewhat similar fashion, achromatic-lesion frequencies, comparable in the 1.5-hr samples, are significantly

TABLE 1. Aberration Frequencies (per Cell) in Human Lymphocytes Given 100 R of X Rays followed by Post-treatment with 5 × 10⁻⁵ M Aphidicolin

Fixation (Post-treatment) Time (hr)	Treatment	Cells Scored	Achromatic Lesions	Chromatid Deletions	Isochromatid Deletions	Chromatid Exchanges
	Control	450	0.05 ± 0.01	0.01 ± 0.01	0.01 ± 0.01	0
1.5	Aphidicolin	450	0.13 ± 0.02	0.09 ± 0.01	0.01 ± 0.01	0
	X rays	450	1.18 ± 0.05	0.95 ± 0.05	0.05 ± 0.01	0.09 ± 0.01
	X rays + aphidicolin	450	3.30 ± 0.09	4.43 ± 0.10	0.12 ± 0.02	0
3.0	Aphidicolin	250	0.33 ± 0.04	0.38 ± 0.04	0.06 ± 0.02	0
	X rays	250	0.26 ± 0.03	0.16 ± 0.03	0.01 ± 0.01	0.01 ± 0.01
	X rays + aphidicolin	170	2.94 ± 0.13	4.89 ± 0.17	0.14 ± 0.03	0

depressed in the 3.0- and 4.5-hr samples. Interestingly, the trend for both aberration categories is toward increased yield for the combined treatment in the latest collection intervals. Had we sampled even later, we might have seen a return to a synergistic effect as is suggested by the curves drawn through the data points in FIGURE 2.

DISCUSSION

These experiments confirm our earlier observations[3] that aphidicolin induces aberrations in G_2 lymphocytes, that post-treatment with aphidicolin results in a large synergistic increase in the production of chromosomal aberrations in lymphocytes X-irradiated during the latter portion of the G_2 phase of the cell cycle, and that exchanges do not occur in the presence of aphidicolin. Dr. R. C. Moore and I have recently studied the effect of various concentrations of aphidicolin on normal "semi-conservative" DNA synthesis in human lymphocytes and in several experiments found it to decrease exponentially (as measured by scintillation counting after exposure of the cells to tritiated thymidine) over several decades of concentration, with minimal effect at about 5×10^{-6} M and 99% inhibition at about 10^{-3} M (unpublished data). At the concentration used in the present experiments, DNA synthesis is about 80% inhibited as measured this way. We have found in addition (also unpublished) that both aberration induction by aphidicolin alone and the synergistic increase in aberration induction by X rays are linear functions of aphidicolin concentration over the same range. As we speculated earlier, the conclusion that these effects result from

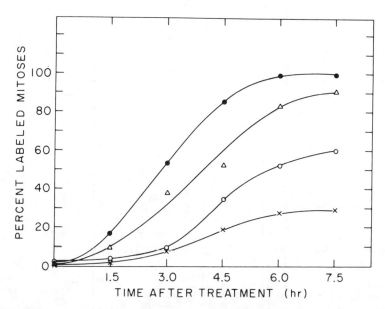

FIGURE 1. Percentage labeled mitoses curves for G_2 human lymphocytes treated with 5×10^{-5} M aphidicolin for 1.5 hr ($\circ$), 50 R of X rays ($\triangle$), or 50 R of X rays followed by 5×10^{-5} M aphidicolin for 1.5 hr ($\times$) and collected over successive 1.5-hr intervals. See text for details. $\bullet$, Solvent control.

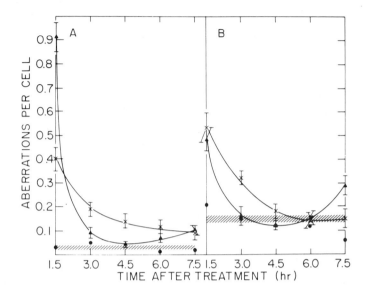

FIGURE 2. Frequencies of chromosomal aberrations in metaphases of G_2 human lymphocytes treated with 5×10^{-5} M aphidicolin for 1.5 hr (●), 50 R of X rays (×), or 50 R of X rays followed by 5×10^{-5} M aphidicolin for 1.5 hr (▲) and collected over successive 1.5-hr intervals. See text for details. Hatched area, mean plus or minus Poisson error of individual values for cells treated with aphidicolin alone. (A) Chromatid aberrations except achromatic lesions. (B) Achromatic lesions.

inhibition of some sort of DNA repair process seems inescapable. Though inhibition of more than one enzyme cannot be ruled out, it seems not unlikely that polymerase α functions as a repair enzyme as well as in normal DNA synthesis. Because only unlabeled mitoses were scored in the present experiments, the cells in which aberrations were induced by aphidicolin alone had, insofar as it is possible to determine, completed their S phase. Thus the mechanism seems most likely to involve inhibition of either some "final assembly" or some "maintenance" function in which too few bases are inserted to be detected autoradiographically.

The rationale of the present experiments lies in the need to determine aberration yields in G_2 cells over a sufficiently long sampling interval to ensure that most of the cells actually in G_2 in the treated population are included in the sample before concluding that two treatments (or two types of cell) generate different responses. This is of course because shifts in the normal progression of cells to metaphase can generate large apparent differences in yield as a consequence of sampling of cells actually in different G_2 substages, possibly of differing sensitivity, even though they arrive at metaphase simultaneously. What is needed, then, amounts to a comparison of the integral of aberration yields over all G_2 cells. Furthermore, in simple cases where aberration yields are consistently different for all sampling intervals and curve shapes are the same, it is possible to ask whether the two curves are different in slope, in intercept, or both. Such information can provide insight into mechanism; for example, a difference in intercept might imply a different number of lesions induced initially, while a difference in slope might imply that lesions are repaired at different rates. We have recently used this approach successfully to explore the G_2 chromosomal radiosensitivity of lymphocytes from persons affected with ataxia telangiectasia.[5]

TABLE 2. Aberration Frequencies in Human Lymphocytes Given 50 R of X Rays followed by a 1.5-hr Post-treatment with 5×10^{-5} M Aphidicolin or Solvent (DMSO) Alone and Fixed at 1.5-hr Intervals

Fixation Time (hr)	Treatment	Cells Scored	Achromatic Lesions	Chromatid Deletions	Isochromatid Deletions	Chromatid Exchanges	Percentage Labeled Mitoses
1.5	Solvent control	200	8	1	0	0	16.5
	Aphidicolin	200	42	4	2	0	4.0
	X rays	161	85	57	7	1	9.0
	X rays + aphidicolin	185	88	142	24	2	2.0
3.0	Solvent control	200	9	3	1	0	53.5
	Aphidicolin	200	30	6	3	0	9.5
	X rays	170	55	18	14	0	47.5
	X rays + aphidicolin	200	31	16	2	0	7.5
4.5	Solvent control	124	2	1	0	0	85.0
	Aphidicolin	161	19	5	0	0	34.5
	X rays	200	36	18	7	2	52.5
	X rays + aphidicolin	200	23	5	3	0	14.5
6.0	Solvent control	100	6	2	0	0	99.0
	Aphidicolin	106	12	1	1	0	52.0
	X rays	140	20	9	6	2	83.0
	X rays + aphidicolin	200	30	8	4	1	28.0
7.5	Solvent control	20	0	0	0	1	99.0
	Aphidicolin	53	3	1	0	0	59.5
	X rays	109	16	9	0	1	91.5
	X rays + aphidicolin	200	58	9	8	2	29.0

The apparent failure of a limited aphidicolin post-treatment to interact synergistically with X irradiation in metaphases collected over intervals when it is no longer present, as in the experiment shown in TABLE 2 and FIGURE 2, is difficult to interpret. Since the experiment was only carried out once, it will naturally have to be repeated before final conclusions are drawn. Nevertheless, the data from the two donors were consistent and those for successive collection intervals appeared to conform well to smooth curves; thus the data seem unlikely to represent a simply capricious result. A more significant problem lies in the fact that the percentages of labeled mitoses in samples of aphidicolin-treated cells never reached the high levels that would suggest that most of the G_2 cells had been sampled (FIGURE 1). For cells treated with aphidicolin alone this does not appear to constitute a real problem, as aberration yields are low and do not appear to change in any consistent way from the earliest to the latest collection interval. For the combined treatment, however, not only did the percentage of labeled cells never exceed about 30%, implying that the experiment may have failed to sample a large cohort of G_2 cells, but the aberration yield appeared to be increasing again during the last two collection intervals after reaching a nadir during the 3.0- to 4.5-hr interval.

Integrating crudely by simply adding up all the aberration yields for all sampling periods from TABLE 2, there is no difference between the overall yields of aberrations in the samples given X rays alone and those given X rays plus aphidicolin (for total aberrations the frequencies of aberrations per cell are 0.47 and 0.46, respectively). It might thus be concluded that aphidicolin is not really increasing the yield of X-ray-induced aberrations at all, but rather somehow causing those cells with aberrations to reach metaphase earlier. On the other hand, in light of the important role of DNA repair systems in the production of chromosomal aberrations,[5,6] it is difficult to discard the idea that the effect is a real one influencing the efficacy with which radiation-induced damage to DNA is repaired. Nevertheless, a definite conclusion must await additional data, particularly for later collection intervals for the combined treatment.

The failure of X-irradiated cells treated continuously with aphidicolin to continue to arrive at metaphase after the first few hours as seen in the experiments summarized in TABLE 1 strongly suggests that the cells irradiated early in G_2 are for some reason prevented from progression through the cell cycle in the absence of polymerase α function. This is clearly not true, or at least not to the same extent, without the prior X irradiation, so whatever block there is would seem to involve unrepaired X-ray damage.

ACKNOWLEDGMENTS

I would like to thank Dr. A. H. Todd and Imperial Chemical Industries, Ltd. for the gift of aphidicolin and Mrs. Beatrice E. Pyatt, Miss Maureen M. Mulcox, and Mr. Michael S. Makar for expert technical assistance.

REFERENCES

1. IKEGAMI, S., T. TAGUCHI, M. OHASHI, M. OGURO, H. NAGAO & Y. MANO. 1978. Aphidicolin prevents mitotic cell division by interfering with the activity of DNA polymerase-α. Nature (London) 275: 458-460.

2. HUBERMAN, J. A. 1981. New views on the biochemistry of eucaryotic DNA replication revealed by aphidicolin, an unusual inhibitor of DNA polymerase α. Cell **23:** 647-648.
3. BENDER, M. A & R. J. PRESTON. 1982. Role of base damage in aberration formation: interaction of aphidicolin and X-rays. Prog. Mutat. Res. **4:** 37-46.
4. SCOTT, D. & H. J. EVANS. 1967. X-Ray-induced chromosomal aberrations in *Vicia faba*: changes in response during the cell cycle. Mutat. Res. **4:** 579-599.
5. BENDER, M. A, J. M. RARY & R. P. KALE. 1985. G_2 chromosomal radiosensitivity in ataxia telangiectasia lymphocytes. Mutat. Res. **152:** 39-47.
6. BENDER, M. A. 1980. Relationship of DNA lesions and their repair to chromosomal production. *In* DNA Repair and Mutagenesis in Eukaryotes. W. M. Generoso, M. D. Shelby & F. J. deSerres, Eds.: 245-265. Plenum Publishing Corp. New York, N.Y.

Oncogenic Effects of Ionizing Radiation[a]

LUDWIK GROSS

Cancer Research Unit
Veterans Administration Medical Center
Bronx, New York 10468

In our experimental studies we observed that following total-body irradiation (150 to 200 R, four times, at weekly intervals, applied to 6- to 8-week-old mice of the C3H strain) 56 out of 116 mice developed leukemia at $8\frac{1}{2}$ months average age and 2 mice developed multicentric parotid gland carcinomas when 6 to 7 months old. None of the 93 untreated controls developed either leukemia or salivary gland tumors.[1]

On the other hand, we have demonstrated in a more recent study[2] that similar exposure of rats, instead of mice, to total-body γ irradiation increased significantly the incidence of solid tumors, such as mammary or ovarian carcinomas, or subcutaneous sarcomas, but it did not increase, to any significant degree, the incidence of leukemia or lymphomas. In an experiment carried out on Sprague-Dawley rats,[b] the incidence of tumors, mostly of the mammary glands (50% of which were carcinomas), increased, following irradiation, from 22 to 93% in females and from 5 to 59% in males. In a similar experiment carried out on Long-Evans rats,[b] the incidence of tumors increased, following irradiation, from 28 to 63% in females and from 10 to 42% in males. There was no significant increase in the incidence of leukemia or lymphomas.

It was reported by Caldwell and his colleagues[3] that military personnel who participated, in 1957, in a nuclear test called "Shot Smoky," developed subsequently a statistically significant increase in the incidence of, and mortality from, leukemia. The implications of this study have now been apparently diminished by the conclusions reached in a more recent study, carried out by the same investigators,[4] pointing out that over a 22-year period there has been no significant increase in other kinds of cancer among the nuclear test participants. On the basis of this finding, the existence of a causal relation between radiation exposure and the increased incidence of leukemia in the "Shot Smoky" participants was questioned, since, according to the authors, presumably not only leukemia, but other tumors also would have developed in persons exposed to ionizing radiation, if radiation exposure was the causative factor.

[a] Supported by the Veterans Administration Research Service, and grants from the American Cancer Society (#RD-183) and the Cancer Research Institute, New York.

[b] Sprague-Dawley and Long-Evans rats were bred in our laboratory by brother-to-sister mating for 19 and 14 years, respectively, prior to their use in this study.[2]

Of particular interest is the fact that in another study of survivors of an atomic bomb explosion, there was a fivefold increase of salivary gland tumors as compared with unexposed controls.[5]

Salivary gland tumors are very rare in humans. They are exceedingly rare in mice. However, they can be readily induced in mice by total-body X-ray irradiation.

Salivary gland tumors are caused in mice by a small DNA virus, the polyoma virus.[6] Apparently, the virus becomes activated following irradiation. This may explain the development of tumors in two of our irradiated mice (for details of our study see Reference 1); none developed in unexposed controls.

The presence of such viruses in either spontaneous or radiation-induced mouse leukemia is not surprising. In a large number of different animal species, the majority of tumors and lymphomas was found to be caused by transmissible oncogenic viruses. It is true that in certain animal species, such as dogs and rats, it has been thus far very difficult to demonstrate the presence of viruses in spontaneous tumors or lymphomas. This is also true for the majority of human tumors and human lymphomas, in which the presence of hypothetical oncogenic viruses has not yet been documented; among the few exceptions to this rule are the recent studies on human HTLV-I virus, isolated by Gallo and his co-workers,[7] and the hepatitis B virus, which causes hepatocellular carcinomas[8] (for review, see Gross[9]).

The possibility should be considered that oncogenic viruses, similar to those observed in animals, may also be responsible for the development of either spontaneous or induced tumors and lymphomas in humans, as well as in those animal species in which their presence has not yet been documented. Some of these oncogenic viruses may be integrated in the genome of the tumor cells and may not be readily detected by electron microscopic examination or by routine attempts of transmission by filtrates. Immunological tests, molecular biology techniques, and other more sophisticated methods than those previously employed, may have to be used in order to demonstrate their presence.

Essentially, therefore, "genetic susceptibility" to the development of tumors or leukemia may be actually related, in animals as well as in humans, to the presence or absence of oncogenic viruses in the hosts. This may explain the selective oncogenic effects of ionizing radiation.

REFERENCES

1. GROSS, L. 1958. Attempt to recover filterable agent from X-ray-induced leukemia. Acta Haematol. **19:** 353-361.
2. GROSS, L. & Y. DREYFUSS. 1979. Spontaneous tumors in Sprague-Dawley and Long-Evans rats and in their F_1 hybrids: carcinogenic effect of total-body X-irradiation. Proc. Natl. Acad. Sci. USA **76:** 5910-5913.
3. CALDWELL, G. G., D. B. KELLEY & C. W. HEATH, JR. 1980. Leukemia among participants in military maneuvers at a nuclear bomb test. A preliminary report. J. Am. Med. Assoc. **244:** 1575-1578.
4. CALDWELL, G. G., D. KELLEY, M. ZACK, H. FALK & C. W. HEATH, JR. 1983. Mortality and cancer frequency among military nuclear test (Smoky) participants, 1957 through 1979. J. Am. Med. Assoc. **250:** 620-624.
5. BELSKY, J. L., K. TACHIKAWA, R. W. CIHAK & T. YAMAMOTO. 1972. Salivary gland tumors in atomic bomb survivors, Hiroshima-Nagasaki, 1957 to 1970. J. Am. Med. Assoc. **219:** 864-868.

6. GROSS, L. 1976. The fortuitous isolation and identification of the polyoma virus. Cancer Res. **36:** 4195-4196.
7. POIESZ, B. J., F. W. RUSCETTI, A. F. GAZDAR, P. A. BUNN, J. D. MINNA & R. C. GALLO. 1980. Detection and isolation of type C retrovirus particles from fresh and cultured lymphocytes of a patient with cutaneous T-cell lymphoma. Proc. Natl. Acad. Sci. USA **77:** 7415-7419.
8. BEASLEY, R. P., L.-Y. HWANG & C.-C. LIN. 1981. Hepatocellular carcinoma and hepatitis B virus: a prospective study of 22,707 men in Taiwan. Lancet **2:** 1129-1133.
9. GROSS, L. 1983. Oncogenic Viruses. 3rd edit. Pergamon Press. Oxford, England.

The Tritium Toxicity Program in the Medical Department at Brookhaven National Laboratory[a]

ARLAND L. CARSTEN

Medical Research Center
Brookhaven National Laboratory
Upton, New York 11973

INTRODUCTION

It is most apropos that during this symposium honoring Dr. E. P. Cronkite that some brief mention be made of the tritium toxicity (TRITOX) program which developed at Brookhaven National Laboratory during his chairmanship of the Medical Department. In addition to being a staunch supporter of the TRITOX program, and an active participant in its planning, Dr. Cronkite served on the NCRP Committee[1] which addressed directly the problem of the possible genetic hazards to man from tritium compounds.

The development of the TRITOX program as related to worldwide fission and fusion energy programs has been previously reviewed[2,3] and it should suffice to say that the world is becoming more dependent upon nuclear energy as a source of electric power and with this reliance comes the possibility of introducing into the environment increasing amounts of tritiated water (HTO).

The initial concept in establishing this program, which began in 1971 and is still active today, was to examine primarily one particular question: "What might be the genetic hazard (as measured by the dominant lethal mutation test) of continued exposure to tritiated water (HTO) at levels approximately 100 times the maximum permissible concentration (3.0 μCi/ml)?" In order to answer this question, it was necessary to establish a rather large monitored tritium facility and a mouse colony for breeding and maintaining a large number of animals on the HTO regimen. It also became evident that there were many unanswered questions concerning the many possible effects of HTO ingestion. Therefore, over the ensuing years a multiparameter examination of somatic, genetic, and cytogenetic effects, as well as questions related to biochemistry and dosimetry resulting from continuous maintenance on an HTO regimen, was undertaken. Since much of the information obtained from this program has been published already,[4-12] only a brief summary of the program, which is outlined in TABLE 1, will be presented at this time.

[a] This work was sponsored in part by the National Cancer Institute, National Institutes of Health and the U.S. Department of Energy under Contract DE-AC02-76CH00016.

MATERIALS AND METHODS

Mice Breeding and Maintenance

With the exception of studies on induction of leukemia, all animals used in these studies were of the Hale-Stoner-Brookhaven (HSB) strain. This is an albino strain which has been maintained in a single colony for more than 20 years in the Medical Department of Brookhaven National Laboratory. The food used is Purina Laboratory Chow (Ralston Purina Co., St. Louis, Mo.). Animals receive this regimen *ad libitum* and tap water acidified to pH 2.4. Breeding partners are established by random selection

TABLE 1. Outline of Brookhaven Tritium Toxicity Program

GENETIC AND REPRODUCTIVE EFFICIENCY
- Dominant Lethal Mutation Rate
- Cytogenetic Studies
- Examination of Ova and Early Embryos

SOMATIC EFFECTS
- Growth (Body Weight)
- Nonspecific Lifetime Shortening
- Bone Marrow Cellularity and CFU-S Content

RELATIVE BIOLOGICAL EFFECTIVENESS (RBE)
- Comparison of HTO and ^{137}Cs Effects

BIOCHEMISTRY AND MICRODOSIMETRY STUDIES
- Rate of Tritium Incorporation
- Site of Tritium Incorporation
- Rate of Tritium Disappearance
- Histone and DNA Turnover Studies
- Cellular Turnover Studies

CARCINOGENESIS
- Induction of Leukemia

---

from animals born during the same week without attention to littermate selection. These animals remain together throughout their reproductive lifetime. To reduce possible litter variation, only first-litter animals from each breeding pair were used for the TRITOX studies.

At 4 weeks of age, animals were removed from the mouse colony and divided into experimental groups. Depending upon the studies involved, the animals were maintained on HTO concentrations ranging from 0.3 to 30.0 μCi/ml HTO or acidified tap water. For long-term studies, half of the control animals were maintained in the tritium facility while the other half were removed to a similar room which contained only mice maintained on tap water. (This was to determine whether animals maintained on tap water in the tritium room as controls would receive a significant inhalation exposure to HTO due to air contamination.) When the first-generation animals reached 8 weeks of age, breedings were done within the various experimental groups resulting in second-generation animals who, together with their parents, had been maintained on either HTO or tap water. Groups of male and female animals from both HTO and control groups were then maintained for long-term observation. From these larger groups, 20 male and 20 female animals were randomly selected and put aside for monthly weighing. At the time of weighing these animals were closely examined for any apparent differences in appearance. The specific methods for other determinations will be discussed separately.

Genetic, Cytogenetic, and Reproductive Efficiency Studies

Dominant Lethal Mutation (DLM) Rate Studies

When second-generation animals assigned to the study reached 8 weeks of age they were divided into four groups for DLM testing.[13] The four groups were as follows: Group 1—males and females maintained on HTO; Group 2—females on HTO, males on tap water; Group 3—males on HTO, females on tap water; Group 4—males and females on tap water (controls). Breeding groups were arranged with one male placed with five females for a 5-day breeding period. Fifteen days after the midpoint of this breeding period, the females were sacrificed, the number of pregnant females was noted, and the ovaries and uterine contents were examined. Ovaries were evaluated for the number of corpora lutea (CL) and the uterine contents were classified as to number of viable embryos (VIA), early embryonic deaths (ED), and late embryonic deaths (LD). Early embryonic deaths were characterized by a dark "mole" or re-sorption site interpreted as death occurring between implantation and approximately 10 days, whereas late embryonic deaths were characterized by a formed but dead embryo. From the four parameters measured, CL, ED, LD, and VIA, the preimplantation loss (PRE) from each mating was calculated:

$$PRE = CL - (VIA + ED + LD).$$

New breeding groups were started each week so that a continuing program of data accumulation took place in all four experimental groups, thus allowing for the detection of possible temporal shifts in the colony.

The results of the DLM evaluations were compared using three statistical tests: (1) Student's t test,[14] a parametric test which assumes normal distribution of the data. In these evaluations, the analysis makes use of the pooled errors of all groups. (2) The rank test developed by Kruskal and Wallis.[15] This is a nonparametric test described as being applicable for a complete random design with any number of populations in which the final analysis is made using a χ^2 test. (3) The final statistical test involves an arcsine transformation which normalizes the data and computes the mutation index for each treatment, which are compared using a χ^2 test.[16]

Cytogenetic Studies

Liver Cytogenetic Studies. In the adult mouse the liver is not a very mitotically active organ. Therefore, individual cells will tend to accumulate injury during continuous radiation exposure. This damage will become visible as chromosome aberrations (CA) when the cells are stimulated to division by partial hepatectomy. To make the CA evaluations, animals were maintained on 0.3 or 3.0 μCi/ml HTO and acidified tap water beginning at weaning and continuing until sacrifice. After approximately 90, 330, 500-560, and 700 days, the animals underwent partial hepatectomy followed after 54 hr by chromosome analysis using previously published methods.[4]

Bone Marrow Cell Evaluation for Induction of Sister Chromatid Exchanges (SECs). Before and at selected times during continuous HTO ingestion (3.0 μCi/ml) mice were evaluated for the induction of SECs in their bone marrow. Selected animals were given continuous BrdUrd infusions for 24 hr using the technique described by Schneider *et al.*[17]

Two hours prior to sacrifice by CO_2 inhalation the animals received an injection of colchicine. Bone marrow cells from the femur and tibia were harvested and evaluated for the induction of SCEs as previously described.[18]

Micronuclei Evaluation in Red Blood Cells. The induction of micronuclei in red blood cells is accepted as a sensitive measure for evaluating cytogenetic effects of various agents. Preliminary studies have been done on animals maintained on HTO (3.0, 7.5, 15.0, and 30.0 μCi/ml) for periods of 5 to 6 weeks, with ingestion begun at approximately 3 weeks of age. At the end of the ingestion period blood samples were taken and the red blood cells evaluated for micronuclei as described by Tice.[19]

Somatic Effects

Nonspecific Lifetime Shortening

Two hundred animals maintained on 3.0 μCi/ml HTO and age-matched controls were followed throughout their lifetime. Animals were examined weekly for gross changes in appearance. Cages were checked daily for deaths. Any observed changes and time of death were noted.

Growth (Body Weight)

From the animals described in the previous paragraph, 20 animals were randomly selected from each group. These animals were weighed monthly and comparisons were made between groups.

Bone Marrow Cellularity and CFU-S Content

The leg bone marrow (femur and tibia) of animals on HTO and tap water was analyzed for total cellularity, relative number of hematopoietic stem cells (CFU-S), and total number of CFU-S. Harvesting of the marrow was done using the quantitative grinding technique of Stoner and Bond.[20] The stem cell evaluation was made using the spleen colony assay as described by Till and McCulloch.[21] In this evaluation a known number of bone marrow cells are injected intravenously (i.v.) into recipient mice who had previously received a lethal (750 rad) whole-body exposure to 250-kVp X rays. After 7 days the recipients are killed, their spleens are fixed in Bouin's solution, and 24 hr later the surface colonies are counted. Details of the technique used in these studies have been previously published.[7]

Relative Biological Effectiveness (RBE) Studies

Over the years there has been considerable debate concerning the assignment of the correct RBE or "Q" for tritium exposure in the form of HTO. To examine this question, comparisons have been made between animals maintained on HTO and those receiving a continuous (22 hr/day) exposure to ^{137}Cs γ rays. The geometry of the γ-ray radiation facility was arranged so that the depth dose within the peritoneal cavity of exposed mice, as measured by implanted thermoluminescence dosimeters, was equal in dose rate to the exposure resulting from the average soft tissue dose in animals maintained on HTO for extended periods.

The measured values for tritium content of soft tissue varied depending upon water content. Taking an average value for several soft tissues, it was found that a value of 0.69 rad per day would be a reasonable estimate of soft tissue absorbed dose for animals maintained on 3.0 μCi/ml HTO. The γ-radiation facility was thus constructed so that the initial dose rate was 0.69 rad per 22-hr day at the beginning of the long-term experiments. Lifetime shortening, induction of DLMs, growth, bone marrow cellularity, CFU-S content, and induction of bone marrow SCEs were compared for the two experimental groups. Two comparative studies were made. In the first, animals received ^{137}Cs γ exposures equivalent to 3.0 μCi/ml of HTO. In the second, a smaller source was used to give a dose equivalent to the continuous ingestion of 0.3 μCi/ml of HTO.

Biochemistry and Microdosimetry Studies

Rate of Tritium Incorporation

A number of determinations were made on the radiation dose delivered to tissues of interest on an activity per gram basis and also on the basis of tritium incorporated into specific subcellular fractions. The pattern of tritium incorporation was determined by analysis of fresh tissue. Animals were sacrificed by cervical dislocation, and tissues placed immediately into weighed counting bottles containing a tissue solvent-scintillator fluid. Tissue weights were then determined and the radiation in the tissue samples was counted using a well-type scintillation counter. The total tritium content was calculated on the basis of wet tissue weight. For determinations of tritium content in subcellular constituents, techniques previously described by Commerford et al.[8] were used. Briefly, chromatin was isolated under conditions designed to minimize degradation. This involved homogenization, pelleting through 2.2 M sucrose, and extraction from nuclear fragments with EDTA followed by lyophilization and resolution in 2 M NaCl. Material obtained in this way represents a complex of DNA,

RNA, histones, and residual protein amounting to approximately 30, 3, 30, and 37%, respectively, of the total weight. These components were extracted in sequence, with the histones removed first on the basis of their solubility in 0.2 M HCl, followed by RNA which becomes acid soluble when heated 18 hr at 37°C in 0.3 M KOH,[22] and finally DNA, which becomes acid soluble when heated 30 min at 90°C in 1 M HClO₄. The remaining acid-soluble material represents residual protein. Tritium content from all fractions is determined using standard liquid scintillation techniques. All counts were corrected for background chemiluminescence.

The rate of tritium disappearance from tissue, cellular and subcellular components was determined in the same manner on animals that had been maintained on HTO for approximately 6 months followed by maintenance on acidified tap water.

Carcinogenesis (Induction of Leukemia)

A known effect of ionizing-radiation exposure in mammals is the development of leukemia. This is currently being investigated in mice of the CBA strain. This strain was chosen because it has a low incidence of spontaneous acute myelocytic leukemia and a high incidence of the same disease after irradiation. Animals have received single whole-body X-ray exposures of 50, 100, 200, or 300 rad (250 kVp, 100 rad/min) at 3 and 9 months of age. In addition, other animals have received external whole-body ¹³⁷Cs γ exposures at dose rates of 1.2 or 1.8 rad/day (5 days/week) until they have accumulated total doses of 300 rad. Additional animals have received fractionated (250-kVp X-ray) exposures (1-3 times/week) resulting in accumulated doses of 50-300 rad.

For comparison, equivalent-aged animals have received either a single injection of HTO or continuous ingestion of 3.0 μCi/ml which result in integrated whole-body doses equal to the X or γ exposures. All animals are examined daily for the first 6 months following exposure and twice daily thereafter to determine their health status. Sick animals that appear to be near death are sacrificed following peripheral blood counts (red blood cells (RBC), white blood cells (WBC), and differential). They are then autopsied and microscopic evaluation is made of the liver, kidney, lung, spleen, mesenteric lymph nodes, femoral bone marrow, and sternum, including surrounding muscle. This project is part of an overall leukemia study being done in collaboration with Dr. E. P. Cronkite.

RESULTS

Due to the relatively long history of the TRITOX program, much of the results have already been published. Therefore whenever such information is available elsewhere, only brief comments will be made with the original reference being cited.

Genetic, Cytogenetic, and Reproductive Studies

Dominant Lethal Mutation Studies

Studies have been completed on animals maintained on 3.0, 1.0, and 0.3 μCi/ml HTO together with animals exposed to equivalent doses of external γ radiation. Data for the 3.0 μCi/ml and the 1.0 μCi/ml animals have been published in References 7 and 23, respectively.

In summary, when both the male and female breeding partners are maintained on 3.0 μCi/ml, a significant reduction in viable embryos ($p < 0.0001$) and a significant increase in early deaths ($p < 0.01$) are observed. Similarly, when only the female is maintained on 3.0 μCi/ml, a significant reduction ($p < 0.01$) in viable embryos is seen.

If both breeding partners are maintained on 1.0 μCi/ml, a significant ($p < 0.01$) reduction in viable embryos is noted. In all other cases for 3.0, 1.0, or 0.3 μCi/ml, no significant effects are observed.

Cytogenetic Studies

Regenerating Liver Studies. Animals maintained on 3.0 μCi/ml HTO for 100, 330, and 500-560 days exhibited a significant increase in the number of abnormal cells in the regenerating livers as compared to animals maintained on acidified tap water. Details of this study have been previously published.[4] Similar effects were not noted in animals maintained on 0.3 μCi/ml.

Bone Marrow Cells. The SCE levels in femoral bone marrow cells of mice maintained on 3.0 μCi/ml HTO for 28 to 261 days were always higher than those in age-matched control groups. In mice drinking HTO the number of SCEs per cell ranged from 2.00 to 4.03 while comparable figures for control animals were 1.70 to 2.81. Significantly (1.0%) higher numbers of SCEs were seen in HTO animals on 81, 163, 192, 247, and 261 days after continuous ingestion of HTO. At 72, 86, and 227 days, the difference was significant at the 5% level. Using a one-way analysis of variance and covariance, the probability that the mean of all the control data is not different from that of the exposed animals is less than 0.0001. Details of this study are reported elsewhere.[18]

Micronuclei Studies in Red Blood Cells. Results of preliminary studies on the induction of micronuclei in animals maintained continuously on HTO for 5 to 6 weeks beginning at age 3 weeks indicated that there was a significant increase in micronuclei ($p < 0.01$) in animals drinking 30.0 μCi/ml HTO. A slight increase was noted in animals maintained on 15.0 μCi/ml; however, no effect was seen at 3.0 or 7.5 μCi/ml. It should be noted that these are preliminary results and the studies are being repeated.

Somatic Effects

Growth (Body Weight)

Continuous ingestion of 3.0 μCi/ml of HTO or equivalent external γ exposure caused no measurable effect on growth as measured by body weight.

Nonspecific Lifetime Shortening

Continuous ingestion of 3.0 μCi/ml of HTO or equivalent external γ exposure caused no measurable effect on nonspecific lifetime shortening. By gross appearance, it was impossible to identify the HTO, γ-ray-exposed, or control animals.

Bone Marrow Cellularity and CFU-S Content

There was no effect on the total number of leg bone marrow cells in any of the animals maintained on HTO or those receiving continuous external γ-ray exposures. In contrast, reductions in the number of bone marrow stem cells (CFU-S) were noted as early as 8-12 weeks in the 3.0 μCi/ml mice and by 24 weeks in the 1.0 μCi/ml animals. In both groups, the stem cell depression continued with some variability throughout the lifetime observation. No effect was measurable in the 0.3 μCi/ml animals, other than a somewhat greater than normal variability in the number of CFU-S per leg. Details of this study have been previously published.[7,9]

Relative Biological Effectiveness (RBE)

In all studies completed to date, there was no significant difference ($p < 0.01$) between animals ingesting HTO and animals receiving equivalent external γ-ray exposures. However, for several of the parameters measured, the effects were somewhat greater for HTO, although not significantly so. This might be interpreted as an indication that the RBE or Q value for HTO may be slightly greater than 1 but less than 2. (It should be noted that in all cases, the reference radiation must be strictly defined.)

Biochemistry and Microdosimetry Studies

When animals were placed on an HTO regimen, tritium concentrations in body water and soft tissues rapidly approached equilibrium levels.[5] When they were removed from the HTO regimen the tritium level in tissue dropped rapidly from 2.02 μCi/ml before withdrawal to 0.07, 0.01, and 0.001 μCi/ml, respectively, 7, 14, and 28 days later. The rate at which nonexchangeable tritium disappears from brain and liver histones indicates a half-life of 117 days (95% confidence limits of 85 to 188 days) for liver histone and 159 days (95% confidence limits of 129 to 208 days) for brain. The data points for the tritium activity in brain fit a straight line with a slope indicating a half-life of 593 days with 95% confidence limits of 376 to 1406 days. In contrast, those for liver show a pronounced curvature indicating the presence in the liver of two cell populations with distinctly different turnover times. These two liver cell populations exhibit half-lives of 12 and 318 days representing 23 and 77% of the total DNA, respectively. The initial specific activity in liver DNA of 0.90 dpm/μg, as we have reported,[23] is in good agreement with an expected value of 0.89, which can be calculated on the basis of previous studies.[24] Further details of these studies have been previously published.[8,11,12]

Carcinogenesis

Studies on the induction of leukemia are still in progress with no definitive results as yet available. On the basis of routine examination, no other malignancies have been found.

SUMMARY

A summary of all the findings to date is given in TABLE 2.

It appears from this information that it is possible to detect somatic, cytogenetic, and genetic effects resulting from exposures at 33 to 100 times the mpc's for HTO. Similar effects also result from exposure to external γ rays at an equivalent dose.

The reduction in bone marrow cells in animals maintaining normal total cellularity is of interest since it demonstrates both the presence of an effect at the primitive cell level and the animal's ability to compensate for this effect by recruiting stem cells from the G_0 resting state. This evidence of damage together with the observed cytogenetic changes leads one to contemplate the possible importance of radiation exposures at these levels for the induction of leukemia or other blood dyscrasias. Studies to investigate this question are now under way.

As predicted on the basis of established principles of radiobiology, exposure to

TABLE 2. Summary of Results of Brookhaven TRITOX Program

	Effect at HTO Concentration (μCi/ml) of:		
	0.3	1.0	3.0
Somatic effects			
Growth	0	0	0
Lifetime shortening	0	0	0
Bone marrow cellularity	0	0	0
Bone marrow CFU-S	0	+	+ +
Genetic effects			
Dominant lethal mutations	0?	+	+ +
Cytogenetic effects			
Marrow sister chromatid exchanges	0?	NA[a]	+
Regenerating liver aberrations	0?	NA	+
Micronuclei in erythroid cells	NA	NA	+

[a]NA—not available.

tritium β rays from HTO ingestion results in measurable effects on several animal systems.

The importance of position of incorporation of H into molecules of biological importance has not been well defined, nor have the low-dose portions of the dose-response curve for several effects of interest. Experiments designed to address these questions and measure H turnover as a means for analysis of cell kinetics in several systems are now under way.

ACKNOWLEDGMENTS

I wish to acknowledge the contributions of the many scientists and technical assistants who over the tenure of the TRITOX program collaborated in the many studies leading to the results reviewed in this paper. A listing of these is as follows: D. Benz, A. Brooks, J. Bullis, S. Commerford, L. Cook, E. P. Cronkite, A. Gremillion, G. Hook, T. Ikushima, K. Jones, H. Kraner, A. Mead, M. Nawrocky, L. Phillips, D. Slatkin, H. Tezuka, K. Thompson, and M. Torelli. In addition I would like to thank Doris Pion and Linda Wasson for their help in the preparation of the manuscript.

REFERENCES

1. NCRP COMMITTEE. 1979. Report No. 63: Tritium and Other Radionuclide Labeled Organic Compounds Incorporated in Genetic Material.
2. CARSTEN, A. L. 1979. Tritium in the environment. *In* Advances in Radiation Biology. **8:** 419-458. Academic Press, Inc. New York, N.Y.
3. FEINENDEGEN, L. E., E. P. CRONKITE & V. P. BOND. 1980. Radiation problems in fusion energy production. Radiat. Environ. Biophys. **18:** 157-183.
4. BROOKS, A. L., A. L. CARSTEN, D. K. MEAD & J. C. RETHERFORD. 1976. The effect of continuous intake of tritiated water (HTO) on the liver chromosomes of mice. Radiat. Res. **68:** 480-489.
5. CARSTEN, A. L. & S. L. COMMERFORD. 1976. Dominant lethal mutations in mice resulting from chronic tritiated water (HTO) ingestion. Radiat. Res. **66:** 609-614.
6. CARSTEN, A. L. & E. P. CRONKITE. 1976. The genetic and hematopoietic effects of long-term tritiated water (HTO) ingestion in mice. (Presented at the IAEC Symposium on Biological Effects of Low Level Radiation Pertinent to Protection of Man and His Environment, Chicago, Ill., November 3-7, 1975, IAEA-SM-202/203.) *In* Biological and Environmental Effects of Low-Level Radiation. **2:** 51-56.
7. CARSTEN, A. L., S. L. COMMERFORD & E. P. CRONKITE. 1977. The genetic and late somatic effects of chronic tritium ingestion in mice. Curr. Top. Radiat. Res. Q. **12:** 212-224.
8. COMMERFORD, S. L., A. L. CARSTEN & E. P. CRONKITE. 1977. The distribution of tritium in the glycogen, hemoglobin and chromatin of mice receiving tritium in their drinking water. Radiat. Res. **72:** 333-342.
9. CARSTEN, A. L. & E. P. CRONKITE. 1979. Comparison of Late Effects of Single x-Ray Exposure, Chronic Tritiated Water Ingestion, and Chronic Cesium-137 Gamma Exposure in Mice. IAEA-SM-237/45. Pp. 269-276. International Atomic Energy Agency. Vienna, Austria.
10. SLATKIN, D. N., A. L. CARSTEN, S. L. COMMERFORD, K. W. JONES & H. W. KRANER. 1979. Genetic Hazard of ^{3}H: Estimation by Oocyte Uptake of ^{2}H. IAEA-SM-237/57. Pp. 231-240. International Atomic Energy Agency. Vienna, Austria.
11. COMMERFORD, S. L., A. L. CARSTEN & E. P. CRONKITE. 1982. Histone turnover within non-proliferating cells. Proc. Natl. Acad. Sci. USA **79:** 1163-1165.
12. COMMERFORD, S. L., A. L. CARSTEN & E. P. CRONKITE. 1982. The turnover of tritium in cell nuclei, chromatin, DNA and histone. Radiat. Res. **92:** 521-529.
13. BATEMAN, A. J. & S. S. EPSTEIN. 1971. Dominant lethal mutations in mammals. *In* Chemical Mutagens. A. Hollaender, Ed. **2:** 541-568. Plenum Press. New York, N.Y.
14. SNEDECOR, G. W. & W. G. COCHRAN. 1976. Statistical Methods. 6th edit., p. 59. Iowa State University Press. Ames, Iowa.
15. STEEL, R. & J. TERRIE. 1960. Principles and Procedures of Statistics. Pp. 406-407. McGraw-Hill. New York, N.Y.
16. SALSBURG, D. S. 1973. Statistical considerations for dominant lethal mutagenic tests. Environ. Health Perspect. **6:** 51-58.
17. SCHNEIDER, E. L., *et al.* Methods in Cell Biology. **20:** 379. Academic Press, Inc. New York, N.Y.
18. IKUSHIMA, T., R. D. BENZ & A. L. CARSTEN. 1985. Cytogenotoxicity of tritium: sister chromatid exchange level in bone marrow cells of mice maintained on tritiated water. Int. J. Radiat. Biol. In press.

19. TICE, R. Personal communication, 1983.
20. STONER, R. D. & V. P. BOND. 1963. Antibody formation by transplanted bone marrow, spleen, lymph node and thymus cells in irradiated recipients. J. Immunol. **91:** 185-192.
21. TILL, J. E. & E. A. McCULLOCH. 1961. A direct measurement of the radiation sensitivity of normal mouse bone marrow cells. Radiat. Res. **14:** 213-219.
22. DAVIDSON, J. N. & R. M. S. SMELLIE. 1952. Phosphorus compounds in the cell. Biochem. J. **52:** 594-599.
23. CARSTEN, A. L., A. BROOKS, S. L. COMMERFORD & E. P. CRONKITE. 1982. Genetic and somatic effects in animals maintained on tritiated water. *In* Proceedings, Tritium Radiobiology and Health Physics. NIRS-M-41. Pp. 101-119. Workshop held at the National Institute of Radiological Sciences, Chiba-shi, Japan.
24. INTERNATIONAL COMMISSION OF RADIOLOGICAL PROTECTION. Publication 26, Vol. 1, No. 3. Adopted January 17, 1977.

Alkylation Repair Activity in the Lung Macrophages of Smokers and Nonsmokers

E.-H. CAO AND R. B. SETLOW

Biology Department
Brookhaven National Laboratory
Upton, New York 11973

A. JANOFF

Pathology Department
School of Medicine
State University of New York at Stony Brook
Stony Brook, New York 11794

Nitrosamines are carcinogenic. Their carcinogenicity has been associated with their enzymatic activation to alkylating agents that react with cellular macromolecules. The biological activities of methylating and ethylating agents are associated with the alkylation of DNA, in particular the alkylation of guanine to yield O^6-alkylguanine. Such altered purines pair with thymine in addition to cytosine and so are mutagenic. The alkylating agents that produce appreciable amounts of O^6-alkylguanine are strong carcinogens and the target tissues tend to be those in which the rate of repair of this product is very slow. We have used a simple assay to measure the ability of extracts of cells to repair O^6-methylguanine (m^6G). In this repair reaction, the methyl group is transferred stoichiometrically from DNA to an acceptor protein. The reaction is quantitated by incubating a cell extract with an exogenous DNA containing [*methyl*-$^3H]m^6G$ and measuring the loss of radioactivity from the DNA or the gain in radioactivity by extract protein. We estimated the m^6G acceptor activity in macrophages obtained by lung lavage of 13 smokers and 8 nonsmokers. The acceptor activities in cell extracts of nonsmokers were, in femtomoles of methyl removed per 200 μg of protein, 50 to 100. These values are similar to those observed for extracts of peripheral blood lymphocytes. On the other hand, macrophage extracts gave values less than 10 in 11 of the smokers and 15 and 25 in the other 2. The low activity in smokers' macrophages is not the result of inhibition of methyl transferase by a component of the extract, since the extracts of smokers' cells do not inhibit the activity in extracts of nonsmokers' cells or of HeLa cells. Preliminary experiments indicate that the low activity in smokers' extracts arises from oxidation reactions in such cells, because treatment of them *in vitro* with the reducing agent dithiothreitol increases the activity by four- to fivefold to 50 to 80% of the activity of similarly treated cells from nonsmokers. The low acceptor activity in the lung macrophages of smokers implies that lung tissue exposed to smoke may also have low repair activity for m^6G. A low repair activity for m^6G would be expected to increase the carcinogenicity of simple nitrosamines in cigarette smoke.

Preliminary Observations on the Correlation of Proliferative Phenomena with *in Vivo* ^{31}P NMR Spectroscopy after Tumor Chemotherapy[a]

LEWIS M. SCHIFFER[b] AND
PAUL G. BRAUNSCHWEIGER[c]

Department of Experimental Therapeutics
AMC Cancer Research Center
Lakewood, Colorado 80214

JERRY D. GLICKSON, WILLIAM T. EVANOCHKO,
AND THIAN C. NG

Comprehensive Cancer Center
University of Alabama in Birmingham
Birmingham, Alabama 35294

INTRODUCTION

The pioneering studies of Gene Cronkite, and his associates, on the methodology, theory, and reality of mammalian cell kinetics are well known. During the initial years of study of animal and human hematopoiesis, there was a tacit assumption that, in addition to dissecting the physiology of proliferating systems, we would eventually use cell kinetic techniques for the management of various hematologic and malignant conditions. This has been very slow in coming to fruition which has been disappointing to many scientists and clinicians. The reasons for it are quite clear, however, and

[a]Supported by grants from Bill L. Walters and the Hill Foundation to the AMC Cancer Research Center and Grant CA13148 to the University of Alabama in Birmingham.

[b]Deceased.

[c]Author to whom correspondence should be addressed: Dr. Paul G. Braunschweiger, AMC Cancer Research Center, 1600 Pierce Street, Lakewood, Colo. 80214.

many were recognized very early. First of all, the study of unperturbed cell kinetics, prior to any treatments, does not appear to have great utility, except, perhaps, in terms of disease prognosis or stratification for treatment. Other reasons to explain this lack of clinical activity are numerous and include the restrictions on the use of certain isotopic compounds in humans, the realization and implications of cellular and tumor heterogeneity, the slow development and acceptance of techniques to study perturbations in solid tumors, and, probably the most important factor, the need to access repeated biopsy specimens for study during perturbation, especially in solid tumors.

Since solid tumors represent well over 90% of the malignancies of man, it was appropriate that some attention be paid to the cell kinetic changes occurring in solid tumors as a result of extensive cytotoxic therapy.

Our group developed a series of *in vitro* techniques by which one could follow the kinetic course of a solid tumor after *in vivo* perturbation.[1,2] In animal tumor systems we showed that the time sequencing of treatment modalities, based on the changing cell kinetics of the tumor, resulted in more efficient tumor volume reduction than either simultaneous treatment administration or treatment given at kinetically inappropriate times.[3-5] In some systems we even obtained complete remissions and cures where none existed before, and with less cytotoxicity.

While acceptable for animal tumor systems, the *in vitro* techniques were not readily transferable to patient care because of the need for multiple tumor biopsies. The need for tissue samples, along with several other problems similar to those mentioned previously, can also be cited for the slow utilization of flow cytometry for clinical patient management.

This theme was developed in detail by one of us (L.M.S.) several years ago, at the meeting of the European Study Group for Cell Proliferation in Aarhus, Denmark. In order to translate the concepts that have been developed in animal systems to human treatment programs, there is an urgent need for noninvasive techniques to study tumor cell biology.

The characteristics of the ideal technique for the noninvasive monitoring of cell proliferation are truly imposing. The method should not require repeated biopsies; it should be amenable to repeated studies at frequent intervals without patient discomfort; it should monitor the proliferative response to the treatment modality; and it should not, in itself, perturb the tumor. Ideally, one would also like to be able to evaluate normal cell proliferation as well.

It appears now that a new technique, ^{31}P nuclear magnetic resonance (^{31}P NMR), may fulfill these rather rigid requirements. However, many studies in animal systems are necessary before it can be applied to the study of human tumors.

The theory and mechanics of ^{31}P NMR have been well described.[6,7] Recently, its use as a noninvasive technique to study *in vivo* metabolic processes has become important.[8,9] We have presented a series of reports on the use of ^{31}P NMR for the evaluation of tumor metabolism in animal systems under a variety of conditions.[10-12] Studies of subcutaneously transplanted mouse tumors and human xenografts detected significant changes in nucleotide triphosphate (NTP), phosphocreatine, and inorganic phosphorus (Pi) as a result of tumor growth and perturbation with chemotherapeutic drugs, radiation, and hyperthermia.

Our collaborative studies were designed to evaluate the changing effects of a noncurative single dose of cyclophosphamide on the ^{31}P NMR resonances from the RIF-1 tumor, and to compare them with the proliferative changes that occur with time after drug administration. They were carried out in the hope of finding a noninvasive correlate with tumor cell proliferation.

METHODS

^{31}P NMR spectra were obtained[10] with a Bruker CXP-200/300 operating at 80.96 MHz. A surface or solenoidal coil was placed adjacent to the subcutaneous tumor in mice otherwise surrounded by a Faraday shield.[13] Control studies confirmed that signals arose only from the tumor. The chemical shift of Pi was measured relative to the phosphocreatine resonance, and the apparent intracellular pH of the tumor was measured from this shift. The relative abundance of metabolites was estimated by the areas beneath the resonances. Spectra from control and treated animals were obtained daily and related to the pretreatment (day 0) values.

RIF-1 tumors were produced in C3H/HeJ female mice by subcutaneous inoculation of 1×10^6 tissue culture cells (obtained from and cultivated by the method of Dr. R. Kallman, Stanford University, Stanford, Calif.).[14] Tumors were utilized when they were approximately 1 cm³ in volume. The baseline cell kinetics[15] for these tumors were: tritiated thymidine labeling index ([3H]TdR LI), 0.17; DNA synthesis time, 7.6 hr; growth fraction by primer dependent DNA polymerase (PDP) assay, 0.41; and cell cycle time, 16 hr.

After transplantation some animals were transported to the University of Alabama in Birmingham for ^{31}P NMR studies, while the ones remaining at AMC Cancer Research Center were entered into the cell kinetics part of the study. Animals were controlled for crowding, and were acclimatized for at least 3 days.

Fourteen days after transplantation the treatment animals were given 150 mg/kg freshly prepared cyclophosphamide, intraperitoneally. This dose was designed to reduce the tumor volume by half. Tumors were measured in two dimensions with calipers and tumor volume or weight was calculated as an oblate ellipsoid. Animals were immobilized for ^{31}P NMR daily with 60 mg/kg pentobarbital, intraperitoneally. Control studies showed no significant effect by pentobarbital on the PDP index.

Cohorts of animals were sacrificed daily for tumor cell kinetic studies. The [3H]TdR LI assay was performed by an *in vitro* technique, the results representing the fraction of cells in S phase.[1] The PDP index assay was also performed *in vitro*,[2] the results representing the fraction of cells in the growth fraction.[16] In both assays labeling indices are determined by autoradiography.

Regrowth delay was determined by subtracting the time in days for control tumors to reach four times pretreatment size from the time required for treated tumors to reach the same end point. For comparison purposes they are expressed as multiples of the doubling time, for that tumor, during the regrowth phase.

RESULTS

Following treatment with cyclophosphamide the average tumor volume decreased to approximately 50% by day 4. Tumor volume did not significantly start to increase again until after day 7 (FIGURE 1).

The [3H]TdR LI decreased from 0.15 to 0.03 after treatment and the number of cells in S phase increased significantly between days 3 and 4. Estimates of the growth fraction by the PDP index showed a similar reduction from 0.41 to 0.15, with proliferative recovery also occurring between days 3 and 4 (FIGURE 2). Studies of proliferation in control tumors showed no such perturbations.

The lower curve in FIGURE 2 represents the tumor regrowth delay caused by the initial dose of cyclophosphamide followed by another dose of 100 mg/kg given at the times indicated. This is an indication of the most efficient time sequencing of this drug combination. Thus, timing two doses of cyclophosphamide between days 4 and 5 seems most efficacious. It can be appreciated that tumor cells resumed proliferation well before obvious tumor regrowth occurred.

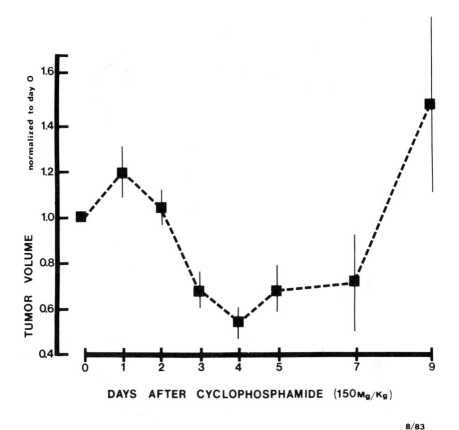

8/83

FIGURE 1. Tumor volume of RIF-1 tumor, normalized to day 0, during the experimental period of 9 days. Cyclophosphamide was administered on day 0. The tumor volume of untreated control animals (data not shown) reached ~ 9.

Turning to the NMR studies (FIGURE 3), it can be noted that the NTP_β/Pi ratio rose significantly between days 1 and 2 after drug administration. This is a result, almost exclusively, of a decrease in the magnitude of the Pi. The lower curves represent the intracellular pH of control and treated animals as measured by the chemical shift of Pi, using the phosphocreatine resonance as a reference point.

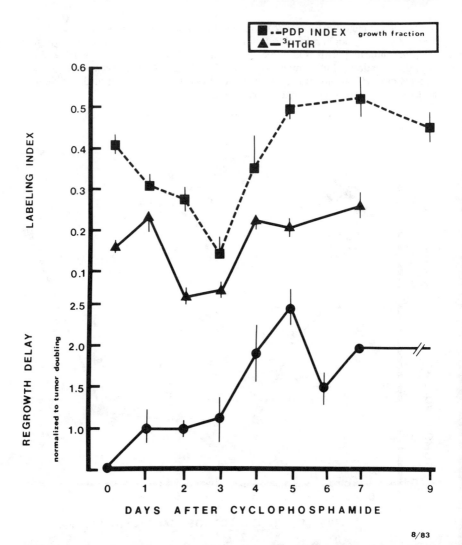

FIGURE 2. Proliferative phenomena of RIF-1 tumor: the [³H]TdR labeling index (▲) and the PDP index (■) during the experimental period of 9 days. Cyclophosphamide was administered on day 0. The regrowth delay, normalized to tumor doubling time, after 150 mg of cyclophosphamide on day 0 and 100 mg of cyclophosphamide on the other days is represented on the lower curve (●).

There was little or no change until, between days 3 and 4, there was a sharp, highly significant rise of 0.6 pH unit. The pH then remained elevated for a number of days. This timing was precisely the same as that of the proliferative changes and just slightly different from the most efficient drug sequencing time.

DISCUSSION

The mechanism of the alkaline pH shift is not entirely clear. In a variety of eucaryotic organisms, as well as mammalian cells, it has been shown that mitosis and proliferation are accompanied by a significant pH rise.[17-19] Furthermore, it is of interest that the optimum pH values for many of the studied nucleoside and nucleotide kinases, and DNA polymerases, are in the alkaline range.[19,20] There is no specific information,

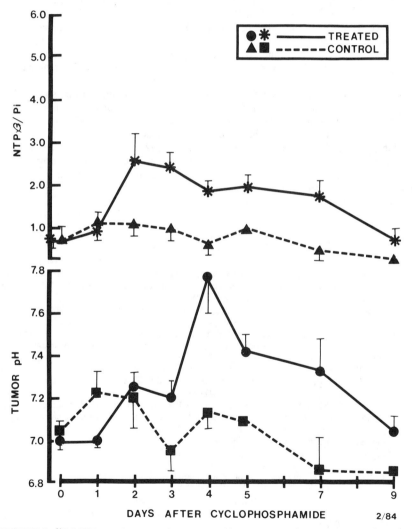

FIGURE 3. ^{31}P NMR studies of RIF-1 tumor. The upper graph represents the ^{31}P NMR NTP$_\beta$/Pi ratio of the treated and control animals during the experimental period of 9 days. The lower graph represents the pH as measured by chemical shift of Pi.

however, on the enzymes of the RIF-1 tumor. There are some uncertainties involved in *in vivo* intracellular pH measurement by ^{31}P NMR, including suitable reference points and assignment of signals. However, *in vitro* comparison studies by NMR and other methods tend to confirm the *in vivo* results obtained by the NMR technique.[9] In only 6 of the 10 treated animals could the pH be evaluated, because of temporary loss of the Pi resonance.

Studies of control, growing tumors demonstrate a decrease in the high-energy phosphates, NTP and phosphocreatine, an increase in the Pi, and a chemical shift of the Pi to a more acidic pH. Our experiments, using clinically applicable, noncurative doses of drug, show retention of NTP resonances, recovery of Pi levels, and a substructure of pH shifts with potential therapeutic implications.

Regardless of the basic mechanisms, the pH change in this system correlates with the acute proliferative increases and the best timing for sequencing the next dose of cyclophosphamide. The proliferative measurements were invasive and required tissue samples, whereas the ^{31}P NMR measurements were noninvasive, nondestructive, and repeatable in the same animals.

This is only one tumor system and only one drug. It remains to be seen if these results can be duplicated in other systems with other treatment modalities. Nevertheless, the results are highly encouraging and lead us to conclude that in tumor model systems ^{31}P NMR may be quite useful for following tumor cell proliferation during therapeutic perturbations. If this proves to be generally so, with the knowledge that the technology to do similar studies with human tumors is now becoming operational, the early vision of using cell kinetics more directly for treatment planning may be realized in the near future.

REFERENCES

1. BRAUNSCHWEIGER, P. G., L. POULAKOS & L. M. SCHIFFER. 1976. *In vitro* labeling and gold activation autoradiography for determination of labeling index and DNA synthesis time of solid tumors. Cancer Res. **36:** 1748-1753.
2. NELSON, J. S. R. & L. M. SCHIFFER. 1973. Autoradiographic detection of DNA polymerase containing nuclei in sarcoma 180 ascites cells. Cell Tissue Kinet. **6:** 45-54.
3. BRAUNSCHWEIGER, P. G. & L. M. SCHIFFER. 1980. Cell kinetically based combination chemotherapy of T1699 mammary tumors with adriamycin and cyclophosphamide. Cancer Res. **40:** 737-743.
4. BRAUNSCHWEIGER, P. G., L. L. SCHENKEN & L. M. SCHIFFER. 1981. Kinetically directed combination therapy with adriamycin and X-irradiation in a mammary tumor model. Int. J. Radiat. Oncol. Biol. Phys. **7:** 747-754.
5. SCHIFFER, L. M. & P. G. BRAUNSCHWEIGER. 1985. Tumor cell kinetic studies in animal models can aid the design of human tumor treatments. *In* Current Controversies in Breast Cancer, Proceedings of the 26th M. D. Anderson Annual Clinical Conference. University of Texas Press. Austin, Tex. In press.
6. GADIAN, D. G. 1982. Nuclear Magnetic Resonance and Its Applications to Living Systems. Oxford University Press. Oxford, England.
7. JAMES, T. L. 1975. Nuclear Magnetic Resonance in Biochemistry: Principles and Applications. Academic Press, Inc. New York, N.Y.
8. SHULMAN, R. G., T. R. BROWN, K. UGURBIL, S. OGAWA, S. M. COHEN & J. A. DEN HOLLANDER. 1979. Cellular applications of ^{31}P and ^{13}C nuclear magnetic resonance. Science **205:** 160-166.
9. GADIAN, D. G. 1983. Whole organ metabolism studied by NMR. Annu. Rev. Biophys. Bioeng. **12:** 69-89.

10. NG, T. C., W. T. EVANOCHKO, R. N. HIRAMOTO, V. K. GHANTA, M. B. LILLY, A. J. LAWSON, T. H. CORBETT, J. R. DURANT & J. D. GLICKSON. 1982. ^{31}P NMR spectroscopy of in vivo tumors. J. Magn. Reson. **49:** 271-286.
11. EVANOCHKO, W. T., T. C. NG, J. D. GLICKSON, J. R. DURANT & T. H. CORBETT. 1982. Human tumors as examined by in vivo ^{31}P NMR in athymic mice. Biochem. Biophys. Res. Commun. **109:** 1346-1352.
12. EVANOCHKO, W. T., T. C. NG, M. B. LILLY, A. J. LAWSON, T. H. CORBETT, J. R. DURANT & J. D. GLICKSON. 1983. In vivo ^{31}P NMR study of the metabolism of murine mammary 16/C adenocarcinoma and its response to chemotherapy, x-radiation and hyperthermia. Proc. Natl. Acad. Sci. USA **80:** 334-338.
13. NG, T. C., W. T. EVANOCHKO & J. D. GLICKSON. 1982. Faraday shield for surface-coil studies of subcutaneous tumors. J. Magn. Reson. **49:** 526-529.
14. TWENTYMAN, P. R., J. M. BROWN, J. W. GRAY, A. J. FRANKO, M. A. SCOLES & R. F. KALLMAN. 1980. A new mouse tumor model system (RIF-1) for comparison of end points. J. Natl. Cancer Inst. **64:** 595-604.
15. BRAUNSCHWEIGER, P. G., H. L. TING & L. M. SCHIFFER. 1982. Receptor dependent antiproliferative effects of corticosteroids in radiation-induced fibrosarcomas and implications for sequential therapy. Cancer Res. **42:** 1686-1691.
16. SCHIFFER, L. M., A. M. MARKOE & J. S. R. NELSON. 1976. Estimation of tumor growth fraction in murine tumors by the primer-available DNA-dependent DNA polymerase assay. Cancer Res. **36:** 2415-2418.
17. GERSON, D. F. & A. C. BURTON. 1977. The relation of cycling of intracellular pH to mitosis in the acellular slime mould Physarum polycephalum. J. Cell. Physiol. **91:** 297-304.
18. GILLIES, R. J. 1981. Intracellular pH and growth control in eukaryotic cells. *In* The Transformed Cell. I. L. Cameron & T. B. Pool, Eds.: 367-395. Academic Press, Inc. New York, N.Y.
19. GERSON, D. F. 1982. The relation between intracellular pH and DNA synthesis rate in proliferating lymphocytes. *In* Intracellular pH: Its Measurement, Regulation and Utilization in Cellular Functions. R. Nuccitelli & D. W. Deamer, Eds.: 375-383. Alan R. Liss, Inc. New York, N.Y.
20. ANDERSON, E. P. 1973. Nucleoside and nucleotide kinases. *In* The Enzymes—Volume IX. P. D. Boyer, Ed.: 49-96. Academic Press, Inc. New York, N.Y.

Cell Kinetic Studies of the Effect of Cytotoxic Drugs on Survival and Proliferation of Ascites and Solid Tumor Cells of the Mouse

B. SCHULTZE,[a] R. FIETKAU, E. SCHÄFER,
AND I. BASSUKAS

Institut für Medizinische Strahlenkunde
Universität Würzburg
D-8700 Würzburg, Federal Republic of Germany

Proliferation of normal and tumor cells in mice and rats has been studied by our group for many years. Cell kinetic parameters of the different cell types and in many cases the mode of growth of these cell types have been elucidated with different cell kinetic methods.[1-8] During recent years, studies of the cytostatic and cytocidal effects of cytotoxic drugs (vincristine (VCR), vinblastine (VLB), 5-fluorouracil (5-FU), Ftorafur (FT), bleomycin (BLM), *cis*-platinum (DDP), 1-β-D-arabinofuranosylcytosine (Ara-C), and cyclophosphamide (CY)) on experimental ascites and solid tumors as well as on normal tissue of the mouse have been our main interest.[9-13] Cell kinetic methods as well as cell counting and caliper measurements were used in these studies. Supplemental experiments were carried out *in vitro* on HeLa cells using cell counts and time-lapse cinematography.[14,15] The latter method provides knowledge on sublethal damage of cells, since—in contrast to *in vivo* conditions—cells can be followed throughout several cycles. Thus, drug-induced damage becoming manifest long after drug application can be revealed by these studies.

Since chemotherapy of malignant human tumors has gained increasing significance in complementing surgery and radiotherapy, better knowledge of the effects of the various cytotoxic drugs should contribute to an improvement of the chemotherapeutic regimens used in the treatment of human tumors, particularly in the combination therapy applied today. Three examples of studies of these effects will be presented here.

QUANTITATIVE STUDIES OF THE EFFECT OF Ara-C ON L 1210 ASCITES TUMOR CELLS

Ara-C, a nucleoside analogue, acts predominantly by inhibiting DNA synthesis via inhibition of DNA polymerase. This inhibiting effect on DNA synthesis is well

[a] Author to whom correspondence should be addressed: Prof. B. Schultze, Institut für Medizinische Strahlenkunde der Universität Würzburg, Versbacher Str. 5, D-8700 Würzburg, Federal Republic of Germany.

demonstrated by the steep decrease of the *labeling index* (LI) of the L 1210 ascites tumor cells to about zero within 1 hr after application of 200 mg/kg Ara-C (FIGURE 1A). After 8 hr the LI increases again and exceeds the control values of the untreated animals after 14 hr; it then decreases to a minimum at 21 hr and finally levels at about the control values. That means that application of Ara-C leads immediately to a complete but reversible block of DNA synthesis which lasts about 8 hr. After release of the block cells arrested in S phase or at the G_1/S border pass more or less synchronously through the cycle.

The *mitotic index* (MI) also decreases to about zero within 1.5 hr after Ara-C application (FIGURE 1B). That means that cells in mitosis at the time of Ara-C application complete mitosis without delay. Almost no mitoses are observed for 10

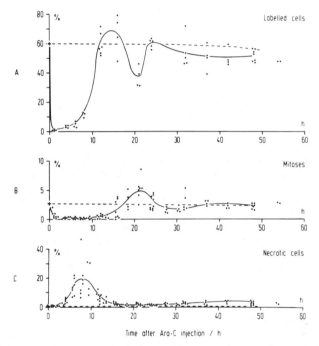

FIGURE 1. Labeling index (A), mitotic index (B), and percentage of necrotic cells (C) of L 1210 ascites tumor cells as a function of time after application of 200 mg/kg Ara-C.

hr, since no cells move out of S. The maximum MI, about twice the control values, is observed 21 hr after Ara-C application; it corresponds to the minimum LI and is due to the synchronous passage through the cycle of those cells released from the block in S phase.

The peak at about 20% *necrotic cells* (compared to 0.5% in the untreated tumor) shows that quite a number of L 1210 cells are killed by this dose of Ara-C, and the early appearance of the peak suggests that these cells die out of interphase (FIGURE 1C). However, to specify the cycle phases where cell death occurs requires an additional double-labeling experiment with [³H]thymidine ([³H]TdR) and [¹⁴C]thymidine ([¹⁴C]TdR) that permits the distinction of the cells in different phases of the cycle due to their different label.

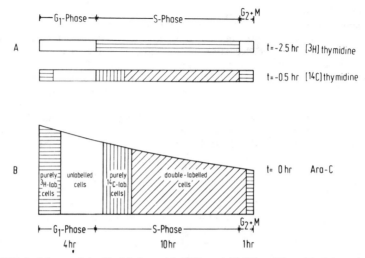

FIGURE 2. Scheme of double labeling with [³H]- and [¹⁴C]thymidine. (A) Schematic representation of the double-labeling method. (B) Age distribution of the differently labeled and unlabeled cells throughout the cycle at the time of Ara-C application.

For this purpose mice received a first injection of [³H]TdR and 2 hr later a second injection of [¹⁴C]TdR. According to the scheme in FIGURE 2A this double labeling leads to a 2-hr-wide subpopulation of purely ¹⁴C-labeled cells at the beginning of S phase and a 2-hr-wide subpopulation of purely ³H-labeled cells in G_1 + mitosis + beginning of G_1. The remaining cells in S are double labeled (8 hr wide) and the remaining cells in G_1 are unlabeled (3 hr wide). FIGURE 2B depicts the age distribution of the differently labeled and unlabeled cells throughout the cycle at the time of Ara-C injection. The effect of Ara-C on cells in different cycle phases was then examined by following the fate of the various categories of differently labeled and unlabeled cells on two emulsion layer autoradiographs as a function of time after Ara-C application (up to 30.5 hr). FIGURE 3A depicts schematically the positions of the differently labeled and unlabeled cell populations throughout the cycle at the time of Ara-C application. In FIGURE 3B-D the percentages of interphase cells (B), mitoses (C), and necrotic cells (D) are plotted as a function of time after Ara-C injection. The percentages in each case are related to *all* cells, including necrotic cells, counted at the different time intervals after drug application.

Purely ¹⁴C-Labeled Cells

These cells which were in early S phase at the time of Ara-C application decrease from 13 to about 1% within 12 hr. Simultaneously a peak of purely ¹⁴C-labeled necrotic cells of about 4% appears. No purely ¹⁴C-labeled mitoses are observed. That means that almost all of these early-S-phase cells are killed by Ara-C.

Double-Labeled Cells

The double-labeled cells that were in S minus the first 2.5 hr and to a small extent (6%) in G_2 at the time of Ara-C application decrease from 39 to about 7% up to 30 hr after drug application. The percentage of double-labeled necrotic cells increases simultaneously to about 5%. This means that the majority of cells that were in S at the time of Ara-C application are killed by this drug. Only a small portion of double-labeled cells, most probably G_2- and some late-S-phase cells, survives and is able to undergo a delayed mitotic division.

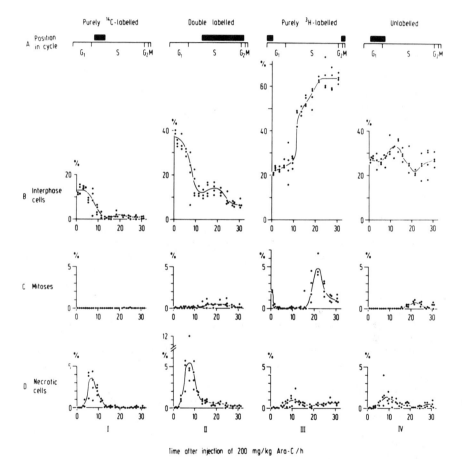

lime after injection of 200 mg/kg Ara-C / h

FIGURE 3. Percentages of interphase cells, mitoses, and necrotic cells for the various categories of labeled and unlabeled cells as a function of time after Ara-C application. (A) Schematic representation of the positions of the differently labeled and unlabeled cells throughout the cycle at the time of Ara-C application. (B)-(D) Results for the different categories of cells plotted as a percentage of the total cell count from one animal.

Purely ^3H-Labeled Cells

The percentage of purely ^3H-labeled cells that were in mitosis and the beginning of G_1 at the time of Ara-C application steeply increases. Since no purely ^3H-labeled mitoses appear prior to about 15 hr, the increase between 10 and 15 hr is a relative one due to the steep decrease in total cell number caused by the massive death of purely ^{14}C- and double-labeled cells. The further increase of purely ^3H-labeled interphase cells is due to the mitotic division of these cells expressed as a mitotic peak of more than 5% about 21 hr after application of Ara-C. Only a few purely ^3H-labeled necrotic cells are observed. Thus, there is only a slight cell loss out of this population.

Unlabeled Cells

The percentage of unlabeled cells that were in G_1 and to a small extent in S at the time of Ara-C injection also shows a relative increase. These cells also divide with some delay. Cell loss out of this population is small, too.

Conclusions

This double-labeling experiment clearly shows that Ara-C mainly kills S-phase cells; cell loss out of the other cycle phases is small. However, quantitative rates of cell loss out of the different cycle phases cannot be derived from this experiment, since the observed percentages of necrotic cells are only relative values; they are linked to a rapidly changing, i.e., decreasing, cell number. In order to obtain absolute cell loss rates out of the different cell compartments a multicompartment model was applied which is based on the results of this double-labeling experiment (for details see Fietkau et al.[16]).

The application of this multicompartment model shows that 54% of all cells are killed by Ara-C within 15 hr after drug application. This agrees well with an approximately 50% decrease in cell number obtained by cell counting. Furthermore, the model shows that 87% of the cells in S at the time of Ara-C application are killed by Ara-C while only 20% of the G_1 cells are killed.

With these absolute cell loss rates derived from the model the measured values in FIGURE 3 can be corrected for cell loss. Applying this correction the decrease of the purely ^{14}C- and double-labeled interphase cells or the increase of the purely ^3H- and unlabeled cells can be quantitatively explained by the peaks of necrotic or mitotic cells, respectively.

Furthermore, with this multicompartment model a mean life span of 1.9 hr has been estimated for the necrotic L 1210 ascites tumor cells killed by Ara-C. This is the first time that the mean life span of necrotic cells has been determined *in vivo*. There is no other way to measure the mean life span of necrotic cells *in vivo*. For this reason there is little data on this subject available in the literature. A value of 8 hr derived from the decrease of ^{125}I activity in the peritoneal cavity following the injection of heat-killed ^{125}I-labeled L 1210 ascites tumor cells is not necessarily comparable with the present result.[17] Devik[18] estimated a mean life span of 2-3 hr or more for necrotic intestinal epithelia after X-ray irradiation. Our group derived a mean life span similar to that derived from the present experiment by using the same double-labeling procedure with L 1210 ascites tumor cells but with other cytotoxic drugs. However, Camplejohn *et al.*[12] found a mean life span of 16-18 hr for necrotic JB-1 ascites tumor cells killed in mitosis by VCR. These differing values suggest that the mean life span of necrotic cells *in vivo* might differ substantially depending on cell type, animal strain, immune status, cytotoxic substance, kind of therapy, and kind of cell death.

CYTOCIDAL EFFECT OF VARIOUS CYTOTOXIC DRUGS ON DIFFERENT ASCITES TUMORS OF THE MOUSE

The cytocidal effect of various cytotoxic drugs is manifested by the necrotic cells observed. However, the number of cells killed by the drug cannot be derived from the number of necrotic cells observed, since—as mentioned above—the mean life span of these necrotic cells is not known. For instance, a peak value of 7% necrotic cells measured after drug application might correspond to a large number of killed cells, if the mean life span of these necrotic cells is short, or it might represent a small number of killed cells, if the mean life span is long.

Up to now there have been only indirect estimates on the number of cells killed by a drug from the increase in survival time of the tumor-bearing animals. These estimates have been based on the observation that the animals die when a certain number of tumor cells is reached presuming that the cycle time of the tumor cells does not change after drug application.

In order to find out how many tumor cells actually are killed by a single dose of the various drugs the number of ascites tumor cells was counted as a function of time after drug application for three different ascites tumors (L 1210, JB-1, Ehrlich). The animals received a single dose of the various drugs 4 days after tumor inoculation, i.e., during exponential growth. FIGURE 4 contains the results. The growth curves of the untreated tumors are plotted as thick lines.

L 1210 Ascites Tumor

In the case of the L 1210 ascites tumor (FIGURE 4A) a single dose of 0.05 mg/kg *VCR* only leads to a retardation of tumor growth. A dose of 200 mg/kg *Ara-C* kills about 65% of all tumor cells within about 16 hr; then the tumor starts to repopulate and reaches the plateau value of the untreated tumors with some delay. A single dose of 13 mg/kg *DDP* kills more than 90% of all tumor cells. One-third of the treated animals die earlier than the untreated controls, and another third are permanently cured and live for more than 1 year without tumor (FIGURE 4D). In the last third the tumor starts to grow again (FIGURE 4A). These animals live three times longer than the untreated controls but then die of ascites tumor. A dose of 8 mg/kg DDP kills about the same amount of cells. Fifteen percent of the animals are permanently cured. In the remaining animals the tumor repopulates. These animals

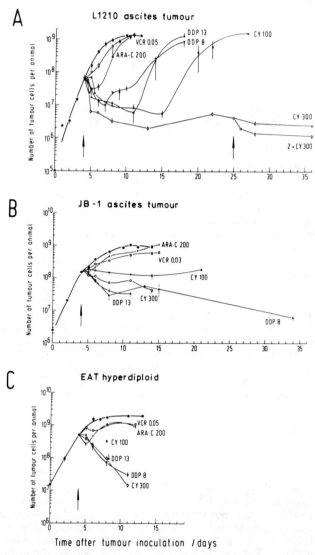

FIGURE 4. Effect of various cytotoxic drugs on different ascites tumors. (A) (C) Number of ascites cells as a function of time after tumor inoculation and drug application. (D)-(F) Survival curves of the tumor-bearing animals.

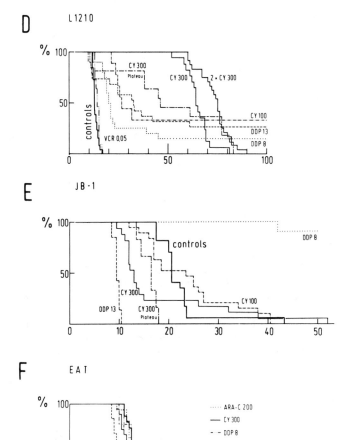

Time after tumour inoculation / days

FIGURE 4. (*Continued.*)

live two times longer than the untreated controls and then die of ascites tumor. *CY,* 100 mg/kg, also kills more than 90% of the tumor cells. One-third of the animals are permanently cured and live more than 1 year tumor free (FIGURE 4D). The other two-thirds live three times longer than the untreated controls but then die of the regrown ascites tumor (FIGURE 4A). A single dose of 300 mg/kg CY kills 97% of the tumor cells. From about 10 days on the cell number reaches the level that is usually found in the peritoneal cavity in normal animals without tumor. These animals no longer have tumor cells. They live for 70-80 days and then die in a cachectic state. The cause of their death is not yet known. There are no macroscopic or microscopic signs of tumor or of other causes of death; there is no depression of the bone marrow and the blood values are normal.

As shown by the survival curves in FIGURE 4D, all of the different treatments—apart from the small dose of VCR—lead to a considerable prolongation of the median survival time which is 12.8 days for the untreated animals. A permanent cure for about 30% of the animals is achieved after application of 100 mg/kg CY and 13 mg/kg DDP.

JB-1 Ascites Tumor

Compared to the L 1210 tumor the portion of JB-1 ascites tumor cells killed by *CY* and *DDP* is much smaller (FIGURE 4B). Similar to the L 1210 tumor, *Ara-C* and *VCR* in the doses applied lead only to a growth retardation. As shown by the survival curves (FIGURE 4E) the sensitivity of these animals to the cytotoxic effect of high doses of DDP and CY is much greater. These animals die earlier than the untreated controls. The median survival time of the animals treated with 100 mg/kg CY is about the same as that of the untreated controls. Only a single dose of 8 mg/kg DDP kills all ascites tumor cells. These animals survive 70-80 days and longer, compared to only 21 days for the untreated animals, and then die of solid tumors.

Ehrlich Ascites Tumor

The same amount of Ehrlich ascites tumor cells is killed by high doses of *CY* and *DDP* as in the case of the L 1210 tumor, namely, more than 90% (FIGURE 4C). However, these animals are very sensitive to the toxic effect of these drugs; they all die earlier than the untreated controls, the median survival time of which is 13 days (FIGURE 4F). The small doses of *VCR* and also *Ara-C* result in a reduction of tumor cell number and in some growth delay.

Conclusions

These results clearly demonstrate that the therapeutic effect of a cytotoxic drug is influenced by quite a number of different factors such as factors originating from the tumor. The different types of tumors derived from the different cell types used in the present study differ in their growth and cell kinetic parameters. The L 1210 tumor is a rapidly growing tumor with a short cycle time ($\sim$14 hr). The cycle time of the other tumors is much longer (30-35 hr). On the other hand, there are factors originating from the host animal. The three different mouse strains used in the present experiment differ considerably in their response to the drugs. Metabolic processes certainly play a role in the different drug sensitivities of the various animal strains. For details see Schäfer *et al.*[19]

PROLIFERATION CHARACTERISTICS OF A SOLID MOUSE TUMOR (ADENOCARCINOMA E0 771) AND THE EFFECT OF CY ON THIS TUMOR

With respect to the frequent use of human tumor material transplanted to nude mice for testing cytotoxic drugs the question arises whether these studies are representative for the response in the tumor patient. The aim of the present study was to find out whether the proliferation characteristics of a mouse tumor change if it is transplanted to nude mice.

Growth and Histology

The solid adenocarcinoma E0 771 usually grows on the C57bl/6j mouse strain. Seven days after transplantation of 1.75×10^5 tumor cells into the right hind leg of the animals an invasively growing tumor of about 0.9 g appears. It shows the histological characteristics of a solid medullary carcinoma without differentiated glandular structures and with central necrotic areas. These necrotic areas increase with increasing tumor growth. From about 10 days after transplantation on, the living tumor tissue remains constant (ca. 2.5 g) although the total tumor mass increases threefold (4 to 12 g) up until the death of the animals.

Tumor growth, histology, and proliferation, as well as the reaction to CY treatment, were studied after transplantation of the tumor to three different mouse strains: the C57 (C57bl/6j), the nude (Balb/c-nu/nu), and the Balb/c. The latter mouse strain has the same genetic substance as the nude mice derived from it.

The take rates of the tumors were 100% in all mouse strains. Seven days after transplantation the same size tumor was found at the implantation site in all three mouse strains. However, tumor growth was the cause of death for all C57 and nude mice but only 25% of the Balb/c mice, while in 75% of the animals spontaneous regression of the tumor occurred.

FIGURE 5 shows the growth curves of the adenocarcinoma E0 771 on the three different mouse strains. The caliper measures, i.e., the derived areas, are positively correlated to the tumor weight. The growth curves for the tumor growing on C57 and on nude mice are very similar and can be described by a Gompertz function. If

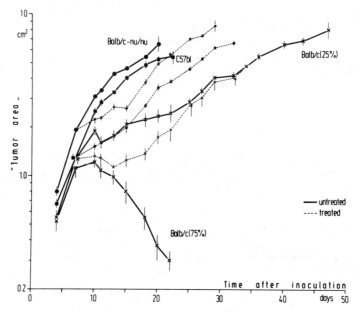

FIGURE 5. Growth curves of a solid tumor (adenocarcinoma E0 771) transplanted to three different mouse strains and the effect of cyclophosphamide on tumor growth.

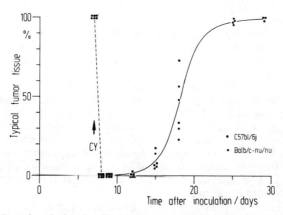

FIGURE 6. Effect of cyclophosphamide treatment on the typical tumor tissue of the adenocarcinoma E0 771.

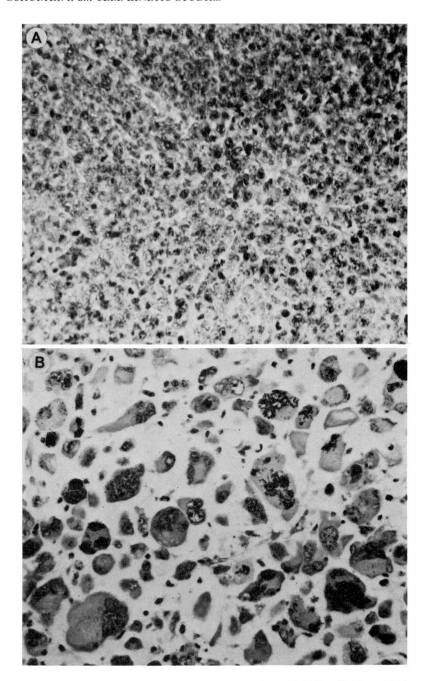

FIGURE 7. Change in nuclear morphology of adenocarcinoma E0 771 cells after cyclophosphamide treatment. (A) Untreated tumor; (B) 11 days after cyclophosphamide treatment. (Magnification for both (A) and (B), ×330.)

the tumor is transplanted to Balb/c mice the growth curve is similar during the first week. During the second week after transplantation, however, the tumor growth slows down and in 75% of the Balb/c mice spontaneous tumor regression occurs. In the remaining 25% of the animals the tumor grows more slowly with a doubling time of about 2 weeks. The median survival time of these animals is about 51 days compared to 22 or 19 days for the tumor-bearing C57 or nude mice, respectively.

Proliferation

Pulse labeling with [^{3}H]TdR 7 days after transplantation to C57 as well as to nude mice results in a quite irregular labeling of the tumor tissue: strongly, less strongly, and weakly labeled areas can be recognized. There is a positive correlation between the mean grain number per nucleus and the LI as well as the MI in the different areas. LI and MI strongly depend on the size of the living tumor tissue and decrease with increasing tumor volume. The persistence of the correlation between mean grain number per nucleus and LI as well as MI suggests that the decrease of the LI and MI is due to a decrease at the growth fraction. Seven days after transplantation the cycle time of the tumor growing on nude mice is shorter (12-13 hr) than that of the tumor growing on C57 mice (16-18 hr) due to a shortening of the G_1 phase; the duration of S, G_2, and M is similar. This difference in the cycle time suggests that the cycle time of human tumor cells transplanted to nude mice might change more drastically.

Cyclophosphamide Treatment

A single dose of 300 mg/kg CY leads to a prolongation of the mean survival time by a factor of 1.25 in the case of the C57 mice and of 1.65 in the case of the nude mice (FIGURE 5). The same treatment, however, has a disastrous effect in the case of the Balb/c mice: instead of spontaneous regression of the tumors in 75% of the animals, tumor regression occurs in only 30%. The remaining 70% of the animals die, not because of the toxicity of the drug, but because of tumor growth. There is no longer spontaneous regression of these tumors due to the influence of the drug on the immune status of the animals.

The treated tumor undergoes characteristic changes in morphology, histology, and cell kinetics. For instance, the population of rapidly and invasively growing tumor cells with the typical characteristics of this tumor decreases immediately after treatment (FIGURE 6). It is replaced by morphologically quite different cells. However, with increasing time after treatment the first population increases again until the tumor finally is repopulated by these typical tumor cells with the characteristics of the untreated tumor (FIGURE 6). The nuclear morphology exhibits the most impressive changes. The volume of the nuclear material often divided into more than one nuclear configuration increases 50-fold (!!) within 3 weeks by passing through several "S phases" with only very few divisions of the karyoplasm (FIGURE 7). For details see Bassukas and Schultze.[20]

SUMMARY

The three studies discussed show that the response of experimental ascites and solid tumors, as well as of the host organism, to a cytotoxic drug can be studied quantitatively with cell kinetic methods. Knowledge of this kind is necessary in the attempt to improve the application of cytotoxic drugs in chemotherapy of tumors which up to now has been based mainly on pure empiricism.

REFERENCES

1. HILSCHER, B., W. HILSCHER & W. MAURER. 1969. Autoradiographische Untersuchungen über den Modus der Proliferation und Regeneration des Samenepithels der Wistarratte. Z. Zellforsch. **94:** 593-604.
2. SCHULTZE, B., V. HAACK, A. C. SCHMEER & W. MAURER. 1972. Autoradiographic investigation on the cell kinetics of crypt epithelia in the jejunum of the mouse. Cell Tissue Kinet. **5:** 131-145.
3. KORR, H., B. SCHULTZE & W. MAURER. 1973. Autoradiographic investigations of glial proliferation in the brain of adult mice. I. The DNA synthesis phase of neuroglia and endothelial cells. J. Comp. Neurol. **150:** 169-176.
4. SCHULTZE, B., B. NOWAK & W. MAURER. 1974. Cycle times of the neural epithelial cells of various types of neuron in the rat. An autoradiographic study. J. Comp. Neurol. **158:** 207-218.
5. KORR, H., B. SCHULTZE & W. MAURER. 1975. Autoradiographic investigations of glial proliferation in the brain of adult mice. II. Cycle time and mode of proliferation of neuroglia and endothelial cells. J. Comp. Neurol. **160:** 477-490.
6. BURHOLT, D. R., B. SCHULTZE & W. MAURER. 1976. Mode of growth of the jejunal crypt cells of the rat: an autoradiographic study using double labelling with 3-H- and 14-C-thymidine in lower and upper parts of crypts. Cell Tissue Kinet. **9:** 107-117.
7. SCHULTZE, B., A. M. KELLERER, C. GROSSMANN & W. MAURER. 1978. Growth fraction and cycle duration of hepatocytes in the three-week old rat. Cell Tissue Kinet. **11:** 241-249.
8. SCHULTZE, B., A. M. KELLERER & W. MAURER. 1979. Transit times through the cycle phases of jejunal crypt cells of the mouse. Analysis in terms of the mean values and the variances. Cell Tissue Kinet. **12:** 347-359.
9. JELLINGHAUS, W., R. MAIDHOF, B. SCHULTZE & W. MAURER. 1975. Experimentelle Untersuchungen und zellkinetische Berechnungen zur Frage der Synchronisation mit Vincristin *in vivo* (Mäuseleukämie L 1210, Krypten-Epithelien der Maus). Z. Krebsforsch. **84:** 161-176.
10. JELLINGHAUS, W., B. SCHULTZE & W. MAURER. 1977. The effect of vincristine on mouse jejunal crypt cells of differing cell age: double labelling autoradiographic studies using ^{3}H- and ^{14}C-TdR. Cell Tissue Kinet. **10:** 147-156.
11. CAMPLEJOHN, R. S., B. SCHULTZE & W. MAURER. 1977. *In vivo* cell synchrony in the L 1210 mouse leukaemia studied with 5-fluorouracil or 5-fluorouracil followed by cold thymidine infusion. Br. J. Cancer **35:** 546-556.
12. CAMPLEJOHN, R. S., B. SCHULTZE & W. MAURER. 1980. An *in vivo* double labelling study of the subsequent fate of cells arrested in metaphase by vincristine in the JB-1 mouse ascites tumour. Cell Tissue Kinet. **13:** 239-250.
13. SCHULTZE, B., W. JELLINGHAUS, G. WEIS, V. MÜLLER & W. MAURER. 1981. Comparing cell kinetic studies of the effect of Ftorafur and 5-fluorouracil on the L 1210 ascites tumor. J. Cancer Res. Clin. Oncol. **100:** 25-40.

14. LENGSFELD, A. M., B. SCHULTZE & W. MAURER. 1981. Time-lapse studies on the effect of vincristine on HeLa cells. Eur. J. Cancer **17:** 307-319.
15. LENGSFELD, A. M., J. DIETRICH & B. SCHULTZE-MAURER. 1982. Accumulation and release of vinblastine and vincristine by HeLa cells: light microscopic, cinematographic, and biochemical study. Cancer Res. **42:** 3798-3805.
16. FIETKAU, R., H. FRIEDE & B. MAURER-SCHULTZE. 1985. Cell kinetic studies of the cytostatic and cytocidal effect of 1-β-D-arabinofuranosyl-cytosine on the L 1210 ascites tumor. Cancer Res. **44:** 1105-1113.
17. HOFER, K. G. & M. HOFER. 1971. Kinetics of proliferation, migration, and death of L 1210 ascites cells. Cancer Res. **31:** 402-408.
18. DEVIK, F. 1968. Quantitative cellular aspects of the epithelium in the small intestine of mice following total-body irradiation: cell death, mitosis and chromosome aberrations. *In* Effects of Radiation on Cellular Proliferation and Differentiation. Pp. 531-539. International Atomic Energy Agency. Vienna, Austria.
19. SCHÄFER, E., B. SCHULTZE & W. MAURER. Comparison of the cytocidal effect of various cytotoxic drugs on different ascites tumors of the mouse. In preparation.
20. BASSUKAS, I. & B. SCHULTZE. Studies on cell proliferation and on the effect of cyclophosphamide on a transplantable solid mouse tumor (adenocarcinoma EO 771). In preparation.

Redifferentiation of Cancer Cells: Bestatin, Estradiol, and Prostaglandin D$_2$

SHINICHI OKUYAMA,[a] HITOSHI MISHINA,[a]
AND TETSUO MAKI[b]

Departments of [a]Radiology and [b]Surgery
Tohoku Rosai Hospital
Sendai, Japan

INTRODUCTION

Several clinical situations in which induction of redifferentiation of cancer cells will be invaluable as soon as such a technique becomes available are: (1) residual cancer cells from the log kill limitation of radiotherapy and/or chemotherapy; (2) probable dissemination of cancer cells at the time of surgery; (3) widespread small metastases; and (4) probable maintenance of induced remissions. On the basis of our past experimental and clinical research,[1-4] we decided to carry out investigations on bestatin.[5,6] We have become convinced of the clinical inducibility of cancer cell redifferentiation with bestatin and appropriate hormones.

Bestatin is a small molecular product of *Streptomyces olivoreticuli*.[7] Through binding to hydrolytic enzymes on the cell surface, it may induce immunostimulation when it binds to lymphocytes as illustrated in FIGURE 1. It may also prevent metastatic settlement of cancer cells in normal tissues[8] through inhibition of hydrolytic enzymes which can be activated as soon as cancer cells approach.[9] What happens to cancer cells when they are sufficiently coated with bestatin molecules? This question served as the starting point for the present investigation on the probable induction of cancer redifferentiation with bestatin.

EXPERIMENTAL AND CLINICAL RESULTS

Bestatin is virtually nontoxic. Cancer cell kill in cell line FM3A of undifferentiated mammary adenocarcinoma of the mouse was marginal at 72 hr of exposure to the agent. Cell counts after 72 hr revealed a reduction in the saturation density (FIGURE 2).[5] This finding seemed to suggest the feasibility of induction of cancer redifferentiation, and a second agent, estradiol, was added to the culture on day 3. Pleomorphic alterations of the bestatin-treated cancer cells were observed as shown in FIGURE 3. There were goblet cell-like, neuron-like, and macrophage-like configurations in addition to others. Enlargement of the individual round cells was also a conspicuous feature. The dose response of FM3A cells to estradiol consisted of an initial sensitive

293

BESTATIN BINDS TO HYDROLYTIC ENZYMES ON CELL SURFACE

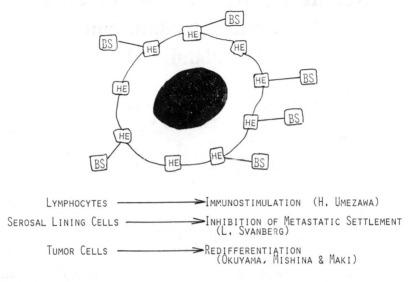

FIGURE 1. Biological significance of bestatin in mammalian cells. BS = bestatin; HE = hydrolytic enzyme.

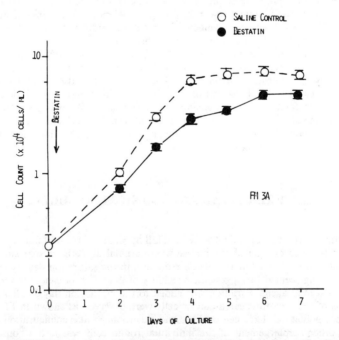

FIGURE 2. Bestatin reduces the saturation density of a cancer cell culture.

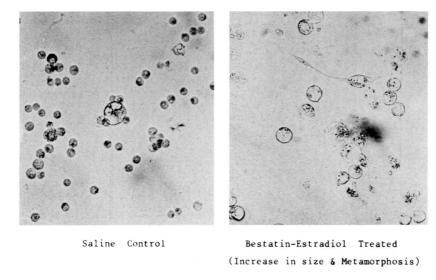

Saline   Control   Bestatin-Estradiol   Treated
(Increase in size & Metamorphosis)

FIGURE 3. Bestatin increases the cell size and induces morphological redifferentiation.

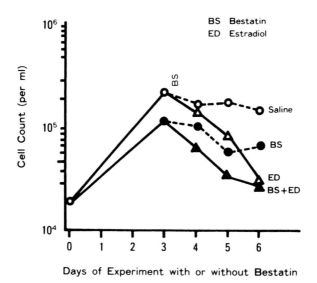

Days of Experiment with or without Bestatin

FIGURE 4. Bestatin-hormone regimen additively increases cell loss at a progressive rate.

phase, a plateau, and a phase of proportional cell kill; the induction of morphologic redifferentiation was feasible with the doses during the plateau phase. From the clinical point of view, reduction of cancer cells is the ultimate goal, so a viable cell count follow-up was carried out (FIGURE 4).

An additive effect on the viable cell count was observed. However, morphological redifferentiation was remarkably accelerated and augmented when bestatin and estradiol were administered consecutively (FIGURE 5). A deliberate dose-response analysis indicated that an optimal response is obtainable using a range of doses of estradiol

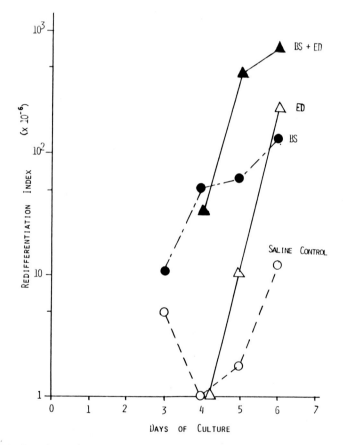

FIGURE 5. Bestatin accelerates and augments morphological redifferentiation, especially when consecutively followed by estradiol.

and a fixed dose of bestatin, and the response to a fixed dose of estradiol is greater, the larger the dose of bestatin. Therefore, it can be surmised that bestatin plays a preparatory function, while estradiol is a developer.

Testosterone was marginally toxic to FM3A cells, and morphological redifferentiation was increased by the consecutive bestatin-testosterone regimen.

The sequence of events was closely followed in a case of multiple skin metastasis from an operated breast cancer in a 74-year-old woman. FIGURE 6A shows a typical

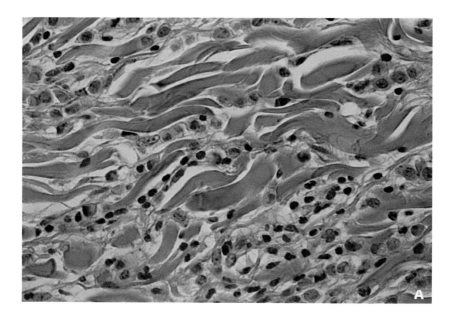

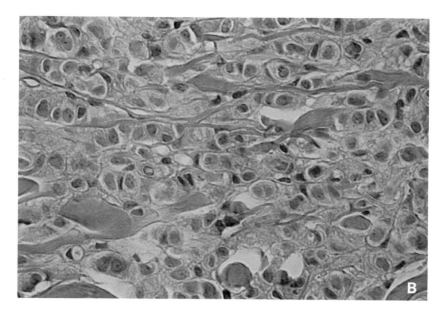

FIGURE 6. Induction of redifferentiation of cancer cells in a case of breast cancer: sheet formation in place of cord formation. The cancer cells became markedly larger than those in the untreated control (both A and B: bioptic materials of skin metastasis). (A) Before treatment. (B) Two weeks before lytic disappearance of the metastases.

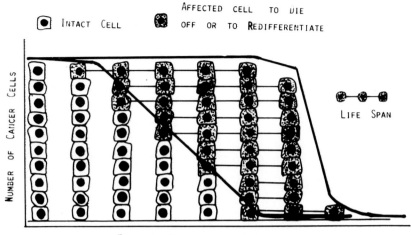

FIGURE 7. Redifferentiation of a tumor vs. tumor regression on effective radiotherapy or chemotherapy. In the former, the affected cells die off rather abruptly when their definite life span is over, while in the latter the affected cells disappear gradually as soon as the sensitive populations start waning.

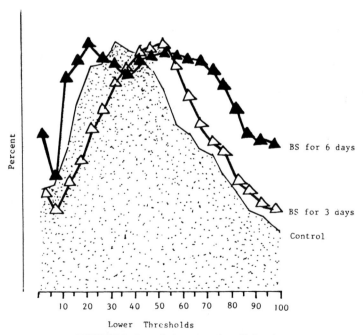

FIGURE 8. Bestatin increases the cellular size.

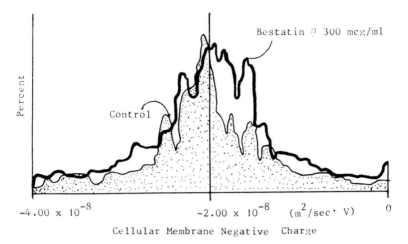

FIGURE 9. Bestatin reduces the membrane negative charge. This may be one of the fundamental alterations that can trigger cancer cells into cessation of proliferation and subsequent redifferentiation.

invasion of cancer cells. The metastatic nodules were essentially unchanged for 1 year in spite of tegafur and Cytoxan. Then bestatin was added to the regimen. Three weeks later, fluoxymesterone was added. Two weeks later, one of the metastases was biopsied. FIGURE 6B shows a sheet of large cancer cells. Cytoplasmic enlargement, nuclear enlargement, and sheet formation rather than tumor cord formation simulating the normal hepatocyte arrangement were characteristic. This sheet formation may represent the return of contact inhibition. During the subsequent 2 weeks, the metastatic nodules were reduced in size and ultimately disappeared. Thus, this lytic contracture of tumors following a period of incubation seemed to suggest a loss of cancer cells via redifferentiation, that is, the acquisition of a limited life span for the cancer cells (FIGURE 7).

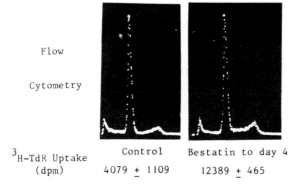

FIGURE 10. A threefold increase in [³H]TdR uptake and slight increase in the proportion of 4n cells: Bestatin increases DNA synthesis, and yet blocks the age progression at the $G_2 + M$ phase.

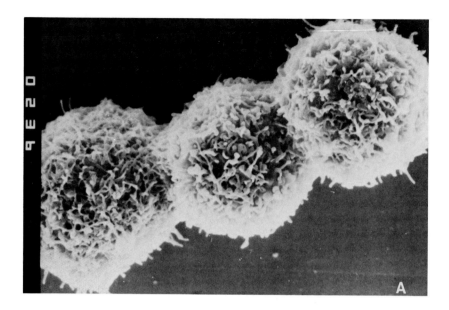

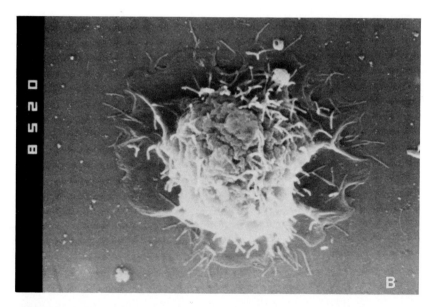

FIGURE 11. Bestatin promotes formation of fine tree-like processes in the presence of estradiol, but eventually leads the cancer cells to degenerate as studied by scanning electron microscopy. (A) Untreated FM3A cells with fine villi on the surface. (B) Fine tree-like processes were formed when consecutively exposed to bestatin and estradiol. (C) Eventual degeneration of bestatin-estradiol-treated cells after a definite life span was consumed.

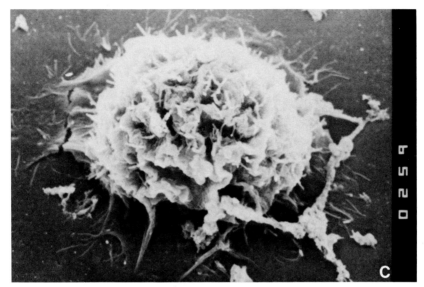

FIGURE 11. (*Continued.*)

How can cancer cells be seduced to redifferentiate and eventually die off after a limited life span? Using the same FM3A cells, the following observations were made: (1) bestatin increased the cell size (FIGURE 8); (2) it reduced the cell membrane negative charge (FIGURE 9); (3) it increased the [^{3}H]thymidine ([^{3}H]TdR) uptake threefold; (4) the treated cells were blocked at the $G_2 + M$ phase as studied by flow fluorocytometry (FIGURE 10); and (5) on the scanning electron microscope, bestatin-treated cancer cells appeared to be roughened on their surface as they apparently lost the fine villi, while cancer cells treated with estradiol developed much finer villi (FIGURE 11). On the consecutive bestatin-estradiol regimen, the finer villi were accompanied by large processes on one hand, and degenerative changes to the surface structures on the other. We may therefore speculate here that redifferentiation of the undifferentiated mammary adenocarcinoma cells is achievable, that these redifferentiated cells die off following a definite life span, and that bestatin plays a preparatory role.

Prostaglandin D_2 kills cancer cells *in vitro.*[10] It controls metastatic phenomena[11,12] probably through alteration in the cellular membrane negative charge.[13] We therefore had a logical reason to look for any signs of cancer redifferentiation in the presence of prostaglandin D_2. FIGURE 12 shows the typical response of FM3A cells when the agent was administered consecutively with bestatin. Additive effects on viable cell count (FIGURE 13) and induction of morphological redifferentiation (FIGURE 14) were confirmed.

The experiments were extended to the M1 leukemia cell line of the mouse. This line is well known for induction of redifferentiation to macrophages and granulocytes. In a dose-response study, the proportion of sensitive populations did not change between 48 and 96 hr of exposure (FIGURE 15). This may suggest the evolution of sensitive cells as the cancer cells advance in cell age. The consecutive bestatin-prostaglandin D_2 regimen increased the nuclear and cytoplasmic volumes (FIGURE

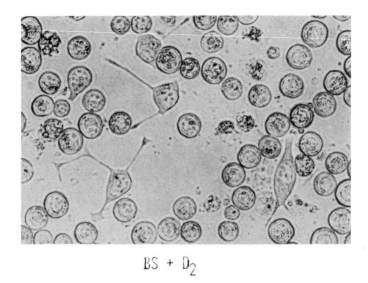

$$BS + D_2$$

FIGURE 12. Bestatin-prostaglandin D_2 regimen can also increase morphological redifferentiation in mammary adenocarcinoma cells.

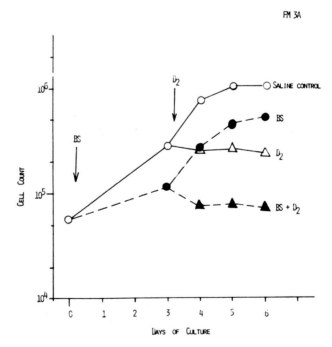

FIGURE 13. Prostaglandin D_2 may prolong the mean life span of cancer cells since it eliminates a fraction of sensitive cells and since it induces redifferentiation in the remaining majority.

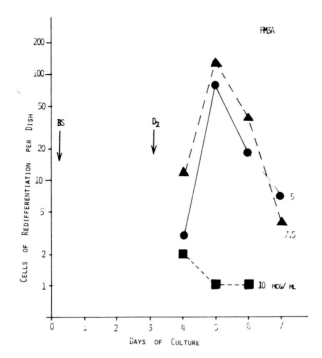

FIGURE 14. Prostaglandin D_2 induces redifferentiation of cancer cells.

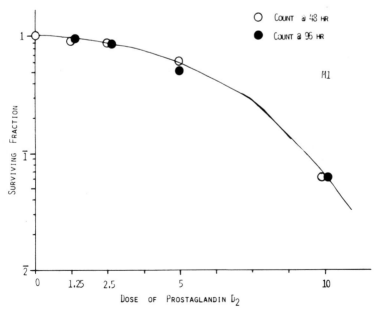

FIGURE 15. Prostaglandin D_2 eliminates cancer cells dose dependently.

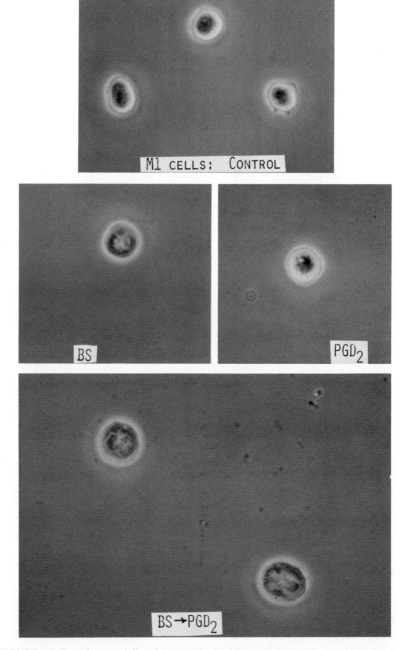

FIGURE 16. Bestatin, especially when combined with prostaglandin D_2, markedly increased the nuclear and cytoplasmic volumes. (Original magnification, $\times 600$; reduced to 80% of original size.)

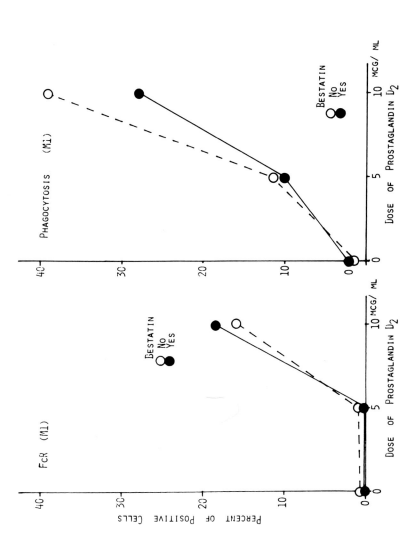

FIGURE 17. Prostaglandin D_2 induced differentiation of Fc receptors and phagocytic function irrespective of bestatin.

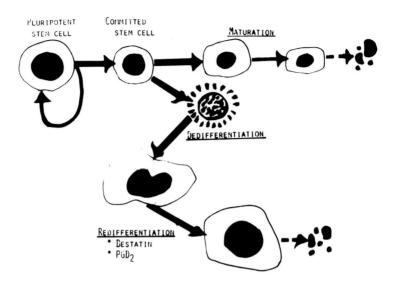

FIGURE 18. Redifferentiation against dedifferentiation and normal maturation.

16). This change is common to both FM3A and M1 cells in response to bestatin alone or in combination. There was no morphological differentiation to macrophages or granulocytes. However, functional differentiation of Fc receptors and phagocytosis occurred (FIGURE 17).

COMMENTS

Cessation of proliferation, acquisition of definite life span, functional to morphological differentiation, and ultimate cell death seem to be the sequence of events when cancer cells are treated with both bestatin alone or in combination with hormones, and prostaglandin D_2 alone or in combination with bestatin. The initial biological alteration can be the reduction of the cellular membrane negative charge which eventually leads to tetraploidy with subsequent redifferentiation. The clinical diagnosis of cancer redifferentiation might be permitted from the prolonged latency with lytic contracture of the tumor (FIGURE 7). Redifferentiation is nothing but an attempt at reversal of dedifferentiation, and it may have nothing to do with the attainment of normal maturation of the cell renewal systems (FIGURE 18).

SUMMARY

The induction of redifferentiation of cancer cells was studied. This was achievable with bestatin, especially in combination with sex hormones or prostaglandin D_2, in murine undifferentiated mammary adenocarcinoma cells *in vitro.* Prostaglandin D_2 also exerted a similar redifferentiating effect on M1 murine leukemia cells and a consecutive bestatin-hormone regimen was effective in endocrine tumors in man. Cancer redifferentiation may one day be developed into a clinical technique.

REFERENCES

1. OKUYAMA, S., T. SATO, K. TAKAHASHI & T. MATSUZAWA. 1978. Gallium modification of cancer biology: experimental studies on V2 rabbit carcinoma. Sci. Rep. Res. Inst. Tohoku Univ. Ser. C **25**: 58.
2. AWANO, T. & T. MATSUZAWA. 1977. Accumulation and biological effects of gallium in malignant cell lines in vitro. Jpn. J. Nucl. Med. **14**: 73.
3. OKUYAMA, S., M. SANO, T. AWANO, S. TAKEDA, K. YAMADA, K. TAKAHASHI & T. MATSUZAWA. 1984. Gallium induces reduction of negative charge of the cell membrane and redifferentiation of cancer cells. Tohoku J. Exp. Med. **142**: 347.
4. OKUYAMA, S. & H. MISHINA. 1983. Principia of cancer therapy. V. Clinical and histopathological criteria for cancer redifferentiation. Sci. Rep. Res. Inst. Tohoku Univ. Ser. C **30**: 31.
5. OKUYAMA, S. & H. MISHINA. 1984. Decrease in saturation density of mammalian carcinoma cell culture during exposure to *bestatin,* a clinically applicable agent. Tohoku J. Exp. Med. **142**: 349.
6. OKUYAMA, S., H. MISHINA & T. MAKI. Consecutive bestatin-hormone regimen for cancer redifferentiation. *In* Proceedings, 13th International Congress on Chemotherapy, Vienna, 28 August-2 September 1983. Part 289, pp. 11-14.
7. UMEZAWA, H. 1978. Recent advances in bioactive microbial secondary metabolites. J. Antibiot. **30**(Suppl.): 138.
8. SVANBERG, L. E. & O. ELISSON. Application of bestatin to the treatment of lung cancer. *In* Proceedings, 13th International Congress on Chemotherapy, Vienna, 28 August-2 September 1983. Symposium 67. Chemo-immunotherapy (Bestatin).
9. BIRBECK, M. S. C. & D. N. WHEATLEY. 1965. Electron microscopic study of the invasion of ascites tumor cells into the abdominal wall. Cancer Res. **25**: 490.
10. FUKUSHIMA, M., T. KATO, R. UEDA, K. OTA, S. NARUMIYA & O. HAYAISHI. 1982. Prostaglandin D_2, a potential antineoplastic agent. Biochem. Biophys. Res. Commun. **105**: 956.
11. FITZPATRICK, F. A. & D. A. STRINGFELLOW. 1979. Prostaglandin D_2 formation by malignant melanoma cells correlates inversely with cellular metastatic potential. Proc. Natl. Acad. Sci. USA **76**: 1765.
12. STRINGFELLOW, D. A. & F. A. FITZPATRICK. 1979. Prostaglandin D_2 controls pulmonary metastasis of malignant melanoma cells. Nature **282**: 76.
13. KONDO, K., T. SHIMIZU & O. HAYAISHI. 1981. Effects of prostaglandin D_2 on membrane potential in neuroblastoma $\times$ glioma hybrid cells as determined with a cyanine dye. Biochem. Biophys. Res. Commun. **98**: 648.

Leukemic Cellular Proliferation: A Perspective[a]

P. C. VINCENT

Kanematsu Research Laboratories
Royal Prince Alfred Hospital
Missenden Road
Camperdown, New South Wales 2050, Australia

The golden age of morphological hematology characterized the appearance of normal and leukemic hematopoietic progenitors, but a century passed before techniques became available to study the proliferative kinetics of these cells. Lack of techniques did not, however, prevent hematologists of the time from speculating about the origin and interrelationships of the cells they saw under the microscope, and many of their conclusions based on deductive reasoning were remarkably accurate. Neumann in Germany and Bizzozero in Italy are credited with being the first, in 1868, to recognize that blood cells were produced in the bone marrow.[1] This conclusion seems all the more remarkable when one considers that other theories of red cell production favored at the time included: disintegration of white cell nuclei; "hemoglobinic degeneration" of white cells; production from fat globules in the liver; formation from protoplasm of scavenger cells, platelets, or other cells; and aggregation of pigmented granules. With the recognition that blood cells were produced in the marrow by a process which continued throughout adult life, the search began for the proliferative relationships between these cells, and for the elusive progenitors from which they arose. The discussions of the time generated more heat than light, the principal argument being between the monophyletic theory espoused by Pappenheim and others and the dualistic theory of Ehrlich, Naegeli, and their supporters.[2] Even as late as 1938, Bloom, writing in Downey's famous *Handbook of Hematology*, was able to summarize 12 different theories of hematopoiesis, belonging to one school or the other, and to add one more of his own[3]; similar discussions can be found in textbooks of the 1940s.[4]

During a period when there was so much debate about the process of normal hematopoietic proliferation, it is hardly surprising that leukemic cellular proliferation was also the subject of untested speculation. The disease leukemia was first described in 1845, the origin of leukemic cells from the marrow recognized by 1870, classification of the leukemias begun by 1900, and radiation recognized as a potential leukemogenic agent in 1911.[5] Nonetheless the concepts of leukemic cellular proliferation were influenced by the stem cell school to which the hematologist belonged, and the interrelationships between leukemic cells and their supposedly normal counterparts were adjusted to fit the relevant theory. Lest we regard these old theories with amused

[a]Research supported by grants from the National Health and Medical Research Council of Australia, the New South Wales State Cancer Council, the Jenny Leukaemia Foundation, and the New South Wales Department of Health.

detachment, however, it is worth remembering that it has been only in the last 10 years that membrane phenotype and enzyme studies have proved what would previously have been thought inconceivable—namely, that in a significant proportion of patients with chronic granulocytic leukemia (CGL) the cells in the acute phase of the disease are indistinguishable from those of acute lymphoblastic leukemia (ALL).[6] This observation, and similar studies using membrane phenotype analysis,[7,8] in turn led to a reappraisal of normal hematopoietic stem cells and finally vindicated Pappenheim's monophyletic theory.

Prior to the late 1950s, most hematologists believed that leukemic cells proliferated more rapidly than normal. In the absence of any method of measuring the proliferative rate of leukemic cells, and faced with the evidence of marrow expansion, organomegaly, and frequent leukocytosis, this interpretation was understandable. It provided the rationale for the development of chemotherapeutic agents selected for their ability to attack dividing cells, and it was perhaps fortunate that the efficacy of the earliest drugs had been established before anything was known of the true nature of leukemic cell proliferation.[9-11] What is now known makes it harder, not easier, to explain why these drugs work as well as they do.

MEASUREMENT OF LEUKEMIC CELL PROLIFERATION

Quantitative analyses of normal and malignant hematopoietic cellular proliferation became possible in the late 1950s as a result of a confluence of disciplines (FIGURE 1). Radiation biology was the first of these, following the events of 1945. Although radiation had been recognized as a probable leukemogen as early as 1911 and radiation effects *in vitro* had been studied in the 1930s,[12] it was not until the period after World War II that recruitment began of a new breed of what could well be called mathematical hematologists, among whom Eugene P. Cronkite was one of the leading figures.[13-17] In addition to analyzing the mechanism of radiation leukemogenesis, radiation biology led to studies of the therapeutic effects of internal or external radiation [including the innovative approach of extracorporeal irradiation of the blood (ECIB)][18-20] and to the development of bone marrow transplantation, and isotopic techniques for analyzing cell proliferation.

Bone marrow transplantation was more than a development leading to the definitive treatment of selected patients with leukemia by the 1970s. The capacity of infused marrow to protect syngeneic animals from radiation, demonstrated in 1950, led to the classical studies by Ford and his colleagues which proved that marrow reconstitution in this situation resulted from the clonal expansion of hematopoietic pluripotential stem cells (HPSC),[21] and to the spleen-colony HPSC assay of Till and McCulloch.[22] Successful human marrow transplantation had to await the elucidation of human transplantation antigens and the recognition of graft-versus-host disease, but in the meantime experimentalists used radiation as a tool to answer many of the questions concerning hematopoietic reconstitution in animals.

ISOTOPIC ANALYSES

Isotopically labeled nucleic acid precursors provided experimental hematologists with a powerful tool for studying normal and leukemic hematopoiesis. Radioactive

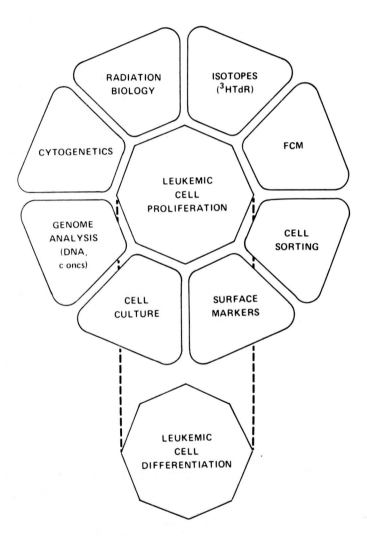

FIGURE 1. Schematic summary of the disciplines that have contributed to the study of leukemic cell proliferation and differentiation.

phosphorus had been used to study leukemic cell proliferation by 1951,[23] and to determine the intravascular survival of leukocytes by 1954.[24] Important contributions were also made using [^{14}C]thymidine and [^{125}I]- or [^{131}I]iododeoxyuridine, but easily the most significant compound was [^{3}H]thymidine ([^{3}H]TdR) developed at Brookhaven National Laboratory and in Belgium in 1956.[25,26] Incorporated specifically by a salvage pathway into cells synthesizing DNA and capable of giving high-resolution autoradiographs, [^{3}H]TdR allowed experimentalists to identify which morphological cell types were proliferating, the proportion of each type synthesizing DNA, the time parameters of the cell cycle and each of its phases, the rate of cell production, the nature of chromosome duplication, and the subsequent fate of the labeled cells.[25-34] In hematopoiesis, for example, it became possible for the first time to establish the qualitative and quantitative relationships between proliferating and maturing nonproliferating pools, and to confirm the orderly movement of cells through the marrow compartments and into the blood,[35-43] previously inferred from traditional morphological studies.

Predictably, [^{3}H]TdR was also used to study cell kinetics in acute leukemia (AL) with somewhat unexpected results.[27,28,32,44-46] Contrary to expectations, AL cells gave the appearance of a population with a low proliferative rate and with relatively few cells synthesizing DNA, as measured by the low overall [^{3}H]TdR labeling index (LI).[27,28,47-50] Further analysis showed that AL cells consisted of heterogeneous populations with different proliferative capacities, with populations of large, usually morphologically typical, blasts having higher LIs than populations of smaller, often atypical, blasts.[50-59] Large proliferative blasts were more frequently found in the marrow than in the blood, but blasts in the blood were able to return to the marrow.[60] Even more significantly, it was shown that nondividing AL cells could resume division[56] and could repair their DNA after ultraviolet (UV) exposure.[61] In this respect, it became apparent that AL resembled the solid tumors, in which it had already been shown that the fraction of cells in cycle was appreciably less than unity.[62] Whether quiescent AL cells are in a true G_0 state—i.e., they are not in cycle but are capable of reentering it—or are merely in a grossly prolonged G_1 phase but still in cycle might be a matter of semantics, but has yet to be decided.

The explanation for the steady expansion of leukemic tissue in AL thus lay not in a greatly increased proliferative rate, but in the relentless reentry of daughter cells into the proliferative pool. Even if this reentry was quantitatively small, and even if leukemic cell death was considerable, it was possible to show by computer modeling that the blast count would steadily increase.[63]

It is interesting to recall that one of the objectives in mind when [^{3}H]TdR was first developed was the possibility of using it as an antileukemic agent, utilizing its ability to deliver a high dose of radiation over a short distance within the nucleus.[33] Some success has been reported using this approach,[64] and Cronkite et al. have recently presented a reappraisal of its potential.[26] The selectively cytocidal effect of a high dose of [^{3}H]TdR has of course been extensively used in vitro as the thymidine suicide technique for deducing the proportions of cells in culture that are synthesizing DNA.[65]

Isotope analyses have also contributed to our understanding of cell proliferation in the chronic leukemias. In CGL the proliferative pattern that emerged was qualitatively remarkably similar to normal granulopoiesis, as defined by studies using diisopropyl fluorophosphate-^{32}P (DF^{32}P) or [^{3}H]TdR. Both blood granulocyte pools, marginated and circulating, were found to be grossly expanded, with some prolongation in blood granulocyte survival,[66] and the proliferative characteristics of CGL myelocytes in blood or marrow were little different from normal.[48,66-68] However, extensive cellular traffic among the spleen, blood, and marrow was demonstrable, and it seemed probable that the spleen was a significant source of immature cells.[67]

In 1967 Dameshek characterized chronic lymphocytic leukemia (CLL) as an accumulative disease of immunologically incompetent lymphocytes.[69] Subsequent kinetic studies showing low [³H]TdR LIs in CLL lymphocytes, slow emergence of labeled cells into the blood, and complex disappearance patterns of reinfused autologous lymphocytes,[70-72] confirmed Dameshek's hypothesis. ECIB, as well as proving to be a useful therapeutic procedure in selected patients with CLL, provided a means by which the complex lymphocyte pools in this disease could be analyzed.[73]

FLOW CYTOMETRY

One could suggest, facetiously perhaps, that flow cytometry (FCM) was devised by experimentalists who had wearied of counting autoradiographs. Certainly, an apprenticeship in [³H]TdR analysis is a good background to appreciate the advantages of the technique, first developed in the 1960s[74] and since refined to the point where FCM-derived histograms of cells stained with DNA-specific dyes are widely used to obtain rapid, accurate estimates of the proportions of cells in each of the phases of the cell cycle.[75-78] It is interesting to compare the advantages and disadvantages of [³H]TdR autoradiography (ARG) and FCM (TABLE 1). FCM has the advantage that larger numbers of cells can be sampled (thus lessening the Poisson counting error) much more quickly than with ARG, but the distinct disadvantage that in most situations it is not possible to tell which cells are being analyzed. In relatively homogeneous populations such as leukemic blasts this is not as critical as in normal marrow, although it would be helpful if FCM techniques could be developed to analyze large and small blasts separately. Contamination of aspirated marrow samples by blood cells is a greater problem with FCM than with [³H]TdR ARG. In normal marrows, contamination with nondividing nucleated blood cells leads to a serious underestimate of the percentage of S-phase cells,[79] while in AL marrows, contamination with predominantly nondividing blood blasts has a similar effect.[78,80] These problems can be overcome, but must be taken into account. FCM has other advantages: it can be used to enumerate cells in the G_0/G_1 and $(G_2 + M)$ phases of the cycle, and it can easily identify aneuploid populations.[78] On the other hand, the S-phase percentage of aneuploid populations cannot be determined by FCM in most cases, due to overlap of aneuploid G_1 cells with diploid S-phase cells and of aneuploid S-phase cells with diploid $(G_2 + M)$ cells (FIGURE 2). Very rarely, the leukemic population is hypertetraploid and it then becomes possible to analyze its kinetic profile separately from that of diploid cells.[81]

If [³H]TdR is given intravenously, it is possible (but not easy) to measure cell cycle times,[29,40] and to follow the fate of labeled cells.[36-38,41-43] By contrast, cycle time analysis is difficult using FCM, although some progress has been made.[82-84] FCM analyses can be obtained quickly enough to be used in treatment planning,[85] whereas this is impossible using [³H]TdR ARG. The existence of G_0 cells can be inferred from [³H]TdR studies,[62] but which of the population of nonlabeling cells they are cannot be decided from autoradiographs. Differential DNA/RNA staining with acridine orange[86] followed by FCM has been described as a way of identifying resting leukemic cells, and indeed subdividing them into functional subclasses.[80,87] The transferrin receptor, recognized by the monoclonal antibody OKT 9, is expressed preferentially on proliferating cells.[88] Whether it will prove possible, however, to distinguish (and separate) quiescent cells by their low density of this receptor has yet to be determined.

The ability to sort cells by any of the properties detected by FCM has been extensively developed.[89] [The acronym FACS (fluorescence-activated cell sorting) applied to this technique is somewhat misleading, since sorting can be equally well achieved using nonfluorescent parameters such as cell size, membrane structure, "time of flight," and so on. Parameter-activated cell sorting (PACS) might be preferable, and has the added advantage of avoiding the commercial associations of "FACS."] PACS has proved valuable in immunology and in membrane phenotype analysis (see below), but has been used less frequently in kinetic studies.[82] Sorting of OKT 9-positive leukemic cells[88] might help our understanding of leukemic cell proliferation.

Finally, TABLE 1 includes an estimate of the capital cost of the equipment for FCM compared with, say, a microscope for [³H]TdR ARG. Even purely analytical FCM instruments are expensive, and the cost more than doubles if a sorting capacity is added.

TABLE 1. Comparison of Kinetic Analyses Using Tritiated Thymidine Autoradiography ([³H]TdR ARG) and Flow Cytometry (FCM)

	[³H]TdR ARG	FCM
Number of cells	10^3	10^5
Counting error	3%	0.3%
Time for: Preparation	Weeks	Hour(s)
Analysis	Days	Minutes
Cell-type recognition	Yes	No
Marrow aspirates	Yes	No
Phases of cell cycle	S, M	All
G_0 vs. G_1 cells	No	Possibly
Detection of aneuploidy	No	Yes
S analysis if aneuploid	Yes	No
Cycle times	Yes[a]	No(?)
Fate of cells	Yes[a]	No
Clinically applicable	No	Yes
Cell sorting	No	Yes
Cost ($)	5,000-10,000	100,000-250,000

[a]With in vivo [³H]TdR only.

MEMBRANE PHENOTYPE ANALYSES

The observation that small mature lymphocytes, of uniform morphological appearance in conventional blood smears, belonged to two distinct populations distinguishable by whether they formed nonimmune rosettes with sheep erythrocytes[90] was the forerunner of an explosive growth of membrane phenotype analysis in immunology and in leukemia research. This growth was accelerated by the development of hybridomas secreting uniquely specific monoclonal antibodies (moab's)[91,92] capable of recognizing membrane antigens previously obscured in the "noise" of even the best conventional antisera. Direct or indirect labeling with fluorescein isothiocyanate (FITC)-conjugated antibodies has enabled rapid analysis of the populations by FCM, and their separation by PACS. In the case of the leukemias, membrane phenotype analyses have contributed particularly to our understanding of ALL,[7,93,94] of CLL,[93,95–97] and of the acute phase of CGL.[7,98] The use of moab's in acute myeloblastic leukemia (AML) has lagged behind, but will undoubtedly catch up.[99] The possibility that moab's might be useful in eliminating leukemic cells from human bone marrow *in vitro* is also being explored.[100]

Membrane phenotype analyses have revealed the sequential interrelationships in leukemic cell proliferation, particularly in ALL, CLL, and CGL. In this sense the qualitative or descriptive assessment they provide is complementary to quantitative measurements using [3H]TdR ARG or FCM. Theoretically at least it should be possible to combine the two techniques to measure the flow rates from one maturative compartment to the next, using, for example, [3H]TdR labeling and PACS sorting of cells labeled with FITC moab's against the relevant antigen. Another approach could be to measure the rate of outflow of [3H]TdR-labeled cells from the proliferating pool identified and sorted by the presence of the transferrin receptor.[88]

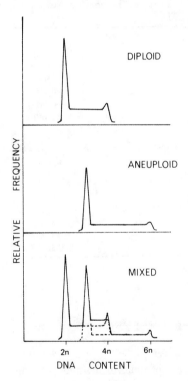

FIGURE 2. Diagrammatic FCM traces showing the effect aneuploid cells have on the S-phase estimate of mixed populations containing diploid and aneuploid cells. Pure diploid or aneuploid populations show a major G_0/G_1 peak and a less pronounced $(G_2 + M)$ peak; cells in S have intermediate amounts of DNA. In the mixed population (bottom panel) the aneuploid G_0/G_1 cells overlap diploid S cells, and diploid $(G_2 + M)$ cells overlap aneuploid S cells.

THE CLONAL NATURE OF LEUKEMIC CELL PROLIFERATION

The presence of the Philadelphia (Ph[1]) chromosome in CGL, first reported by Nowell and Hungerford in 1960,[101] was the first evidence that leukemia in man could result from the proliferation of a clone derived from a single cell which had undergone genetic rearrangement. Subsequent studies have confirmed this conclusion, and it is now known that: (1) the Ph[1] chromosome involves a translocation of material from the long arm of chromosome 22, usually (but not always) to chromosome 9; (2) all hematopoietic cells in CGL arise from the same—i.e., Ph[1] positive—cell line; and (3) B lymphocytes in CGL are also Ph[1] positive.[102,103] Glucose-6-phosphate dehydrogenase (G6PD) isoenzyme analyses have confirmed these findings.[104,105] The presence of Ph[1]-positive, isoenzyme-identical, B lymphocytes in CGL, predicted from membrane phenotype analyses of CGL in the blastic phase,[6,7,98] is probably the best evidence for the existence of pluripotential hemopoietic stem cells in man, originally proposed by Pappenheim as his monophyletic theory.

Nonrandom cytogenetic abnormalities are found in some, but by no means all, cases of acute leukemia (for reviews, see References 102, 106, and 107). The 15:17 translocation, for example, is found in 40% of patients with acute promyelocytic leukemia (APL) and the 8:21 translocation in 15% of those with AML.[102] G6PD isoenzyme studies have also confirmed the clonal nature of the blast cell population in AML, but in contrast with the situation in CGL, red cells do not appear to arise from the same clone.[104]

Recent studies have shown that human oncogenes (c-oncs) tend to be located at or near breakpoints involved in translocations in leukemias.[108,109] In CGL, for example, the c-abl sequence located on chromosome 9 has been shown to be reciprocally translocated to chromosome 22.[110] The rearrangement in Burkitt's lymphoma is particularly interesting, since the 8:14 translocation frequently found in this disorder has been shown to involve the insertion of a c-myc gene from 8q24 into the immunoglobulin μ-chain gene.[111,112] The c-mos oncogene, also found on chromosome 8, has been localized to 8q22,[113] which is also the breakpoint in the 8:21 translocation seen in a proportion of patients with AML.[108] Two other findings strengthen the view that c-oncs might be related to leukemogenesis. First, they have been implicated as possible regulators of cell proliferation, either by tyrosine phosphorylation[114] or by production of growth factors[115]; and second, c-onc genes have been shown to be amplified in human leukemic cells.[116,117]

Although these cytogenetic and oncogene studies shed a great deal of light on the clonal origin and possible proliferative abnormalities of leukemic cells, many questions remain to be answered. For example, in a minority of patients with CGL the Ph[1] chromosome results from a translocation to a chromosome other than number 9; how does this fit in with the reciprocal c-abl translocation? Again, while the 15:17 and 8:21 translocations of APL and AML, respectively, are frequent abnormalities, they are by no means invariably found. Are APLs or AMLs which lack these markers different diseases? Or is the leukemogenic event more subtle, and are the translocations secondary, albeit frequent, consequences? What triggers c-onc expression or amplification? Finally and perhaps most intriguingly, given that this presumably occurs in a single cell to begin with, how does this confer a proliferative advantage on that cell?

STEM CELLS IN LEUKEMIA

By the early 1970s, sufficient experimental data had accumulated to provide a reasonably clear picture of the role of stem cells in normal hematopoiesis.[118,119] A small pool of pluripotential stem cells,[22] capable of self-renewal, with a low proliferative activity but a vast proliferative potential feeds into pools of second-generation stem cells, each committed to one line of hematopoiesis or lymphopoiesis,[120-122] which in turn feed into recognizable cell compartments which amplify the input and promote cellular maturation.[41-43] Amplification probably occurs at the level of the second-generation stem cells as well,[119,123] along with a progressive loss of "stemness." The second-generation cells are also the key points at which normal hematopoietic regulators such as erythropoietin[124,125] and monocyte-derived colony stimulating activity[126] act.

Normal hematopoiesis requires a continuous input of stem cells in order to provide for the one-way traffic of cells moving through the recognizable marrow compartments into the blood. Even with extensive amplification, the magnitude of this input is considerable. What is not known is whether established leukemic hematopoiesis involves a similar continual stem cell input.[44-46] The cytogenetic and isoenzyme data reviewed above point clearly to the clonal origin of leukemia, almost certainly as a result of genetic rearrangement in a normal hematopoietic stem cell,[127] but once the disease is established it is quite conceivable that continual reentry of blasts into cycle could account for leukemic cell expansion, even in the presence of considerable cell death, without the need for further stem cell input[46,63] (FIGURE 3). Attempts to study leukemic stem cells using the granulocyte-monocyte (CFU-C) colony technique revealed that in the great majority of patients with AL, colonies either failed to grow or were replaced by small clusters of cells.[128,129] Eventually, appropriate conditions were defined to allow the growth of AL cells in culture,[130,131] and the ability of these cells to form colonies on subculture was demonstrated.[130] Whether this capacity for self-renewal *in vitro* proves that leukemic colony forming cells are true stem cells is, however, still open to question. In particular, it is not clear whether this population

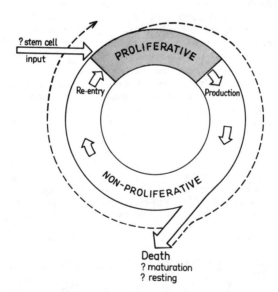

FIGURE 3. Reentry of nonproliferating blasts into the proliferative pool is sufficient to account for a progressive expansion of leukemic cell numbers (shown by the broken line), even with significant cell loss (by cell death, possible maturation, or removal to a quiescent phase). The magnitude and significance of a continuous stem cell input are unknown. (Reprinted by permission from: Leukemia. Chapter 6: Cell Kinetics of the Leukemias. 1983. F. W. Gunz & E. S. Henderson, Eds. Grune & Stratton. New York, N.Y.)

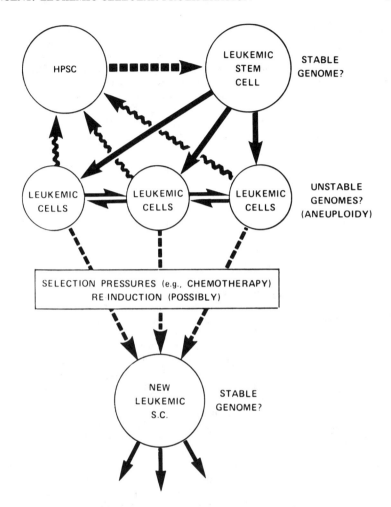

FIGURE 4. Model of possible leukemic stem cell evolution. Leukemic stem cells originate by transformation of a normal hematopoietic stem cell (HPSC) and give rise to leukemic cells which inhibit any residual normal HPSC. Leukemic cells may have unstable genomes and under selection pressures (such as chemotherapy) could give rise to new leukemic stem cells.

functions as a leukemic stem cell pool *in vivo,* but if it does it would have far-reaching implications for treatment.

Recent studies have shed light on the effect of leukemic stem cells on normal hematopoietic progenitors, and have partly explained the failure of normal marrow function characteristic at least of AL. Morris *et al.* were the first to show that leukemic cells co-cultured with normal marrow inhibited CFU-C.[132] Broxmeyer and his colleagues subsequently reported that leukemic cell extracts, or media conditioned by short-term leukemic cell cultures, contained a potent specific inhibitor of normal CFU-C.[133,134]

FIGURE 4 presents one model in which the leukemic stem cell originates by transformation of a normal hematopoietic stem cell and gives rise to recognizable leukemic blasts. These in turn inhibit residual normal stem cells and are themselves subject to selection pressures such as chemotherapy. It is possible that cells within this population have unstable genomes—as evidenced, for example, by the frequency of random chromosome abnormalities in AL. All too frequently, drug-resistant relapse occurs, presumably by mutation of existing blasts or by selection of innately resistant cells from within a persisting stem cell pool. Considerable progress has been made in understanding the reasons for resistance to antimetabolites. In the case of methotrexate resistance, for example, amplification of genes coding for dihydrofolate reductase occurs in homogeneously staining regions and in double minute chromosomes of resistant cells.[135,136]

LEUKEMIC CELL PROLIFERATION AND CHEMOTHERAPY

All the antileukemic drugs in use today—with the possible exception of steroids—were developed for their ability to inhibit or preferably kill proliferating cells.[44–46,137–142] In a given patient, two questions which follow from this are: (1) Does the effectiveness of a given drug or regimen relate to the proliferative characteristics of leukemic blasts? (2) Can the proliferative behavior of the cells be modified to increase the effectiveness of therapy?

The answer to the first question is that most workers have been unable to show any relationship between the proportion of leukemic S-phase cells (measured either as the [³H]TdR LI, or by FCM) and the likelihood of response to treatment, while a few have reported better responses in patients with higher marrow LIs and others a better ultimate survival in patients whose marrow S-phase cells were initially low (for a list of relevant references, see Reference 46).

Occasional successes have been reported following maneuvers designed either to increase the numbers of cells in cycle (by recruiting quiescent cells[143–145]) or to increase the proportions in a phase of the cycle more susceptible to subsequent chemotherapy (by synchronizing leukemic cell division[81,143,145–148]). These approaches have, however, failed to gain wide acceptance.[142] One problem has been that these agents will also of course synchronize normal cells (FIGURE 5), and it has been impossible in most instances to distinguish this effect from any synchronization induced in leukemic cells.[81] If normal and leukemic cells are synchronized in step with each other, subsequent treatment may have an enhanced myelosuppressive effect. A second problem has been that results cannot be obtained quickly enough from [³H]TdR ARG to decide the timing of subsequent therapy, which must obviously coincide with an enhanced number of either synchronized or recruited cells to be of any use. The use of FCM analysis could, however, overcome this problem.[81,149]

A completely different approach to the treatment of AL, namely, to attempt to induce differentiation of leukemic cells, was suggested by Sachs[150,151] following early observations that defective differentiation is almost certainly related to the ability of leukemic cells to reenter the cell cycle.[52,53] The effect of low doses of cytosine arabinoside (Ara-C), one of the agents capable of inducing differentiation in vitro, is currently being evaluated after an earlier promising report.[152] The results are encouraging, particularly in patients with hypocellular marrows.[153,154] One interesting finding is the possibility that patients refractory to conventional doses of Ara-C might respond to the drug in low dose.

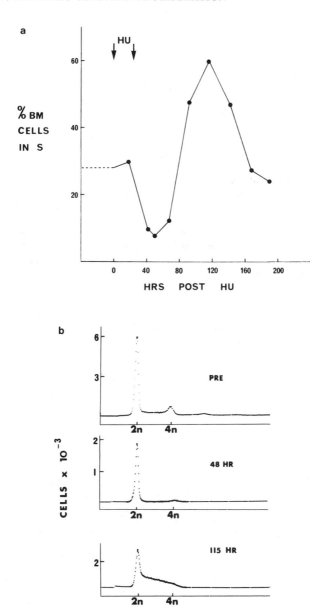

FIGURE 5. Effect of hydroxyurea on normal sheep bone marrow cells: synchronization of normal marrow cells in sheep following two doses of hydroxyurea (HU) 80 mg/kg 24 hr apart. (a) Percentage of marrow S-phase cells (determined by FCM) with time from the first dose of HU. (b) FCM traces before HU, and at 48 and 115 hr after HU. The increased proportion of S-phase cells at 115 hr shows the skewed distribution expected in a synchronized population, the majority of the cells being in early S phase.

CONCLUSION

A variety of disciplines have contributed to our understanding of leukemic cell proliferation. Radiation biology, radioactive isotopes, and flow cytometry have provided the means by which the proliferative activity of leukemic blasts can be determined, and the mathematical models with which the results can be analyzed. Cytogenetics, isoenzyme studies, membrane phenotype analyses, and cell culture studies have defined the clonal nature of leukemic cell proliferation, and more recently work on oncogenes, combined with refined cytogenetic studies, has begun to shed light on leukemogenesis and on the proliferative defects of leukemic cells.

Advances in our understanding of leukemic and normal hematopoietic cell proliferation have proceeded in parallel, each contributing to the other. Much remains to be learned, and some of the future developments which might be anticipated include: (1) improved means for studying hematopoietic pluripotential stem cells (HPSC) in man, including, for example, culture techniques and specific monoclonal antibodies; (2) improved understanding of the cellular and humoral regulation of hematopoiesis; (3) identification and enumeration of leukemic G_0 cells and definition of what triggers them into cycle; (4) determination of cellular proliferative characteristics in individual patients promptly enough to allow the data to be used in planning treatment; (5) identification and prevention of the clonal expansion of resistant leukemic cells; (6) counteraction of the effect of leukemic cells on normal HPSC; (7) refinement of methods for inducing leukemic cell maturation *in vivo;* (8) definition of the role of oncogenes in normal and leukemic cells with determination of the genetic controls of proliferation and differentiation and the role of gene expression; and (9) further elucidation of the heterogeneity of leukemic cells within and between patients, using, for example, monoclonal antibodies.

REFERENCES

1. TAVASSOLI, M. 1980. Bone marrow: the seedbed of blood. *In* Blood, Pure and Eloquent. M. M. Wintrobe, Ed.: 57-79. McGraw-Hill Book Co. New York, N.Y.
2. LAJTHA, L. G. 1980. The common ancestral cell. *In* Blood, Pure and Eloquent. M. M. Wintrobe, Ed.: 81-95. McGraw-Hill Book Co. New York, N.Y.
3. BLOOM, W. 1938. Lymphocytes and monocytes: theories of hematopoiesis. *In* Handbook of Hematology. H. Downey, Ed.: 375-435. Paul B. Hoeber Inc. New York, N.Y.
4. HADEN, R. L. 1946. Principles of Hematology. Lea & Febiger. Philadelphia, Pa.
5. GUNZ, F. W. 1983. Leukemia in the past. *In* Leukemia. 4th edit. F. W. Gunz & E. S. Henderson, Eds.: 3-11. Grune & Stratton. New York, N.Y.
6. JANOSSY, G., M. ROBERTS & M. F. GREAVES. 1976. Target cells in chronic myeloid leukaemia and its relationship to acute lymphoid leukaemia. Lancet 2: 1058-1061.
7. JANOSSY, G., M. F. GREAVES, R. SUTHERLAND, J. DURRANT & C. LEWIS. 1977. Comparative analysis of membrane phenotypes in acute lymphoid leukemia and in lymphoid blast crisis of chronic myeloid leukemia. Leuk. Res. 1: 289-300.
8. GREAVES, M. F. 1981. Analysis of the clinical and biological significance of lymphoid phenotypes in acute leukemia. Cancer Res. 41: 4752-4766.
9. FARBER, S., L. K. DIAMOND, R. D. MERCER, R. F. SYLVESTER, JR. & J. A. WOLFF. 1948. Temporary remissions in acute leukemia in children produced by folic acid antagonist, 4-aminopteroyl-glutamic acid (aminopterin). N. Engl. J. Med. 238: 787-793.
10. GALTON, D. A. G. & M. TILL. 1955. Myleran in chronic myeloid leukaemia. Lancet 1: 425-430.

11. ELLISON, R. R., R. T. SILVER & F. L. ENGLE, JR. 1959. Comparative study of 6-chloropurine and 6-mercaptopurine in acute leukemia in adults. Ann. Intern. Med. **51:** 322-338.

12. OSGOOD, E. E. 1940. Effects of irradiation of leukemic cells in marrow cultures. Proc. Soc. Exp. Biol. Med. **45:** 131-135.

13. CRONKITE, E. P., W. MOLONEY & V. P. BOND. 1960. Radiation leukemogenesis: an analysis of the problem. Am. J. Med. **28:** 673-682.

14. CRONKITE, E. P. 1964. The diagnosis, treatment, and prognosis of human radiation injury from whole-body exposure. Ann. N.Y. Acad. Sci. **114:** 341-349.

15. FLIEDNER, T. M., G. A. ANDREWS, E. P. CRONKITE & V. P. BOND. 1964. Early and late cytologic effects of whole body irradiation on human marrow. Blood **23:** 471-487.

16. CRONKITE, E. P., V. P. BOND & R. A. CONARD. 1964. The hematology of ionizing radiation. *In* Atomic Medicine. 4th edit. C. F. Behrens & E. R. King, Eds.: 170-202. The Williams & Wilkins Co. Baltimore, Md.

17. CRONKITE, E. P. 1967. Radiation-induced aplastic anemia. Semin. Hematol. **4:** 273-277.

18. OSGOOD, E. E. 1951. Titrated, regularly spaced radioactive phosphorus or spray roentgen therapy of leukemias. Arch. Intern. Med. **87:** 329-348.

19. CRONKITE, E. P., A. D. CHANANA & H. SCHNAPPAUF. 1965. Extracorporeal irradiation of blood and lymph in animals. N. Engl. J. Med. **272:** 456-461.

20. SCHIFFER, L. M., A. D. CHANANA, E. P. CRONKITE, M. L. GREENBERG, D. D. JOEL, H. SCHNAPPAUF & P. A. STRYCKMANS. 1966. Extracorporeal irradiation of the blood. Semin. Hematol. **3:** 154-167.

21. FORD, C. E., J. L. MANERTON, D. W. H. BARNES & J. F. LOUTIT. 1956. Cytological identification of radiation-chimaeras. Nature **177:** 452-454.

22. TILL, J. E. & E. A. MCCULLOCH. 1961. A direct measurement of the radiation sensitivity of normal mouse bone marrow cells. Radiat. Res. **14:** 213-222.

23. OSGOOD, E. E., J. G. LI, H. TIVEY, M. L. DUERST & A. J. SEAMAN. 1951. Growth of human leukemic leucocytes *in vitro* and *in vivo* as measured by uptake of P^{32} in desoxyribose nucleic acid. Science **114:** 95-98.

24. OTTESEN, J. 1954. On the age of human white cells in peripheral blood. Acta Physiol. Scand. **32:** 75-93.

25. TAYLOR, J. H., P. S. WOODS & W. L. HUGHES. 1957. The organization and duplication of chromosomes as revealed by autoradiographic studies using tritium-labeled thymidine. Proc. Natl. Acad. Sci. USA **43:** 122-128.

26. CRONKITE, E. P., R. G. FAIRCHILD & M. E. MILLER. 1983. Are there unexploited possibilities for the therapeutic use of radioactive and stable isotopically labeled DNA precursors and extracorporeal irradiation of the blood in treatment of leukemia? Blood Cells **9:** 107-123.

27. CRONKITE, E. P., T. M. FLIEDNER, V. P. BOND, J. R. RUBINI, G. BRECHER & H. QUASTLER. 1959. Dynamics of hemopoietic proliferation in man and mice studied by H^3-thymidine incorporation into DNA. Ann. N.Y. Acad. Sci. **77:** 803-820.

28. BOND, V. P., T. M. FLIEDNER, E. P. CRONKITE, J. R. RUBINI, G. BRECHER & P. K. SCHORK. 1959. Proliferative potentials of bone marrow and blood cells studied by *in vitro* uptake of H^3-thymidine. Acta Haematol. **21:** 1-15.

29. QUASTLER, H. & F. G. SHERMAN. 1959. Cell population kinetics in the intestinal epithelium of the mouse. Exp. Cell Res. **17:** 420-438.

30. CRONKITE, E. P., T. M. FLIEDNER, V. P. BOND, J. R. RUBINI, G. BRECHER & H. QUASTLER. 1959. Dynamics of hemopoietic proliferation in man and mice studied by H^3-thymidine incorporation into DNA. Prog. Nucl. Energy Ser. 6 **2:** 92-105.

31. CRONKITE, E. P., V. P. BOND, T. M. FLIEDNER & S-A. KILLMANN. 1960. The use of tritiated thymidine in the study of haemopoietic cell proliferation. *In* Ciba Foundation Symposium on Haemopoiesis. G. E. W. Wolstenholme & M. O'Connor, Eds.: 70-92. J. & A. Churchill Ltd. London, England.

32. RUBINI, J. R., V. P. BOND, S. KELLER, T. M. FLIEDNER & E. P. CRONKITE. 1961. DNA synthesis in circulating blood leukocytes labeled *in vitro* with H^3-thymidine. J. Lab. Clin. Med. **58:** 751-762.

33. FEINENDEGEN, L. E. 1967. Tritium-Labeled Molecules in Biology and Medicine. Academic Press, Inc. New York, N.Y.

34. CLEAVER, J. E. 1967. Thymidine Metabolism and Cell Kinetics. North-Holland Publishing Co. Amsterdam, the Netherlands.
35. STOHLMAN, F., JR. 1962. Erythropoiesis. N. Engl. J. Med. **267:** 342-348, 392-399.
36. CRONKITE, E. P. & T. M. FLIEDNER. 1964. Granulocytopoiesis. N. Engl. J. Med. **270:** 1347-1352, 1403-1408.
37. FLIEDNER, T. M., E. P. CRONKITE & J. S. ROBERTSON. 1964. Granulocytopoiesis. I. Senescence and random loss of neutrophilic granulocytes in human beings. Blood **24:** 402-414.
38. FLIEDNER, T. M., E. P. CRONKITE, S-A. KILLMANN & V. P. BOND. 1964. Granulocytopoiesis. II. Emergence and pattern of labeling in neutrophilic granulocytes in humans. Blood **24:** 683-700.
39. CRONKITE, E. P., T. M. FLIEDNER, P. STRYCKMANS, A. D. CHANANA, J. CUTTNER & J. RAMOS. 1965. Flow patterns and rates of human erythropoiesis and granulocytopoiesis. Ser. Haematol. **5:** 51-64.
40. STRYCKMANS, P., E. P. CRONKITE, J. FACHE, T. M. FLIEDNER & J. RAMOS. 1966. Deoxyribonucleic acid synthesis time of erythropoietic and granulopoietic cells in human beings. Nature **211:** 717-720.
41. CRONKITE, E. P. & P. C. VINCENT. 1969. Granulocytopoiesis. Ser. Haematol. **II:** 3-43.
42. VINCENT, P. C. 1977. Granulocyte kinetics in health and disease. Clin. Haematol. **6:** 695-717.
43. CRONKITE, E. P. 1979. Kinetics of granulocytopoiesis. Clin. Haematol. **8:** 351-370.
44. CRONKITE, E. P. 1968. Kinetics of leukemic cell proliferation. *In* Perspectives in Leukemia. W. Dameshek & R. M. Dutcher, Eds.: 158-186. Grune & Stratton. New York, N.Y.
45. CLARKSON, B. D. 1969. Review of recent studies of cellular proliferation in acute leukemia. *In* Human Tumor Cell Kinetics. National Cancer Institute Monograph No. 30, pp. 81-119.
46. VINCENT, P. C. 1983. Kinetics of leukemia and control of cell division and replication. *In* Leukemia. 4th edit. F. W. Gunz & E. S. Henderson, Eds.: 77-117. Grune & Stratton. New York, N.Y.
47. GAVOSTO, F., G. MARAINI & A. PILERI. 1960. Proliferative capacity of acute leukaemia cells. Nature **187:** 611-612.
48. KILLMANN, S. A., E. P. CRONKITE, J. S. ROBERTSON, T. M. FLIEDNER & V. P. BOND. 1963. Estimation of phases of the life cycle of leukemic cells from labeling in human beings *in vivo* with tritiated thymidine. Lab. Invest. **12:** 671-684.
49. MAUER, A. M. & V. FISHER. 1963. *In vivo* study of cell kinetics in acute leukaemia. Nature **197:** 574-576.
50. CLARKSON, B., T. OHKITA, K. OTA & J. FRIED. 1967. Studies of cellular proliferation in human leukemia. I. Estimation of growth rates of leukemic and normal hematopoietic cells in two adults with acute leukemia given single injections of tritiated thymidine. J. Clin. Invest. **46:** 506-529.
51. GAVOSTO, F., A. PILERI, C. BACHI & L. PEGORARO. 1964. Proliferation and maturation defect in acute leukaemia cells. Nature **203:** 92-94.
52. KILLMANN, S-A. 1965. Proliferation activity of blast cells in leukemia and myelofibrosis. Morphological differences between proliferating and non-proliferating blast cells. Acta Med. Scand. **178:** 263-280.
53. MAUER, A. M. & V. FISHER. 1966. Characteristics of cell proliferation in four patients with untreated acute leukemia. Blood **28:** 428-445.
54. SAUNDERS, E. F., B. C. LAMPKIN & A. M. MAUER. 1967. Variation of proliferative activity in leukemic cell populations of patients with acute leukemia. J. Clin. Invest. **46:** 1356-1363.
55. WAGNER, H. P. & H. COTTIER. 1967. Blast cell proliferation in a child with untreated acute leukaemia: results of a preliminary study using tritiated thymidine for pulse-labelling in vivo. Eur. J. Cancer **3:** 343-348.
56. SAUNDERS, E. F. & A. M. MAUER. 1969. Reentry of nondividing leukemic cells into a proliferative phase in acute childhood leukemia. J. Clin. Invest. **48:** 1299-1305.
57. CLARKSON, B., J. FRIED, A. STRIFE, Y. SAKAI, K. OTA & T. OHKITA. 1970. Studies of cellular proliferation in human leukemia. III. Behavior of leukemic cells in three adults with acute leukemia given continuous infusions of ³H-thymidine for 8 or 10 days. Cancer **25:** 1237-1260.

58. GREENBERG, M. L., A. D. CHANANA, E. P. CRONKITE, G. GIACOMELLI, K. R. RAI, L. M. SCHIFFER, P. A. STRYCKMANS & P. C. VINCENT. 1972. The generation time of human leukemic myeloblasts. Lab. Invest. **26:** 245-252.
59. CHEUNG, W. H., K. R. RAI & A. SAWITSKY. 1972. Characteristics of cell proliferation in acute leukemia. Cancer Res. **32:** 939-942.
60. TAROCCO, R. P., A. PILERI, A. PONZONE & F. GAVOSTO. 1972. Bone marrow return and division of circulating acute lymphoblastic leukaemia cells. Acta Haematol. **47:** 277-282.
61. STRYCKMANS, P., G. DELALIEUX, J. MANASTER & M. SOCQUET. 1970. The potentiality of out-of-cycle acute leukemic cells to synthesize DNA. Blood **36:** 697-703.
62. MENDELSOHN, M. L. 1962. Autoradiographic analysis of cell proliferation in spontaneous breast cancer of C3H mouse. III. The growth fraction. J. Natl. Cancer Inst. **28:** 1015-1029.
63. MAUER, A. M., C. F. EVERT, JR., B. C. LAMPKIN & N. B. McWILLIAMS. 1973. Cell kinetics in human acute lymphoblastic leukemia: computer simulation with discrete modeling techniques. Blood **41:** 141-154.
64. GREENBERG, M. L., A. D. CHANANA, E. P. CRONKITE, L. M. SCHIFFER & P. A. STRYCKMANS. 1966. Tritiated thymidine as a cytocidal agent in human leukemia. Blood **28:** 851-859.
65. BECKER, A. J., E. A. McCULLOCH, L. SIMINOVITCH & J. E. TILL. 1965. The effect of different demands for blood cell production on DNA synthesis by hemopoietic colony-forming cells of mice. Blood **26:** 296-308.
66. ATHENS, J. W., S. O. RAAB, O. P. HAAB, D. R. BOGGS, H. ASHENBRUCKER, G. E. CARTWRIGHT & M. M. WINTROBE. 1965. Leukokinetic studies. X. Blood granulocyte kinetics in chronic myelocytic leukemia. J. Clin. Invest. **44:** 765-777.
67. OGAWA, M., J. FRIED, Y. SAKAI, A. STRIFE & B. D. CLARKSON. 1970. Studies of cellular proliferation in human leukemia. VI. The proliferative activity, generation time, and emergence time of neutrophilic granulocytes in chronic granulocytic leukemia. Cancer **25:** 1031-1049.
68. VINCENT, P. C., E. P. CRONKITE, M. L. GREENBERG, C. KIRSTEN, L. M. SCHIFFER & P. A. STRYCKMANS. 1969. Leukocyte kinetics in chronic myeloid leukemia. I. DNA synthesis time in blood and marrow myelocytes. Blood **33:** 843-850.
69. DAMESHEK, W. 1967. Chronic lymphocytic leukemia—an accumulative disease of immunologically incompetent lymphocytes. Blood **29:** 566-584.
70. SCHIFFER, L. M. 1968. Kinetics of chronic lymphocytic leukemia. Ser. Haematol. **1(3):** 3-23.
71. ZIMMERMAN, T. S., H. A. GODWIN & S. PERRY. 1968. Studies of leukocyte kinetics in chronic lymphocytic leukemia. Blood **31:** 277-291.
72. BREMER, K., T. M. FLIEDNER & P. SCHICK. 1973. Kinetic differences of autotransfused, ^{3}H-cytidine labeled blood lymphocytes in leukemic and nonleukemic patients with malignant lymphomas. Eur. J. Cancer **9:** 113-124.
73. SCHIFFER, L. M., A. D. CHANANA, E. P. CRONKITE, M. L. GREENBERG, S. OKUYAMA, K. R. RAI, J. S. ROBERTSON, P. A. STRYCKMANS & P. C. VINCENT. 1967. A readily accessible compartment of lymphocytes in chronic lymphocytic leukemia: examination by 3 techniques. Physiologist **10:** 299.
74. KAMENTSKY, L. A., M. R. MELAMED & H. DERMAN. 1965. Spectrophotometer: new instrument for ultrarapid cell analysis. Science **150:** 630-631.
75. BARLOGIE, B., G. SPITZER, J. S. HART, D. A. JOHNSTON, T. BUCHNER, J. SCHUMANN & B. DREWINKO. 1976. DNA histogram analysis of human hemopoietic cells. Blood **48:** 245-258.
76. KRISHAN, A., S. W. PITMAN, M. H. N. TATTERSALL, K. D. PAIKA, D. C. SMITH & E. FREI III. 1976. Flow microfluorometric patterns of human bone marrow and tumor cells in response to cancer chemotherapy. Cancer Res. **36:** 3813-3820.
77. NICOLINI, C., F. KENDALL, C. DESAIVE, R. BASERGA, B. CLARKSON & J. FRIED. 1976. Physical-chemical characterization of living cells by laser-flow microfluorometry. Cancer Treatment Rep. **60:** 1819-1827.
78. BARLOGIE, B., A. M. MADDOX, D. A. JOHNSTON, M. N. RABER, B. DREWINKO, M. J. KEATING & E. J. FREIREICH. 1983. Quantitative cytology in leukemia research. Blood Cells **9:** 35-55.

79. ZBROJA, R. A., J. WASS, P. C. VINCENT & G. A. R. YOUNG. Fragment filtration—a method for the accurate determination of flow cytometric kinetic data from bone marrow aspirates. Exp. Hematol. In press.

80. HIDDEMANN, W., T. BUCHNER, M. ANDREEFF, B. WORMANN, M. R. MELAMED & B. D. CLARKSON. 1982. Cell kinetics in acute leukemia. A critical reevaluation based on new data. Cancer 50: 250-258.

81. VINCENT, P. C., G. A. R. YOUNG, J. WASS & R. A. ZBROJA. 1982. Differential synchronization of leukemic cells *in vivo* by hydroxyurea. Leuk. Res. 6: 243-250.

82. GRAY, J. W., J. H. CARVER, Y. S. GEORGE & M. L. MENDELSOHN. 1977. Rapid cell cycle analysis by measurement of the radioactivity per cell in a narrow window in S phase (RCS$_i$). Cell Tissue Kinet. 10: 97-109.

83. BECK, H. P. 1978. A new analytical method for determining duration of phases, rate of DNA synthesis and degree of synchronization from flow-cytometric data on synchronized cell populations. Cell Tissue Kinet. 11: 139-148.

84. ZIETZ, S. 1980. FP$_i$ analysis. I. Theoretical outline of a new method to analyze time sequences of DNA histograms. Cell Tissue Kinet. 13: 461-471.

85. BURKE, P. J., J. E. KARP, H. G. BRAINE & W. P. VAUGHAN. 1977. Timed sequential therapy of human leukemia based upon the response of leukemic cells to humoral growth factors. Cancer Res. 37: 2138-2146.

86. TRAGANOS, F., Z. DARZYNKIEWICZ, T. SHARPLESS & M. R. MELAMED. 1977. Simultaneous staining of ribonucleic and deoxyribonucleic acids in unfixed cells using acridine orange in a flow cytofluorometric system. J. Histochem. Cytochem. 25: 46-56.

87. DARZYNKIEWICZ, Z., F. TRAGANOS & M. R. MELAMED. 1980. New cell cycle compartments identified by multiparameter flow cytometry. Cytometry 1: 98-108.

88. SUTHERLAND, R., D. DELIA, C. SCHNEIDER, R. NEWMAN, J. KEMSHEAD & M. GREAVES. 1981. Ubiquitous cell-surface glycoprotein on tumor cells is proliferation-associated receptor for transferrin. Proc. Natl. Acad. Sci. USA 78: 4515-4519.

89. KANENTSKY, L. A. & M. R. MELAMED. 1967. Spectrophotometric cell sorter. Science 156: 1364-1365.

90. JONDAL, M., G. HOLM & H. WIGZELL. 1972. Surface markers on human T and B lymphocytes. I. A large population of lymphocytes forming nonimmune rosettes with sheep red blood cells. J. Exp. Med. 136: 207-215.

91. KÖHLER, G. & C. MILSTEIN. 1975. Continuous cultures of fused cells secreting antibody of predefined specificity. Nature 256: 495-497.

92. HOFFMAN, R. A., P. C. KUNG, W. P. HANSEN & G. GOLDSTEIN. 1960. Simple and rapid measurement of human T lymphocytes and their subclasses in peripheral blood. Proc. Natl. Acad. Sci. USA 77: 4914-4917.

93. MINOWADA, J. 1983. Immunology of leukemic cells. *In* Leukemia. 4th edit. F. W. Gunz & E. S. Henderson, Eds.: 119-139. Grune & Stratton. New York, N.Y.

94. PEIPER, S. C. & S. A. STASS. 1982. Markers of cellular differentiation in acute lymphoblastic leukemia. Arch. Pathol. Lab. Med. 106: 3-8.

95. CATOVSKY, D., M. CHERCHI, D. BROOKS, J. BRADLEY & H. ZOLA. 1981. Heterogeneity of B-cell leukemias demonstrated by the monoclonal antibody FMC7. Blood 58: 406-408.

96. KETTMAN, J. R., R. G. SMITH, J. W. UHR, E. S. VITETTA, R. SHEEHAN, F. S. LIGLER & E. P. FRENKEL. 1983. Quantitative monitoring of lymphoid malignancies. Blood Cells 9: 21-33.

97. RAI, K. R., E. P. CRONKITE, A. SAWITSKY, P. CHANDRA & J. STEINBERG. Studies in chronic lymphocytic leukemia: blood lymphocyte surface characteristics and immunologic functional status of patients and correlation with clinical stage. Ann. N.Y. Acad. Sci. (this volume).

98. GREAVES, M. F., W. VERBI, B. R. REEVES, A. V. HOFFBRAND, H. C. DRYSDALE, L. JONES, L. S. SACKER & I. SAMARATUNGA. 1979. "Pre-B" phenotypes in blast crisis of Ph^1 positive CML: evidence for a pluripotential stem cell "target." Leuk. Res. 3: 181-191.

99. KILLMANN, S-A., R. ANDREASEN, P. BIEBERFELD & L. OLSSON. Analyses of acute myeloid leukemias with monoclonal antibodies. Unpublished manuscript.

100. BAST, R. C., JR., J. RITZ, J. M. LIPTON, M. FEENEY, S. E. SALLAN, D. G. NATHAN & S. F. SCHLOSSMAN. 1983. Elimination of leukemic cells from human bone marrow using monoclonal antibody and complement. Cancer Res. 43: 1389-1394.

101. NOWELL, P. C. & D. A. HUNGERFORD. 1960. Chromosome studies on normal and leukemic human leukocytes. J. Natl. Cancer Inst. **25:** 85-93.
102. ROWLEY, J. D. 1980. Chromosome abnormalities in cancer. Cancer Genet. Cytogenet. **2:** 175-198.
103. MARTIN, P. J., V. NAJFELD, J. A. HANSEN, G. K. PENFOLD, R. J. JACOBSON & P. J. FIALKOW. 1980. Involvement of the B-lymphoid system in chronic myelogenous leukaemia. Nature **287:** 49-50.
104. FIALKOW, P. J., J. W. SINGER, J. W. ADAMSON, R. L. BERKOW, J. M. FRIEDMAN, R. J. JACOBSON & J. W. MOOHR. 1979. Acute nonlymphocytic leukemia. Expression in cells restricted in granulocytic and monocytic differentiation. N. Engl. J. Med. **301:** 1-5.
105. FIALKOW, P. J. 1983. Clonal development and stem cell origin of leukemias and related disorders. *In* Leukemia. 4th edit. F. W. Gunz & E. S. Henderson, Eds.: 63-76. Grune & Stratton. New York, N.Y.
106. SANDBERG, A. A. 1980. The Chromosomes in Human Cancer and Leukemia. Elsevier. New York, N.Y.
107. GARSON, O. M. 1980. Cytogenetics of leukemic cells. *In* Leukemia. 4th edit. F. W. Gunz & E. S. Henderson, Eds.: 167-195. Grune & Stratton. New York, N.Y.
108. ROWLEY, J. D. 1983. Human oncogene locations and chromosome aberrations. Nature **301:** 290-291.
109. HAMLYN, P. & K. SIKORA. 1983. Oncogenes. Lancet **2:** 326-330.
110. DE KLEIN, A., A. G. VAN KESSEL, G. GROSVELD, C. R. BARTRAM, A. HAGEMEIJER, D. BOOTSMA, N. K. SPURR, N. HEISTERKAMP, J. GROFFEN & J. R. STEPHENSON. 1982. A cellular oncogene is translocated to the Philadelphia chromosome in chronic myelocytic leukaemia. Nature **300:** 765-767.
111. DALLA-FAVERA, R., M. BREGNI, J. ERIKSON, D. PATTERSON, R. C. GALLO & C. M. CROCE. 1982. Human c-*myc onc* gene is located on the region of chromosome 8 that is translocated in Burkitt lymphoma cells. Proc. Natl. Acad. Sci. USA **79:** 7824-7827.
112. TAUB, R., I. KIRSCH, C. MORTON, G. LENOIR, D. SWAN, S. TRONICK, S. AARONSON & P. LEDER. 1982. Translocation of the c-*myc* gene into the immunoglobulin heavy chain locus in human Burkitt lymphoma and murine plasmacytoma cells. Proc. Natl. Acad. Sci. USA **79:** 7837-7841.
113. NEEL, B., S. C. JHANWAR, R. S. K. CHAGANTI & W. S. HAYWARD. 1982. Two human c-*onc* genes are located on the long arm of chromosome 8. Proc. Natl. Acad. Sci. USA **79:** 7842-7846.
114. BISHOP, J. M. 1982. Retroviruses and cancer genes. Adv. Cancer Res. **37:** 1-32.
115. WATERFIELD, M. D., G. T. SCRACE, N. WHITTLE, P. STROOBANT, A. JOHNSSON, A. WASTESON, B. WESTERMARK, C-H. HELDIN, J. S. HUANG & T. F. DEUEL. 1983. Platelet-derived growth factor is structurally related to the putative transforming protein p28 sis of simian sarcoma virus. Nature **304:** 35-39.
116. COLLINS, S. & M. GROUDINE. 1982. Amplification of endogenous *myc*-related DNA sequences in a human myeloid leukaemia cell line. Nature **298:** 679-681.
117. DALLA-FAVERA, R., F. WONG-STAAL & R. G. GALLO. 1982. *Onc* gene amplification in promyelocytic leukaemia cell line HL-60 and primary leukaemic cells of the same patient. Nature **299:** 61-63.
118. LOUTIT, J. F. 1968. Versatile haemopoietic stem cells. Br. J. Haematol. **15:** 333-336.
119. LAJTHA, L. G., L. V. POZZI, R. SCHOFIELD & M. FOX. 1969. Kinetic properties of haemopoietic stem cells. Cell Tissue Kinet. **2:** 39-49.
120. PLUZNIK, D. H. & L. SACHS. 1965. The cloning of normal "mast" cells in tissue culture. J. Cell. Comp. Physiol. **66:** 319-324.
121. BRADLEY, T. R. & D. METCALF. 1966. The growth of mouse bone marrow cells in vitro. Aust. J. Exp. Biol. Med. Sci. **44:** 287-299.
122. MCLEOD, D. L., M. M. SHREEVE & A. A. AXELRAD. 1974. Improved plasma culture system for production of erythrocytic colonies in vitro: quantitative assay method for CFU-E. Blood **44:** 517-534.
123. QUESENBERRY, P. & L. LEVITT. 1979. Hematopoietic stem cells. N. Engl. J. Med. **301:** 755-760.
124. WAGEMAKER, G., V. E. OBER-KIEFTENBURG, A. BROUWER & M. F. PETERS-SLOUGH. 1977. Some characteristics of in vitro erythroid colony and burst-forming units. *In*

Experimental Hematology Today. S. J. Baum & G. D. Ledney, Eds.: 103-110. Springer-Verlag. New York, N.Y.

125. Iscove, N. N. & F. Sieber. 1975. Erythroid progenitors in mouse bone marrow detected by macroscopic colony formation in culture. Exp. Hematol. **3:** 32-43.

126. Kurland, J. & M. A. S. Moore. 1977. The regulatory role of the macrophage in normal and neoplastic hematopoiesis. *In* Experimental Hematology Today. S. J. Baum & G. D. Ledney, Eds.: 51-62. Springer-Verlag. New York, N.Y.

127. Killmann, S-A. 1968. Acute leukemia: development, remission/relapse pattern, relationship between normal and leukemic hemopoiesis, and the 'sleeper-to-feeder' stem cell hypothesis. Ser. Haematol. **1**(3): 103-128.

128. Moore, M. A. S., G. Spitzer, N. Williams, D. Metcalf & J. Buckley. 1974. Agar culture studies in 127 cases of untreated acute leukemia: the prognostic value of re-classification of leukemia according to in vitro growth characteristics. Blood **44:** 1-18.

129. Vincent, P. C., R. Sutherland, M. Bradley, D. Lind & F. W. Gunz. 1977. Marrow culture studies in adult acute leukemia at presentation and during remission. Blood **49:** 903-912.

130. Buick, R. N., M. D. Minden & E. A. McCulloch. 1979. Self-renewal in culture of proliferative blast progenitor cells in acute myeloblastic leukemia. Blood **54:** 95-104.

131. Park, C. H., M. Amare, M. A. Savin, J. W. Goodwin, M. M. Newcomb & B. Hoogstraten. 1980. Prediction of chemotherapy response in human leukemia using an *in vitro* chemotherapy sensitivity test on the leukemic colony-forming cells. Blood **55:** 595-601.

132. Morris, T. C. M., T. A. McNeill & J. M. Bridges. 1974. Effect of leukaemic cells on the in vitro growth of normal bone marrow colony forming cells. Br. J. Haematol. **28:** 148-149.

133. Broxmeyer, H. E., N. Jacobsen, J. Kurland, N. Mendelsohn & M. A. S. Moore. 1978. In vitro suppression of normal granulocytic stem cells by inhibitory activity derived from human leukemia cells. J. Natl. Cancer Inst. **60:** 497-511.

134. Broxmeyer, H. E., E. Grossbard, N. Jacobsen & M. A. S. Moore. 1978. Evidence for a proliferative advantage of human leukemia colony-forming cells in vitro. J. Natl. Cancer Inst. **60:** 513-521.

135. Balaban-Malenbaum, G. & F. Gilbert. 1977. Double minute chromosomes and the homogeneously staining regions in chromosomes of a human neuroblastoma cell line. Science **198:** 739-741.

136. Wolman, S. R., M. L. Craven, S. P. Grill, B. A. Domin & Y-C. Cheng. 1983. Quantitative correlation of homogeneously stained regions on chromosome 10 with dihydrofolate reductase enzyme in human cells. Proc. Natl. Acad. Sci. USA **80:** 807-809.

137. Cronkite, E. P. 1970. Acute leukemia: is there a relationship between cell growth kinetics and response to chemotherapy? *In* Proceedings of the Sixth National Cancer Conference. R. N. Grant, Coordinator: 113-117. J. B. Lippincott Co. Philadelphia, Pa.

138. Skipper, H. E. 1971. Kinetic behavior versus response to chemotherapy. Natl. Cancer Inst. Monogr. **34:** 2-14.

139. van Putten, L. M. & P. Lelieveld. 1976. The effects of cytostatic drugs and radiotherapy on the cell cycle. *In* Scientific Foundations of Oncology. T. Symington & R. L. Carter, Eds.: 136-145. William Heinemann Medical Books Ltd. London, England.

140. Perry, S. 1976. Cell kinetics and cancer therapy: history, present status and challenges. Cancer Treatment Rep. **60:** 1699-1704.

141. Marsh, J. C. 1976. The effects of cancer chemotherapeutic agents on normal hematopoietic precursor cells: a review. Cancer Res. **36:** 1853-1882.

142. Tannock, I. 1978. Cell kinetics and chemotherapy: a critical review. Cancer Treatment Rep. **62:** 1117-1133.

143. Lampkin, B. C., T. Nagao & A. M. Mauer. 1971. Synchronization and recruitment in acute leukemia. J. Clin. Invest. **50:** 2204-2214.

144. Burke, P. J. & A. H. Owens, Jr. 1971. Attempted recruitment of leukemic myeloblasts to proliferative activity by sequential drug treatment. Cancer **28:** 830-836.

145. Mauer, A. M., S. B. Murphy & F. A. Hayes. 1976. Evidence for recruitment and synchronization in leukemia and solid tumors. Cancer Treatment Rep. **60:** 1841-1844.

146. Lampkin, B. C., T. Nagao & A. M. Mauer. 1969. Synchronization of the mitotic cycle in acute leukaemia. Nature **222:** 1274-1275.

147. ERNST, P., A. FAILLE & S-A. KILLMANN. 1973. Perturbation of cell cycle of human leukaemic myeloblasts *in vivo* by cytosine arabinoside. Scand. J. Haematol. **10:** 209-218.
148. KREMER, W. B., W. R. VOGLER & Y. K. CHAN. 1976. An attempt at synchronization of marrow cells in acute leukemia. Cancer **37:** 390-402.
149. WATSON, J. V. & I. W. TAYLOR. 1977. Cell cycle analysis in vitro using flow cytofluorimetry after synchronization. Br. J. Cancer **36:** 281-287.
150. SACHS, L. 1977. Control of normal cell differentiation in leukemia. Isr. J. Med. Sci. **13:** 654-665.
151. SACHS, L. 1978. The differentiation of myeloid leukaemia cells: new possibilities for therapy. Br. J. Haematol. **40:** 509-517.
152. HOUSSET, M., M. T. DANIEL & L. DEGOS. 1982. Small doses of Ara-C in the treatment of acute myeloid leukaemia: differentiation of myeloid leukaemia cells? Br. J. Haematol. **51:** 125-129.
153. CASTAIGNE, S., M. T. DANIEL, H. TILLY, P. HERAIT & L. DEGOS. 1983. Does treatment with Ara-C in low dosage cause differentiation of leukemic cells? Blood **62:** 85-86.
154. VINCENT, P. C., M. BUCK, G. A. R. YOUNG & W. J. BENSON. 1985. Low-dose Ara-C in acute non-lymphoblastic leukaemia. Aust. N.Z. J. Med. **15:** 10-15.

DISCUSSION OF THE PAPER

D. BOGGS (*University of Pittsburgh Medical School, Pittsburgh, Pa.*): I would like to provide an historical perspective to the discovery that blastic transformation in chronic myelocytic leukemia (CML) could also be lymphoid. About a decade ago such a notion was considered rather unbelievable. I thought I had seen a case of lymphoblastic conversion in CML and I mentioned this to Dr. Fred Stohlman, Jr. (since deceased) who was then the Editor of *Blood*. Dr. Stohlman asked me to write an editorial for the journal to suggest a hypothesis relating CML conversion to lymphoblastic leukemia to the theory that leukemic cells were involved at the stem cell level. Just before my editorial was published in *Blood* (**44** (1974): 449-453), a paper by Dr. Ron McCaffrey (*N. Engl. J. Med.* **292** (1975): 775-780) presented conclusive evidence of lymphoblastic conversion in CML based on terminal deoxynucleotidyl transferase (TdT) positivity of leukemic cells. This paper was obviously in press when my editorial was written. As Dr. McCaffrey is in the audience, I wonder if he would comment on this.

R. MCCAFFREY (*Boston University Medical Center, Boston, Mass.*): We had a series of patients with acute lymphoblastic leukemia (ALL) who all had TdT-positive cells. We started to believe that we had a lymphoblast-specific marker until we got to the next patient who had blastic transformation of CML and whose leukemic cells were found to be TdT positive. We discussed this observation with Dr. Stohlman who showed us a copy of Dr. Boggs' editorial. Thus, in biological interpretation of our observations, we based our reasoning on that editorial.

BOGGS: This whole concept that transformation of CML could also be lymphoblastic was then considered quite ridiculous. I was in the process of writing a chapter on CML for the 7th edition of *Wintrobe's Clinical Hematology*. Dr. Wintrobe thought it was nonsense to suggest that CML would convert to lymphoblastic leukemia and I had to delete that part from my writing. However, as is well known, by the time the 7th edition came out, the idea was already widely accepted.

A Cooperative Study of Polycythemia Vera[a]

LOUIS R. WASSERMAN

Polycythemia Vera Study Group
Mount Sinai School of Medicine
New York, New York 10029

Patients with untreated polycythemia vera (PV) have a 50% chance of surviving approximately 18 months from the time of diagnosis, whereas about half the patients undergoing "phlebotomy-only" treatment die in 3-8 years.[1] The Polycythemia Vera Study Group (PVSG) was founded in 1967 with the stated objective of determining the optimal treatment for polycythemia vera. Much has been learned about the difficulties of conducting a randomized study over a 17-year period of a disease that is rare, long-term, and undergoes numerous changes. The study is still not finished.

Early in the study it became obvious that uniform diagnostic parameters had to be established so that there could be no faulting of the diagnosis. The parameters for entry into the study were carefully listed and a decision tree evolved distinguishing among the absolute, secondary, and spurious polycythemias.[2] Patients who met predetermined diagnostic criteria were phlebotomized to a normal hematocrit. If the hematocrit rose to 55% within 1 year or by 10% above the post-phlebotomy value within 3 months, the patient was randomized to one of the three treatment regimens. The initial phlebotomies were incorporated into the protocol to ensure that only patients in the active, proliferative stage of the disease were entered into the study.

Patients who had an elevated red cell mass, normal arterial oxygen saturation, and splenomegaly were considered to have PV and were eligible for study. Patients having an increased red cell mass and normal arterial oxygen saturation without splenomegaly were also considered to have PV and were eligible for study if they had any two of the following four criteria: thrombocytosis, leukocytosis, elevated leukocyte alkaline phosphatase, and an elevated serum B_{12} or unbound B_{12} binding capacity.[3] On the basis of results of a more extensive evaluation, the basic PVSG diagnostic criteria were found to have a false positive rate of less than 0.5%. Between 1967 and 1974, a total of 431 fully eligible patients were randomized to one of the three treatment regimens of the first protocol. Patients still alive and on study have, therefore, been followed for a minimum of 9 to a maximum of 16 years. The Group's first study, PVSG-01, is a long-term trial, still ongoing, in which previously untreated patients have been randomized to treatment with phlebotomy alone, or myelosuppression with either ^{32}P or chlorambucil supplemented by phlebotomy.[3] Accrual has stopped and all patients have been followed to death since 1974. While all three regimens substantially prolong survival, which is not significantly different statistically in the three groups, treatment with phlebotomy alone is associated with an excess of early, severe

[a]Supported in part by United States Public Health Service Grant CA-10728 from the National Cancer Institute to the Polycythemia Vera Study Group.

thrombotic complications compared to the two myelosuppressive regimens (FIGURE 1). The excess is particularly striking in patients over age 70, in those with a high phlebotomy requirement, and in those with a history of prior thrombosis. On the other hand, ^{32}P and chlorambucil regimens are associated with a significant excess of acute leukemia and cancer of the gastrointestinal tract and skin.[4]

Survival analysis indicated that through the first 3 years of the study, the probability of survival for eligible patients randomized to phlebotomy alone was poorer than that for patients randomized to the other two groups and significantly less than that expected for the general U.S. population (FIGURE 1).

Approximately 60% of deaths in the phlebotomy group are attributable to either thrombotic episodes or cerebrovascular accidents. Not a single patient older than 75 who was randomized to phlebotomy alone survived more than $2\frac{1}{2}$ years. For a non-PV population of the same age one would expect that after 3 years there would be at least a 75% survival.

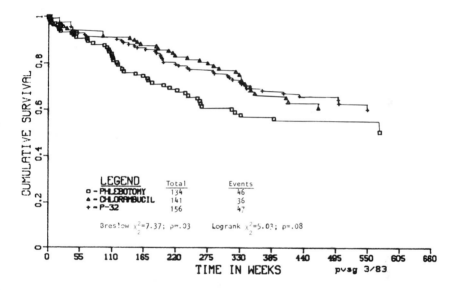

FIGURE 1. Thrombosis-free cumulative survival.

At the inception of the study, experience with chemotherapeutic drugs in the long-term treatment of PV was limited so the Group undertook a number of "efficacy" trials comparing the effectiveness of various chemotherapeutic agents by means of relatively short-term crossover studies utilizing preexisting case material not suitable for the long-term study. A few favorable reports on the use of Myleran had appeared. Chlorambucil had been used successfully in a small number of cases at Mount Sinai Hospital and was the drug finally selected for study in the treatment of PV.

As the study progressed, it seemed obvious on careful observation that chlorambucil-treated cases showed a severalfold increase in the incidence of acute leukemia as compared with phlebotomy- or radioactive-phosphorus-treated cases (TABLE 1, FIGURE 2). A relationship between dose rate and incidence of leukemia was noted. The relative risk of developing leukemia was four or five times greater the more

TABLE 1. Incidence of Leukemia (per 100 Patients/Year) in Each Treatment Group within Years following Randomization

Years on Study	Treatment Group		
	Phlebotomy	Chlorambucil	^{32}P
≤1	0.0	0.0	0.0
1-2	0.0	0.0	0.0
2-3	1.1	4.3	0.8
3-4	0.0	2.0	0.9
4-5	0.0	2.7	1.1
5-6	0.0	6.3	2.9
6-7	0.0	3.3	2.3
7-8	0.0	4.8	0.0
8-9	0.0	8.7	0.0
9-10	0.0	0.0	0.0
10-11	0.0	0.0	—
11-12	0.0	0.0	—
Number in group:	134	141	156

frequent the drug administration. After a number of years, the PVSG discontinued chlorambucil treatment on the careful deliberations of the Group membership as well as the recommendations of a panel of consultants.

One hundred fifty-four deaths have been recorded thus far. Thirty-eight percent of the randomized patients are still alive and under active follow-up. Thrombotic events, acute leukemia, other neoplasms, hemorrhage, and complications of myelofibrosis accounted for 75% of deaths reported among patients on active study.[4]

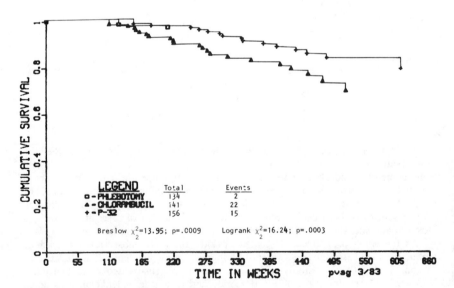

FIGURE 2. Leukemia-free cumulative survival.

Survival curves based on all deaths reported indicate that survival is somewhat poorer among patients treated with chlorambucil than patients on the other two treatments (FIGURE 3). Median survival time is currently 9.1 years on chlorambucil, 11.8 years on ^{32}P, and has not been reached on phlebotomy. Examination of cause of death by treatment regimen suggests that thrombotic events are the cause of 41% of deaths on the phlebotomy regimen and 26-29% of deaths on the myelosuppressive regimens.

On the other hand, acute leukemia was the major cause of death on chlorambucil (31% of deaths), while 17-18% of deaths on myelosuppressive treatment and 9% of deaths on phlebotomy were attributed to other malignant diseases.

One hundred twenty-nine thrombotic events have been reported (FIGURE 1). Thrombosis-free survival remains significantly poorer for patients treated with phlebotomy than for patients treated with either of the myelosuppressive regimens which

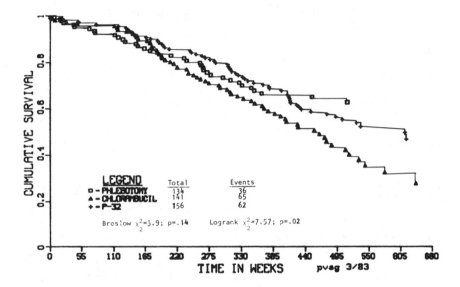

FIGURE 3. Cumulative survival.

have identical incidences of thrombosis. This is due primarily to the high incidence of thrombotic complications on phlebotomy during the first 3 years after randomization. The individuals who survived the initial thrombotic event have had a second or subsequent thrombosis. The case fatality rate from a subsequent thrombosis is 35%. Treatment with phlebotomy, per se, was the major factor associated with incidence of thrombosis. In addition, prior thrombosis and advanced age appear to be associated with incidence of thrombosis. Patients treated with phlebotomy alone have an increased risk of thrombosis.

Because of the negative slope of the survival curve of the phlebotomy-treated cases for the first 3 years, a derivative study was undertaken to see if the survival curve could be influenced by antiaggregating agents. A PVSG randomized study comparing phlebotomy plus Persantine and aspirin with ^{32}P was completed; data from 83 eligible patients who had been randomized to each arm of the study were evaluable. At the close of the study, both groups had been followed for a maximum of 3.4 years and a median of 1.2 years. There is certainly no suggestion of benefit from the use of aspirin/Persantine.[5] The average relative risk of thrombosis on the phlebotomy/aspirin/Persantine treatment was 3.6 times that observed among patients treated with radioactive phosphorus. When compared with corresponding data for the first 2 years of the initial protocol, the incidence of thrombotic events among patients receiving aspirin/Persantine and phlebotomy in the current study was virtually identical to that among patients treated with phlebotomy alone in the preceding study. Hence, there is no evidence either within this study or from a comparison of this protocol with our earlier study that aspirin/Persantine significantly reduced the incidence of thrombotic complications in patients with PV. Although there was no apparent benefit with respect to thrombotic complications from aspirin/Persantine therapy, there was a significant increase in hemorrhagic complications. Six of the patients receiving phlebotomy plus aspirin/Persantine had severe gastrointestinal hemorrhages requiring hospitalization and transfusion. There were no such events among patients treated with ^{32}P. Moreover, the overall cumulative failure rate, including severe thrombotic complications, hemorrhage, and death, was 8 times greater on the phlebotomy/aspirin/Persantine treatment than among patients treated with ^{32}P.

There were 50 cases of nonhematologic malignancies in the three groups: 8 instances in the phlebotomy-treated group, 22 in the chlorambucil-treated group, and 20 in the ^{32}P-treated group. The incidence of such cancers is significantly less on the phlebotomy regimen than on either of the two myelosuppressive regimens. Differences among the three groups are largely attributable to gastrointestinal (GI) and skin cancers, the incidence of other malignancies being similar. The data suggest that malignant transformation may occur in rapidly proliferating tissues (e.g., bone marrow, GI tract, skin) as a long-term consequence of various types of myelosuppressive therapy.[4]

When the current study was initiated, little was known about the leukemogenic potential of chemotherapeutic agents in PV. It was anticipated that chlorambucil might demonstrate the myelosuppressive benefits previously attributed to ^{32}P without the leukemogenic effects. The opposite was noted, however, in that the agent produced a greater risk of acute leukemia. Although there have been more cases of acute leukemia in the chlorambucil group almost from the study's inception, this excess is now highly significant and cannot be explained in any other way (TABLE 1).

The risk of acute leukemia in chlorambucil-treated patients is 2.3 times greater than that in patients treated with ^{32}P and 13.5 times greater than that in patients treated with phlebotomy. Since chlorambucil treatment has been discontinued, the Group's goal of determining optimum treatment has not been achieved as yet. It must await further studies with hydroxyurea and other agents yet to be selected.

Hydroxyurea (Hydrea), a metabolic inhibitor of ribonucleoside reductase, is a potent nonalkylating myelosuppressive agent. It has been used in the treatment of chronic granulocytic leukemia, some solid tumors, and in selected cases of psoriasis. To date, it has not been shown to be leukemogenic in humans. Careful titration of the dose of Hydrea (15-30 mg/kg/day) results in control of the disease. Hydrea is an effective agent in the management of PV, is useful in both young and old patients, and is useful in the treatment of thrombocytosis associated with PV. When combined with phlebotomy, control of the disease may be readily achieved.

Finally, in treating PV patients the following general principles must be followed:

1. All cases have to be followed carefully and must have periodic clinical and hematologic examinations.

2. Phlebotomy must be used only in young patients, Hydrea and phlebotomy for patients under 50, and ^{32}P for those over 70.

3. The tolerance of each patient to the myelosuppressive agents must be titrated.

4. The blood must be maintained at normal levels by using a potpourri of treatments.

5. When marked thrombocytosis (platelet count above $600,000/ml^3$) is noted, hydroxyurea should be used.

6. Finally, elective surgery during the course of PV should be delayed until the blood volume and platelet count are within normal limits for at least 2 months.

The patient with PV, when properly treated with ^{32}P or other myelosuppressive agents, has a normal life expectancy. The danger of complications due to uncontrolled or poorly managed PV is greater by far than the hypothetical risk of inducing leukemia.

REFERENCES

1. VIDABAEK, A. 1950. Polycythemia vera: course and prognosis. Acta Med. Scand. **138:** 179-187.
2. BERLIN, N. I. 1975. Diagnosis and classification of the polycythemias. Semin. Hematol. **XII:** 5-17.
3. WASSERMAN, L. R. 1976. Treatment of polycythemia vera. Semin. Hematol. **XIII:** 167-188.
4. BERK, P. D., J. D. GOLDBERG, M. N. SILVERSTEIN, A. WEINFELD, P. B. DONOVAN, J. T. ELLIS, S. A. LANDAW, J. LASZLO, Y. NAJEAN, A. V. PISCIOTTA & L. R. WASSERMAN. 1981. Increased incidence of acute leukemia in polycythemia vera associated with chlorambucil therapy. N. Engl. J. Med. **304:** 441-447.
5. TARTAGLIA, A. P., J. D. GOLDBERG, M. N. SILVERSTEIN, C. DRESCH, I. TATARSKY, A. V. PISCIOTTA, G. B. FAGUET, D. S. ROSENTHAL, M. CONJALKA, P. B. DONOVAN, P. D. BERK & L. R. WASSERMAN. 1981. Aspirin and persantine do not prevent thrombotic complications in patients with polycythemia vera treated with phlebotomy. Blood **58:** 240a. (Abstract.)

DISCUSSION OF THE PAPER

G. CHIKKAPPA (*Veterans Administration Medical Center, Albany, N.Y.*): Some *in vitro* studies show that red cells which are microcytic and hypochromic are more rigid and have greater difficulty in circulation than normal cells. Dr. Wasserman, your clinical data suggest that the phlebotomy-group patients have more thrombotic complications than the patients in the other treatment groups. Have you studied the effects of iron supplementation in these patients?

L. R. WASSERMAN: It is true that some of the patients are symptomatic from iron deficiency. We did treat many of them initially with supplemental iron and found that such treatment did not influence the results. Another question we are asked occasionally is whether chlorambucil was a good choice as an alkylating drug in this study. In Europe, two studies are currently in progress in which busulfan is being compared with ^{32}P. When we were planning this study very little information was available on the use of chemotherapeutic drugs but we knew that busulfan therapy was associated with severe thrombocytopenia and there were reports of cases of induction of leukemia with this drug. That is why we chose chlorambucil. Although I recognize that some people say busulfan does not cause leukemia, I have seen cases where it has and others have too.

Inhibition of Late Splenic Extra-Colony Formation by Mitobronitol

E. GULYA,[a] E. KELEMEN,[b] AND I. HOLLÓ[b]

[a]Korvin Otto Hospital
[b]First Department of Medicine
Semmelweis University
Budapest, Hungary

We have studied the influence of mitobronitol (Myelobromol, dibromomannitol) on spleen colony formation. It has previously been demonstrated that extra colonies can be produced in the spleens of supralethally irradiated recipients by bone marrow derived from 5-fluorouracil-treated donor mice.[1] We observed that donor marrow subjected to both 5-fluorouracil and mitobronitol failed to induce extra colonies in recipients' spleens. This inhibition could be explained by additional mitobronitol injury increasing that already caused by 5-fluorouracil. Therefore, a different alkylating agent was given to 5-fluorouracil-treated donor mice. Unlike mitobronitol, cyclophosphamide, a non-cell-cycle-specific alkylating agent, injected into the 5-fluorouracil-treated donor did not inhibit extra-colony formation in the recipient. If the fluorouracil effect is due to sparing of pre-CFU-S cells, as suggested by Hodgson and Bradley,[1] mitobronitol may injure this latter compartment too.[2]

REFERENCES

1. HODGSON, G. S. & R. BRADLEY. 1979. Nature **281**: 381.
2. GULYA, E., E. KELEMEN & I. HOLLÓ. 1983. Exp. Hematol. **11**(Suppl. 14): 104.

Mitobronitol: An Alkylating Agent That Does Not Induce Extra Leukemia Cases if Applied as Pulse Therapy for Polycythemia Vera

E. KELEMEN

First Department of Medicine
Semmelweis University
Budapest, Hungary

S. TURA

Department of Hematology
University of Bologna
Bologna, Italy

During a 14-year period, 70 Hungarian and 55 Italian polycythemia vera (PV) patients received mitobronitol (Myelobromol, dibromomannitol: DBM) *pulse therapy* (a total of 1500-3500 mg DBM, during 3 to 5 days), on two to four occasions a year. Patients did not receive any other cytostatic agents. There were no clinical problems of pulse-therapy-induced cytopenia, which have been seen on rare occasions with the usual prolonged DBM therapy.

DBM pulse therapy is not ideal because: (a) remissions endure for a few months only; (b) they are not sufficiently prolonged, i.e., *low normal* peripheral blood counts (in two-thirds or all of the main hemopoietic systems) are not achieved in at least half of the patients; and (c) supplementary initial phlebotomies must sometimes be performed. However: (1) both primary and secondary *drug resistance* occur rarely, (2) *hemopoietic regeneration* was always undisturbed, even after 17 to 39 pulses (given to 10 selected patients) during 6 to 13 years of DBM pulse therapy; and (3) it appears to be considerably safe, as regards *drug-induced leukemia*. In fact, although the literature holds that DBM is an alkylating agent, only two cases of acute nonlymphocytic leukemia developed among more than 100 DBM patients observed for 5 years or longer, which appears to be in accord with the rate of spontaneous leukemia developing in PV; i.e., *extra leukemia cases did not appear to develop*. In any event, compared with the well-known chlorambucil trial of the PV Study Group, this low leukemia rate for an alkylating agent is remarkable.

The following questions arose in the course of this study: Are the above-mentioned advantages of DBM pulse therapy attributable to pulse therapy versus prolonged one? Is chlorambucil-induced acute leukemia the consequence of its prolonged administration rather than of its alkylating power? These important questions need to be investigated further on a larger number of patients.

Studies in Chronic Lymphocytic Leukemia: Blood Lymphocyte Surface Characteristics and Immunologic Functional Status of Patients and Correlation with Clinical Stage[a]

KANTI R. RAI,[b,c] EUGENE P. CRONKITE,[c,d]
ARTHUR SAWITSKY,[b,c] PRADEEP CHANDRA,[c,e]
AND JOSEPH STEINBERG[b]

[b]Division of Hematology/Oncology
Long Island Jewish-Hillside Medical Center
New Hyde Park, New York 11042

[c]School of Medicine
State University of New York at Stony Brook
Stony Brook, New York 11794

[d]Medical Department
Brookhaven National Laboratory
Upton, New York 11973

[e]Veterans Administration Hospital
Brooklyn, New York 11209

INTRODUCTION

In the mid-1960s chronic lymphocytic leukemia (CLL) started to attract the attention of clinical investigators for three reasons:

1. The exceptional ease of diagnosis:
   In clinical medicine, the diagnosis of CLL was perhaps one of the easiest from a clinician's viewpoint. Usually the report of a routine blood count alerted the physician to a possible diagnosis of CLL if an absolute lymphocytosis was present. There were two minimum requirements for diagnosis of CLL:

[a]Work supported by funds from the Helena Rubinstein Foundation, Inc., the National Leukemia Association, the Rosenstiel Foundation, the United Leukemia Fund, the Wayne Goldsmith Leukemia Fund, and a special grant from Doyle Dane Bernbach, Inc.

(a) a persistent absolute lymphocytosis in blood ($\geq$ 5000 lymphocytes/mm³), which could not be explained from any other cause, with morphologically mature-looking cells; and

(b) an increase in the proportion of mature lymphocytes on a smear of bone marrow aspirate ($\geq$ 40% of all nucleated cells).

2. The exceptionally variable prognosis:

It was recognized that there was an extremely wide range of duration of survival among patients diagnosed as having CLL. Some patients died within 6 months after a diagnosis of CLL was made, while others were alive and well 10 to 15 years after such a diagnosis. This wide range became a source of considerable frustration to the clinician in the decision-making process of the management of an individual patient.

3. Increased interest in the lymphocyte as the effector cell of the immune system:

The fascination for the lymphocyte started to gather momentum in the mid-1960s. D. A. G. Galton[1] delivered the Burroughs-Wellcome Lecture at the University of Manitoba in Winnipeg, Canada on October 4, 1965 in which he said: "It is now necessary to re-examine CLL . . . in the light of the rapidly accumulating knowledge concerning the life history and functions of lymphocytes. . . . The picture that emerges is that of a gradual accumulation of aged lymphocytes . . . because these lymphocytes fail to transform." Less than a year later, on August 24, 1966, W. Dameshek[2] delivered the Henry M. Stratton Lecture at a meeting of the International Society of Hematology in Sydney, Australia in which he said: "CLL, far from being simply a very chronic, very dull disease, has many facets which may help to illuminate the pathogenesis of a variety of immunologic aberrations. . . . CLL is an accumulative disease of lymphocytes, the latter are immunologically incompetent."

CLINICAL STAGING AND CORRELATION WITH BODY CELL MASS

Because of the observations of Galton,[1] Dameshek,[2] and many others,[3-5] we were able to propose the following criteria for clinical staging of CLL:

Stage 0: Lymphocytosis only (blood $\geq$ 5000 lymphocytes/mm³ and marrow $\geq$ 40%).

Stage I: Lymphocytosis + enlarged nodes.

Stage II: Lymphocytosis + enlarged spleen and/or liver (with or without enlarged nodes).

Stage III: Lymphocytosis + anemia (< 11 g% hemoglobin), with or without enlarged nodes, spleen, and liver.

Stage IV: Lymphocytosis + thrombocytopenia (< 100,000 platelets/mm³), with or without anemia and enlarged nodes, spleen, and liver.

Phillips *et al.*[6] demonstrated that this method of clinical staging was a reliable index of prognosis. The data in TABLE 1 provide median duration of survival of 125 patients studied by us[7] and classified according to clinical stage at the time of diagnosis. Although this clinical staging was proposed on a largely empirical basis, we subsequently demonstrated that there was a correlation between clinical stage and total body cell mass.[8] An estimate of total body cell mass was derived from the measurement of body burden of ^{40}K by Brookhaven's Whole Body Counter which measures the γ emissions of radioisotopes. There is a fixed ratio of ^{40}K to total potassium; therefore,

TABLE 1. Median Duration of Survival according to Stage at Diagnosis

Stage at Diagnosis	No. of Patients	Median Survival (months)
0	22	> 150
I	29	101
II	39	71
III	21	19
IV	14	19
Overall (all stages)	125	71

measurement of ^{40}K in the body enables us to determine total body potassium (TBK). Since potassium is essentially an intracellular ion, TBK provides a reliable index of total body cell mass. From a nomogram of expected or predicted total body potassium for an individual's sex, height, weight, etc. (TBKp or Kp), and the actually measured TBK for that individual, we calculate the ratio of TBK/Kp.[8] FIGURE 1 depicts TBK/Kp for normal controls and for patients in different clinical stages of CLL. These data demonstrate that there is a progressively increased total body cell mass with increasing clinical stage. In patients with CLL, we believe it is reasonable to assume that increased cell mass can be attributable, to a large extent if not entirely, to an increased number of lymphocytes. These observations provide data confirming the notion first proposed by Galton[1] and Dameshek[2] that in CLL there is a progressive accumulation of lymphocytes.

LYMPHOCYTE SURFACE CHARACTERISTICS IN B-CELL CLL

CLL is a disease characterized by an expansion or accumulation of B lymphocytes.[9-13] Using the standard methodology of identifying T cells by rosetting with sheep erythrocytes (S-RBC rosettes) and B cells by demonstrating lymphocyte surface immunoglobulin (sIg), the approximate normal ratio of T:B cells is 75:25. In classical B-cell CLL this ratio is reversed to nearly 25:75 as shown in TABLE 2. The data in

TABLE 2. Cell Surface Markers in CLL

CLL Stage	No. of Patients	Median Absolute Lymphocyte Count (per mm³)	Mean Percentage T Cells[a] ± SEM	Mean Percentage B Cells[b] ± SEM
0	19	10,600	25 ± 5	66 ± 5
I	26	27,000	20 ± 3	67 ± 4
II	29	20,000	21 ± 5	70 ± 4
III	10	77,000	18 ± 6	70 ± 7
IV	9	86,000	13 ± 3	66 ± 7
Normal controls	50	2,200	65 ± 15	18 ± 7

[a]T cells were identified by rosetting with sheep erythrocytes.
[b]B cells were identified by demonstrating lymphocyte surface immunoglobulin.

TABLE 2 indicate that the absolute lymphocyte count in blood is increased in CLL, but this increase is progressively more pronounced with increased clinical stage. The relative proportion of B cells and the absolute number of B cells are increased in all stages of CLL; the proportion of T cells is decreased in all stages of CLL, but because of an absolute overall lymphocytosis in the blood, the absolute number of T cells may not be decreased, it may be normal or elevated. There does not appear to be a statistically significant correlation between relative or absolute numbers of B or T cells and the clinical stage of CLL. The immunoglobulins on the surface of the majority of B cells in B-cell CLL (B-CLL) were found to be IgM and IgD. These immuno-

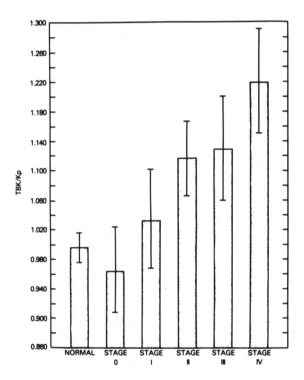

FIGURE 1. Ratio of total body potassium (TBK) to predicted normal total body potassium (Kp) in CLL and normal subjects. The bar graphs show the mean TBK/Kp for normal subjects 40 years of age or older, and for CLL patients in Stages 0, I, II, III, and IV. The vertical bracket at the top of each bar indicates ± 1 SD. Reproduced from Reference 30 with the permission of Plenum Publishing Corporation.

globulins were monoclonal with respect to light chains; i.e., they had either kappa or lambda light chains, but not both.

We studied the T cells in B-CLL to determine the relative proportions of helper-inducer T cells and suppressor-cytotoxic T cells.[14] In man the normal ratio is approximately 1.5 or 2:1 (helper:suppressor). We used T-cell monoclonal antibodies of the Leu system (Becton-Dickinson) in which Leu-1 provides an index of Pan T cells; Leu-2a, suppressor-cytotoxic T cells; and Leu-3a, helper-inducer T cells. TABLE 3 provides a summary of our data according to clinical stage. These data indicate a marked decrease in the proportion of helper T cells in CLL in all stages, except Stage

0. The number of patients studied in Stage 0 was rather small; therefore, we cannot tell at this time if the relatively normal mean value of 41% helper T cells will remain in the same range with a larger sample size. Although we believe the decrease of the helper:suppressor ratio from normal (1.5:1) to 0.7:1 is primarily due to a decreased number of helper T cells, there also is a contribution from a somewhat increased proportion of suppressor T cells. We did not observe a significant correlation between clinical stage and the extent of reversal of helper:suppressor ratios of T lymphocytes. Our observations on T-cell abnormalities in B-cell CLL are consistent with the findings of other investigators.[15–22]

TABLE 3. T-Cell Subpopulations in CLL (Mean Values)

Clinical Stage	No. of Patients	Percentage Pan T Cells[a]	Percentage Suppressor T Cells[b]	Percentage Helper T Cells[c]
0	6	53	30	41
I	14	48	45	25
II	13	36	40	18
III	7	40	22	17
IV	6	35	32	17

[a]Index of Pan T cells provided by Leu-1.
[b]Index of suppressor T cells provided by Leu-2a.
[c]Index of helper T cells provided by Leu-3a.

IMMUNE FUNCTION IN CLL

Serum Immunoglobulin Levels (B-Cell Function)

It is well known that hypogammaglobulinemia[23] occurs in 50-75% of patients with CLL. This abnormality becomes more manifest as the disease advances to late stages. Our data on serum immunoglobulin levels according to clinical stage of CLL are shown in TABLE 4. These results demonstrate that IgG, IgA, and IgM are all markedly decreased in the more advanced stages of CLL (Stages III and IV), and hypogammaglobulinemia of one or the other immunoglobulins may be noted in the earlier stages as well.

Delayed Hypersensitivity Reactivity (T-Cell Function)

We used delayed hypersensitivity reactivity as an index of T-cell function. Four recall antigens were injected intracutaneously at separate sites in the forearms of patients with CLL: Old Tuberculin (PPD), Mumps, Candida, and Streptokinase-Streptodornase (SKSD). At 48 hr after the injection, diameters of induration were measured and qualitatively interpreted as follows: 0 = no induration, erythema only was read as nonreactive; + = up to 5 mm; + + = 6 to 15 mm; and + + + = 16

TABLE 4. Serum Immunoglobulin Levels according to Clinical Stage in CLL

Clinical Stage	No. of Patients	Median Immunoglobulin Level (mg%)		
		IgG	IgA	IgM
0	10	920	109	66
I	15	900	98	46
II	28	720	105	38
III	9	570	50	33
IV	9	600	70	60
	Normal range:	800-1800	90-450	60-280

mm or more. The results expressed as maximum response observed in patients classified according to clinical stage are shown in TABLE 5. All patients in Stage 0 had normal skin reactivity; there were no patients with anergy. Among 8 patients in Stage I, 2 had minimal response (+) and 6 had induration of ≥ 16 mm diameter. Of 20 patients in Stage II, 6 were either anergic or had only minimal response and the other 14 had normal reactions. On the other hand, in the advanced stages (III and IV), 7 out of 10 patients were either anergic or had only minimal response. It is evident, therefore, that cellular immunity (T-cell function) is markedly diminished in the advanced stages, while in the early stages of CLL, this function is well preserved. These results, as well as the work of numerous other investigators, demonstrate that from a functional consideration, there is evidence of abnormality both of B and T lymphocytes in B-cell CLL.

T-CELL INTERACTION IN B-CELL FUNCTION

Although we generally consider the functions of B cells and of T cells as somewhat distinct entities—B cells are necessary for humoral antibody production and T cells are necessary for cellular immunity—we have recently begun to realize that B-cell function is dependent upon T-cell interaction. By mechanisms not yet fully defined,

TABLE 5. Skin Delayed Hypersensitivity Reactions

Clinical Stage	No. of Patients	Maximum Response (% of Patients)			
		+ + +	+ +	+	0
0	9	67	33	0	0
I	8	75	0	25	0
II	20	55	15	10	20
III and IV	10	20	10	30	40
Overall (all stages)	47	53	15	15	17

there is a certain degree of balance in the activity of helper T cell versus suppressor T cell in the eventual end points of B-cell functions. Gupta and Good[24] observed that increased suppressor-T-cell activity and decreased helper-T-cell activity contribute to a basic biosynthetic defect which results in secretion of free light chains rather than an intact immunoglobulin molecule from the eventual B-cell activity. Similarly, several investigators have started to study the mechanism of development of anemia in CLL by studying patients who have pure red cell anemia (PRCA) with CLL.[25-29] These studies suggest that T lymphocytes exert some control over erythropoiesis, regulatory helper-T-cell activity is decreased, and suppressor-T-cell activity is increased in patients with PRCA in association with CLL.

FUTURE DIRECTIONS FOR RESEARCH

Two possible directions for future investigations became apparent following recognition that both B and T cells have defective function in B-CLL: (1) Is the site of leukemogenesis of the lymphocyte closer to the stem cell and not somewhere along the B-cell maturation pathway as was previously believed? (2) Is it possible that there is no intrinsic defect in the T cell in B-CLL and whatever abnormality is observed is only secondary to the progressively increasing B-cell tumor load which interferes with T-cell function? Until further work is performed to pursue these lines of investigation, we believe it is necessary to study both B and T cells to assess the extent of loss of immune function in B-CLL.

REFERENCES

1. GALTON, D. A. G. 1966. The pathogenesis of chronic lymphocytic leukemia. Can. Med. Assoc. J. **94:** 1005-1010.
2. DAMESHEK, W. 1967. Chronic lymphocytic leukemia—an accumulative disease of immunologically incompetent lymphocytes. Blood **29:** 566-584.
3. BOGGS, D. R., S. A. SOFFERMAN, M. M. WINTROBE & G. E. CARTWRIGHT. 1966. Factors influencing the duration of survival of patients with chronic lymphocytic leukemia. Am. J. Med. **40:** 243-254.
4. SILVER, R. T. 1969. The treatment of chronic lymphocytic leukemia. Semin. Hematol. **6:** 344-356.
5. ZIPPIN, C., S. J. CUTLER, W. J. REEVES & D. LUM. 1973. Survival in chronic lymphocytic leukemia. Blood **42:** 367-384.
6. PHILLIPS, E. A., S. KEMPIN, S. PASSE, V. MIKÉ & B. CLARKSON. 1977. Prognostic factors in chronic lymphocytic leukemia and their implications for therapy. Clin. Haematol. **6:** 203-222.
7. RAI, K. R., A. SAWITSKY, E. P. CRONKITE, A. D. CHANANA, R. N. LEVY & B. PASTERNACK. 1975. Clinical staging of chronic lymphocytic leukemia. Blood **46:** 219-234.
8. CHANDRA, P., A. SAWITSKY, A. D. CHANANA, G. CHIKKAPPA, S. H. COHN, K. R. RAI & E. P. CRONKITE. 1979. Correlation of total body potassium and leukemic cell mass in patients with chronic lymphocytic leukemia. Blood **53:** 594-603.
9. JOHANSSON, B. & E. KLEIN. 1970. Cell surface localized IgM-kappa immunoglobulin reactivity in a case of chronic lymphocytic leukaemia. Clin. Exp. Immunol. **6:** 421-428.
10. GREY, H. M., E. RABELLINO & B. PIROFSKY. 1971. Immunoglobulins on the surface of lymphocytes. IV. Distribution in hypogammaglobulinemia, cellular immune deficiency, and chronic lymphatic leukemia. J. Clin. Invest. **50:** 2368-2375.

11. PREUD'HOMME, J. L. & M. SELIGMANN. 1972. Surface bound immunoglobulins as a cell marker in human lymphoproliferative diseases. Blood **40:** 777-794.
12. WILSON, J. D. & A. D. F. HURDLE. 1973. Surface immunoglobulins on lymphocytes in chronic lymphocytic leukaemia and lymphosarcoma. Br. J. Haematol. **24:** 563-569.
13. SALSANO, F., S. S. FROLAND & J. B. NATVIG. 1974. Same idiotype of B-lymphocyte membrane IgD and IgM. Formal evidence for monoclonality of chronic lymphocytic leukemia cells. Scand. J. Immunol. **3:** 841-846.
14. KANTER, R., J. STEINBERG, K. R. RAI, R. E. CALHOON & A. SAWITSKY. 1982. T-cell determinants in B-cell CLL. Clin. Res. **30:** 351A.
15. CATOVSKY, D., E. MILLANI, A. OKOS & D. A. G. GALTON. 1974. Clinical significance of T-cells in chronic lymphocytic leukaemia. Lancet **2:** 751-752.
16. CHIORAZZI, N., S. M. FU, G. MONTZERI, H. G. KUNKEL, K. RAI & T. GEE. 1979. T-cell helper defect in patients with chronic lymphocytic leukemia. J. Immunol. **122:** 1087-1090.
17. PLATSOUCAS, C. D., S. KEMPIN, A. KARANAS, B. CLARKSON, R. A. GOOD & S. GUPTA. 1980. Receptors for immunoglobulin isotype on T and B lymphocytes from untreated patients with chronic lymphocytic leukaemia. Clin. Exp. Immunol. **40:** 256-263.
18. CATOVSKY, D., F. LAURIA, E. MATUTES, R. FUB, V. MARBUAN, S. TURA & D. A. G. GALTON. 1981. Increase in T gamma lymphocytes in B cell chronic lymphocytic leukaemia. II. Correlation with clinical stage and findings in B prolymphocytic leukaemia. Br. J. Haematol. **47:** 539-544.
19. PLATSOUCAS, C. D., M. GALINSKI, S. KEMPIN, L. REICH, B. CLARKSON & R. A. GOOD. 1982. Abnormal T lymphocyte subpopulations in patients with B cell chronic lymphocytic leukemia: an analysis by monoclonal antibodies. J. Immunol. **129:** 2305-2311.
20. KAY, N. E., J. D. JOHNSON, R. STANEK & S. D. DOUGLAS. 1979. T-cell subpopulations in chronic lymphocytic leukemia: abnormalities in distribution and in *in vitro* maturation. Blood **54:** 540-544.
21. FAGUET, G. B. 1979. Mechanisms of lymphocyte activation. The role of suppressor cells in proliferative responses of chronic lymphocytic leukemia lymphocytes. J. Clin. Invest. **63:** 67-74.
22. FOA, R., D. CATOVSKY, F. LAURIA, M. N. ZAFAR & D. A. G. GALTON. 1981. T-lymphocytes in B-cell chronic lymphocytic leukaemia. Haematologica **66:** 105-116.
23. FIDDES, P., R. PENNY & J. V. WELLS. 1972. Clinical correlations with immunoglobulin levels in chronic lymphocytic leukaemia. Aust. N.Z. J. Med. **2:** 346-350.
24. GUPTA, S. & R. A. GOOD. 1981. Clinical significance of human lymphocyte subpopulations. *In* Contemporary Hematology/Oncology. R. Silber, A. S. Gordon, J. LoBue & F. Muggia, Eds. **2:** 153-226. Plenum Publishing Corp. New York, N.Y.
25. MANGAN, K. F., G. CHIKKAPPA & P. C. FARLEY. 1982. T gamma (T) cells suppress growth of erythroid colony-forming units in vitro in the pure red cell aplasia of B-cell chronic lymphocytic leukemia. J. Clin. Invest. **70:** 1148-1156.
26. MANGAN, K. F., G. CHIKKAPPA, W. B. SCHARFMAN & J. F. DESFORGES. 1981. Evidence for reduced erythroid burst (BFU-E) promoting function of T lymphocytes in the pure red cell aplasia of chronic lymphocytic leukemia. Exp. Hematol. (Copenhagen) **9:** 489-498.
27. NAGASAWA, R., T. ABE & T. NAKAGAWA. 1981. Pure red cell aplasia and hypogammaglobulinemia associated with T-cell chronic lymphocytic leukemia. Blood **57:** 1025-1031.
28. HOFFMAN, R., S. KOPEL, S. D. HSU, N. DAINIAK & E. D. ZANJANI. 1978. T cell chronic lymphocytic leukemia: presence in bone marrow and peripheral blood of cells that suppress erythropoiesis in vitro. Blood **52:** 255-260.
29. YOO, D., L. E. PIERCE & L. S. LESSIN. 1983. Acquired pure red cell aplasia associated with chronic lymphocytic leukemia. Cancer **51:** 844-850.
30. RAI, K. & A. SAWITSKY. 1981. Studies in clinical staging, lymphocyte function, and markers as an approach to the treatment of chronic lymphocytic leukemia. *In* Contemporary Hematology/Oncology. R. Silber, A. S. Gordon, J. LoBue & F. Muggia, Eds. **2:** 227-262. Plenum Publishing Corp. New York, N.Y.

Genetically Induced Enzyme Anomalies: Insights into Normal Cellular Processes[a]

DONALD E. PAGLIA[b,d] AND WILLIAM N. VALENTINE[c,d]

[b]Division of Surgical Pathology, Department of Pathology
[c]Department of Medicine
University of California
Center for Health Sciences
Los Angeles, California 90024

[d]Veterans Administration Center
Los Angeles, California 90073

Genetically induced defects of single enzymes within complex metabolic sequences provide unique natural experiments, the consequences of which often yield valuable insights into normal metabolic processes. Studies of such defects in human erythrocytes have been especially revealing, since these cells have rigidly restricted metabolic options with essentially no capacity to engage in oxidative phosphorylation or to synthesize structural or enzymatic proteins beyond the reticulocyte stage.

Because of the special properties of hemoglobin, the erythrocyte's primary functions of gas transport and exchange are performed without energy expenditure, but energy is required for other processes if the cell is to maintain functional integrity throughout its normal 120-day life span. These processes include: (a) cation pumping across the membrane against electrochemical gradients; (b) maintenance of hemoglobin iron in the functional ferrous state; (c) phosphorylation of various substrates to initiate and maintain glycolysis, and to synthesize glutathione (GSH) and other compounds such as phosphoribosylpyrophosphate (PRPP); (d) participation in reactions related to membrane phospholipids; and (e) protection of hemoglobin and other essential structural and enzymatic proteins from irreversible oxidation.

These energy requirements are fulfilled almost entirely by glycolysis, and the energy generated is stored in complementary reservoirs of high-energy phosphates (ATP and 2,3-diphosphoglycerate (2,3-DPG)) and reducing compounds (GSH and the pyridine cofactors, NADH and NADPH).

For proper maintenance, both of these energy pools require effective degradation of glucose to lactate, either anaerobically through the Embden-Meyerhof pathway for ATP, 2,3-DPG, and NADH, or oxidatively through the pentose phosphate shunt for NADPH and GSH (FIGURE 1). This critical dependence on glycolysis is dramatically demonstrated by the deleterious effects of various enzymopathies that are now known to result in hemolytic syndromes.[1-4] Hereditary deficiency states have been identified for 8 of the 11 enzymes of the Embden-Meyerhof pathway, the mutase of the Rapaport-Luebering shunt, and 5 of the enzymes operative in GSH generation or main-

[a]Supported by USPHS Grant HLB-12944 from the National Institutes of Health.

tenance. Virtually all are associated with shortened erythrocyte life spans and induce either chronic or episodic (stress-induced) hemolytic anemia, depending upon which energy pool is affected.

Most erythrocyte enzyme deficiencies are heterogeneous disorders with mutant alleles governing production of diverse isozymes which may be distinguished on the basis of biochemical characteristics. Studies of mutant pyruvate kinase isozymes, for example, have shown that premature hemolysis results not only from insufficient catalytic activity or enzyme instability, but also from decreased avidity for substrate or nucleotide cofactor, from an inability to respond to allosteric activation by fructose-1,6-diphosphate, or from abnormal inhibition by a reaction product (ATP), demonstrating the complex interdependence of these various metabolic components.

Glycolysis serves to generate the proper energy state of the adenine or pyridine nucleotides, but other reactions are necessary to maintain dynamic equilibria among these compounds, particularly within the adenine nucleotide pool. In normal erythrocytes, most of the adenine nucleotides are present as ATP (85-90%) with less

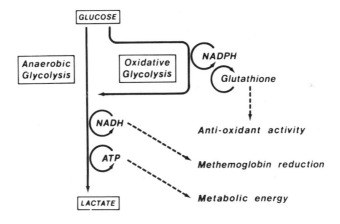

FIGURE 1. Generation of energy by glycolysis in mature erythrocytes.

present as ADP (10-15%) and AMP (1-3%); all are in rapid equilibrium mediated by an active adenylate kinase (AK) (FIGURE 2). AMP is in particular jeopardy, since it may be irreversibly deaminated to inosine monophosphate (IMP) or dephosphorylated to diffusible adenosine, allowing escape of purine base which cannot be synthesized *de novo*.

Several families have now been identified with varying degrees of erythrocyte AK deficiency hereditarily transmitted as an autosomal recessive trait.[5-10] It appears to be a heterogeneous disorder with a wide range of clinical severity that does not necessarily correlate with the amount of residual AK. However, significantly shortened erythrocyte life span does occur in most cases, sometimes producing life-threatening hemolytic anemia, so the crucial role of the enzyme in normal cell metabolism seems assured.

The latter conclusion is supported by other experiments of nature in which erythrocytes possess an overabundance or a deficiency of adenosine deaminase (ADA). Two families are known in which relatively mild chronic hemolysis is associated with decreased concentrations of adenine nucleotides (25-50% of normal) and hyperactive

ADA (50-100 times normal).[11-15] The enzyme is structurally normal by all conventional biochemical criteria, implicating a defect in genetic control of ADA production in erythroid precursors, transmitted as an autosomal dominant trait. Conversely, many instances of severe combined immunodeficiency disease are associated with decreased ADA activity. Although erythrocytes with ADA deficiency do not appear to be adversely affected, they do accumulate enormous quantities of adenine nucleotides, especially the deoxy forms.

These two hereditary abnormalities demonstrate that hyperactive ADA depletes the adenine nucleotide pool, while ADA deficiency expands it. These could be logical complementary events only if adenosine kinase (AdoK) activity were an essential

ADENINE NUCLEOTIDE POOL

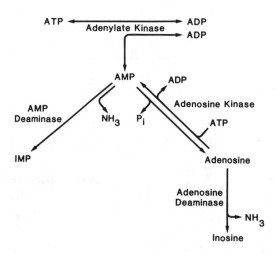

FIGURE 2. Erythrocyte adenine nucleotide interactions with potential degradative and salvage pathways. AMP may be dephosphorylated to adenosine by nonspecific phosphatases or by 5′-nucleotidase activity.

salvage pathway for maintaining the adenine nucleotide pool in normal erythrocytes. Plasma adenosine can be assimilated by circulating erythrocytes, both by passive diffusion and by a facilitated transport system in the membrane. The relative activities and kinetic characteristics of ADA and AdoK determine the fate of the nucleoside, which can either be deaminated to inosine or phosphorylated to AMP (FIGURE 2). The higher activity of ADA and its close physical association with the membrane transport system favor deamination of available (~ 1 μM) plasma adenosine. At low substrate concentrations, however, phosphorylation may predominate because of the 20-fold greater substrate affinity possessed by AdoK.

Thus, a balanced competition for adenosine exists between ADA and AdoK. If that balance is altered by markedly increased or decreased ADA activity, the consequences are manifested by absolute changes in the content of the adenine nucleotide pool.

One of the most revealing experiments of nature, in terms of elucidating normal cellular processes, has involved defects of erythrocyte pyrimidine nucleotidase (PyrNase). Indeed, the very existence of this highly specific enzyme was discovered through studies of several families with an unusual hemolytic syndrome later determined to result from its deficiency.[16] The syndrome was characterized by chronic hemolytic anemia, inherited as an autosomal recessive trait, in which affected erythrocytes (a) retained only 5-10% of normal PyrNase activity, (b) accumulated immense quantities of uridine and cytidine compounds, and (c) exhibited prominent basophilic stippling with Wright's stain. Elevated GSH concentrations and decreased activities of PRPP-synthetase (ribosephosphate pyrophosphokinase (RPK)) were also consistently found, but are considered to be indirect epiphenomena.

Unlike the ubiquitous 5'-nucleotidases found throughout nature, which are variably effective both with purine and pyrimidine nucleotides, the PyrNase found in mature erythrocytes appeared to be restricted to pyrimidine substrates when assayed at physiological pH[16–19]:

$$\left.\begin{array}{c} UMP \\ CMP \end{array}\right\} + H_2O \xrightarrow[\text{5'-Nucleotidase}]{\text{Pyrimidine}} \left\{\begin{array}{c} Uridine \\ Cytidine \end{array}\right\} + P_i.$$

Such substrate specificity is an expected, if not inevitable, evolutionary development: a nucleotidase also capable of dephosphorylating AMP would impose a constant deleterious drain on the adenine nucleotide pool and should be quickly eliminated by natural selective processes. The unique restriction to pyrimidine substrates allows this nucleotidase to dephosphorylate RNA degradation products to diffusible nucleosides during reticulocyte maturation without jeopardizing the essential energy pool of adenine nucleotides[16]:

$$RNA \xrightarrow{\text{Ribonucleases}} \underbrace{AMP \quad + \quad GMP}_{\substack{\text{Purine} \\ \text{Nucleotides}}} \quad + \quad \underbrace{UMP \quad + \quad CMP}_{\substack{\text{Pyrimidine} \\ \text{Nucleotides}}}.$$

Pyrimidine compounds may accumulate sufficiently in affected cells to expand the total nucleotide pool to more than five times that present in normal erythrocytes. The adenine nucleotides are often decreased in concentration and are at a competitive disadvantage against increased pyrimidine analogues, both conditions probably contributing to the induction of hemolysis in older cell cohorts. Feedback inhibition of RNA catabolism results in aggregation of undegraded or partially degraded ribosomal material, producing the basophilic stippling that is the morphologic hallmark of the disorder.

The common denominator of basophilic stippling and the enzyme's exquisite sensitivity to heavy-metal inactivation led to elucidation of its role in lead-induced hemolytic anemia. PyrNase is inactivated both *in vitro* and *in vivo* by concentrations of lead too low to have significant effects on a large number of other erythrocyte enzymes of glucose, nucleotide, and glutathione metabolism.[20] At lead concentrations of approximately 200 μg/dl packed red cells, PyrNase activities are suppressed to levels comparable to those observed in the severe hereditary deficiency state. Intracellular pyrimidine nucleotides and basophilic stippling then become detectable along with a hemolytic process that is distinct from the anemia due to ineffective heme or globin biosynthesis.[21,22] Thus, the syndrome due to severe hereditary deficiency of

PyrNase is recapitulated almost precisely by cases of acquired hemolytic anemia secondary to severe acute lead toxicity.

Recently, evidence has emerged to indicate that PyrNase is accompanied by one or more additional isozymes of 5'-nucleotidase in human erythrocytes.[23,24] Again, hereditary deficiency states provided the otherwise unobtainable natural experiment to reveal the presence of separate isozymes. Subjects who were severely deficient in PyrNase, which traditionally is measured with uridine or cytidine 5'-monophosphates (UMP, CMP), were found to have normal activity with thymidine and other deoxyribonucleotide substrates (dTMP, dUMP, dIMP).[23-25]

Studies in five unrelated families allowed identification of a distinct isozyme with deoxyribonucleotidase (dNase) activity.[25] This isozyme cross-reacts with the corresponding ribonucleotide substrates and probably contributes the slight ($<10\%$) residual activity seen in virtually all reported cases of severe PyrNase deficiency.

The dNase isozyme may have a physiologic function in DNA degradation comparable to that presumed for PyrNase in ribosomal RNA catabolism. This further suggests that a significant degree of karyolysis accompanies nuclear pyknosis and pitting in maturing erythroblasts, requiring dephosphorylation of resultant deoxyribonucleotides to diffusible nucleosides to clear them from the cytosol.[24,25]

Another hemolytic syndrome, so far identified in only one individual, has suggested a link between certain metabolic activities in the erythrocyte and important phospholipid components of the membrane. Affected erythrocytes in this case contained selective increases in CDP-choline that were 15-25 times greater than amounts found in normal cells, equivalent to 20-30% of the total adenine nucleotide content.[26] No other abnormal compounds or defective enzymes, including PyrNase, were detectable.

Selective accumulation of CDP-choline seems most compatible with an inherited deficiency of choline phosphotransferase in erythroid precursors, a hypothesis as yet unproven. FIGURE 3 diagrams a number of reactions centered around CDP-choline. All of the enzymes shown, except for choline phosphotransferase, have now been identified in human erythrocytes.[26] Since no quantitative or qualitative alterations in membrane phospholipids of affected cells have been demonstrable, it seems likely that

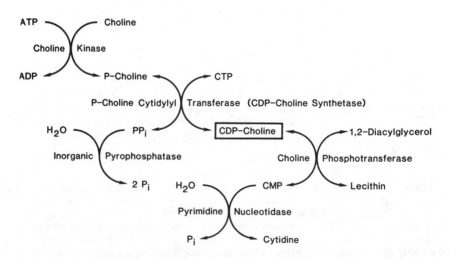

FIGURE 3. Selected reactions in phospholipid metabolism.

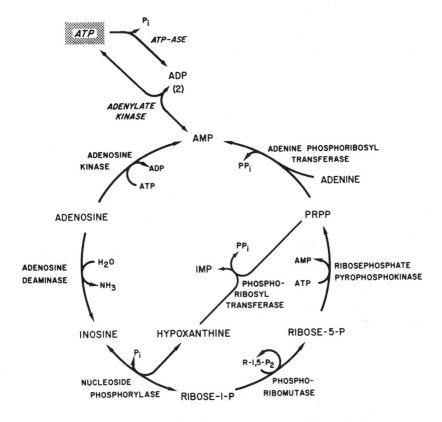

FIGURE 4. Erythrocyte pathways of adenine nucleotide metabolism.

some other mechanism is involved in induction of hemolysis, perhaps similar to the competitive interferences hypothesized to occur in PyrNase deficiency. This case provides support for the normal maintenance of membrane lecithin by passive exchange with plasma components or by acylation of lysolecithin,[27] and it contradicts the hypothesis that hemolysis in PyrNase deficiency is due to deleterious effects of CDP-choline on membrane phospholipid synthesis.[28,29]

Review of these and other genetically induced deficiencies of specific enzymes related to nucleotide metabolism allows compilation of the metabolic pathways shown in FIGURE 4. The lack of apparent deleterious effects in marked deficiency of adenine phosphoribosyltransferase[30] indicates that direct incorporation of adenine into the nucleotide pool is not a salvage mechanism as crucial to cell survival as adenosine phosphorylation. Other apparently nondeleterious conditions include marked deficiencies of nucleoside phosphorylase (seen in some cases of immunodeficiency disease) and hypoxanthine-guanine phosphoribosyltransferase (in Lesch-Nyhan syndrome),[31] and either deficiency[32] or hyperactivity[33, 34] of PRPP-synthetase (RPK). These observations indicate that mature erythrocytes primarily rely on adenosine salvage and avoidance of AMP dephosphorylation to maintain their limited complement of adenine nucleotides.

Studies of biochemical perturbations resulting from such hereditary defects have added substantially to our understanding of normal red cell metabolism and have provided additional insights into the pathophysiology of underlying hemolytic mechanisms.

EPILOGUE

The senior author (D.E.P.) would like to add a personal note in recognition of this special International Conference on Hematopoietic Cellular Proliferation to honor Dr. Eugene Cronkite. It is especially gratifying to be able to present evidence for the existence of a unique enzyme system, possibly pertinent to the final stages of erythroid maturation, that is predicated on thymidine nucleotidase and related deoxynucleotidase activities. It was my privilege, during my formative years as Dr. Cronkite's first technologist at Brookhaven National Laboratory, to assist in the earliest attempts to obtain autoradiographs from tissues labeled with a new entity at that time, generated by Dr. Walter "Pete" Hughes, known as tritiated thymidine.

It seems especially appropriate to close a personal ring 27 years later by dedicating my contribution to the discovery and elucidation of thymidine nucleotidase and its isozymes to the man who urged me into those first tentative steps along the rocky road to creative science: mentor, friend, and colleague, Eugene Pitcher Cronkite.

ACKNOWLEDGMENTS

The studies that originated in the authors' laboratory depended upon the technologic contributions of Shirley Gordon, Richard Brockway, and Misae Nakatani. Alicia Araiza and Carol Appleton assisted in the preparation of the manuscript.

REFERENCES

1. BEUTLER, E. 1978. Hemolytic Anemia in Disorders of Red Cell Metabolism. Plenum. New York, N.Y.
2. VALENTINE, W. N. 1979. The Stratton lecture: hemolytic anemia and inborn errors of metabolism. Blood 54: 549.
3. VALENTINE, W. N. & D. E. PAGLIA. 1980. The primary cause of hemolysis in enzymopathies of anaerobic glycolysis: a viewpoint. Blood Cells 6: 819.
4. MIWA, S. 1983. Hereditary disorders of red cell enzymes in the Embden-Meyerhof pathway. Am. J. Hematol. 14: 381.
5. SZEINBERG, A., S. GAVENDO & D. CAHANE. 1969. Erythrocyte adenylate kinase deficiency. Lancet i: 315.
6. SZEINBERG, A., D. KAHANA, S. GAVENDO, J. ZAIDMAN & J. BEN-EZZER. 1969. Hereditary deficiency of adenylate kinase in red blood cells. Acta Haematol. 42: 111.
7. BOIVIN, P., C. GALAND, J. HAKIM, D. SIMONY & M. SELIGMAN. 1971. Un nouvelle érythroenzymopathie. Anémie hémolytique congénitale non sphérocytaire et déficit héréditaire en adénylate-kinase érythrocytaire. Presse Med. 79: 215.

8. KENDE, G., I. BEN-BASSAT, F. BROK-SIMONI, F. HOLTZMAN & B. RAMOT. 1982. Adenylate kinase deficiency associated with congenital nonspherocytic hemolytic anemia. *In* Abstracts of the Joint Meeting of the 19th Congress of the International Society of Haematology and the 17th Congress of the International Society of Blood Transfusion. P. 48. Akadémiai Nyomda. Budapest, Hungary.

9. MIWA, S., H. FUJII, K. TANI, K. TAKAHASHI, T. TAKIZAWA & T. IGARASHI. 1983. Red cell adenylate kinase deficiency associated with hereditary nonspherocytic hemolytic anemia: clinical and biochemical studies. Am. J. Hematol. **14:** 325.

10. BEUTLER, E., D. CARSON, H. DANNAWI, L. FORMAN, W. KUHL, C. WEST & B. WESTWOOD. 1983. Metabolic compensation for profound erythrocyte adenylate kinase deficiency. A hereditary enzyme defect without hemolytic anemia. J. Clin. Invest. **72:** 648.

11. PAGLIA, D. E., W. N. VALENTINE, A. P. TARTAGLIA & F. GILSANZ. 1976. Perturbations in erythrocyte adenine nucleotide metabolism: a dominantly inherited hemolytic disorder with implications regarding normal mechanisms of adenine nucleotide preservation. Blood **48:** 959.

12. VALENTINE, W. N., D. E. PAGLIA, A. P. TARTAGLIA & F. GILSANZ. 1977. Hereditary hemolytic anemia with increased red cell adenosine deaminase (45- to 70-fold) and decreased adenosine triphosphate. Science **195:** 783.

13. PAGLIA, D. E., W. N. VALENTINE, A. P. TARTAGLIA, F. GILSANZ & R. S. SPARKES. 1978. Control of red blood cell adenine nucleotide metabolism. Studies of adenosine deaminase. *In* The Red Cell. G. J. Brewer, Ed.: 319. Liss. New York, N.Y.

14. MIWA, S., H. FUJII, N. MATSUMOTO, T. NAKATSUJI, S. ODA, H. ASANO, S. ASANO & Y. MIURA. 1978. A case of red-cell adenosine deaminase overproduction associated with hereditary hemolytic anemia found in Japan. Am. J. Hematol. **5:** 107.

15. FUJII, H., S. MIWA & K. SUZUKI. 1980. Purification and properties of adenosine deaminase in normal and hereditary hemolytic anemia with increased red cell activity. Hemoglobin **4:** 693.

16. VALENTINE, W. N., K. FINK, D. E. PAGLIA, S. R. HARRIS & W. S. ADAMS. 1974. Hereditary hemolytic anemia with human erythrocyte pyrimidine 5'-nucleotidase deficiency. J. Clin. Invest. **54:** 866.

17. PAGLIA, D. E. & W. N. VALENTINE. 1975. Characteristics of a pyrimidine-specific 5'-nucleotidase in human erythrocytes. J. Biol. Chem. **250:** 7973.

18. TORRANCE, J. D., D. WHITTAKER & E. BEUTLER. 1977. Purification and properties of human erythrocyte pyrimidine 5'-nucleotidase. Proc. Natl. Acad. Sci. USA **74:** 3701.

19. PAGLIA, D. E. & W. N. VALENTINE. 1980. Hereditary and acquired defects in the pyrimidine nucleotidase of human erythrocytes. Curr. Top. Hematol. **3:** 75.

20. PAGLIA, D. E., W. N. VALENTINE & J. G. DAHLGREN. 1975. Effects of low-level lead exposure on pyrimidine 5'-nucleotidase and other erythrocyte enzymes. Possible role of pyrimidine 5'-nucleotidase in the pathogenesis of lead-induced anemia. J. Clin. Invest. **56:** 1164.

21. VALENTINE, W. N., D. E. PAGLIA, K. FINK & G. MADOKORO. 1976. Lead poisoning. Association with hemolytic anemia, basophilic stippling, erythrocyte pyrimidine 5'-nucleotidase deficiency, and intraerythrocytic accumulation of pyrimidines. J. Clin. Invest. **58:** 926.

22. PAGLIA, D. E., W. N. VALENTINE & K. FINK. 1977. Lead poisoning. Further observations on erythrocyte pyrimidine-nucleotidase deficiency and intracellular accumulation of pyrimidine nucleotides. J. Clin. Invest. **60:** 1362.

23. SWALLOW, D. M., I. AZIZ, D. A. HOPKINSON & S. MIWA. 1983. Analysis of human erythrocyte 5'-nucleotidases in healthy individuals and a patient deficient in pyrimidine 5'-nucleotidase. Ann. Hum. Genet. **47:** 19.

24. PAGLIA, D. E., W. N. VALENTINE, A. S. KEITT, R. A. BROCKWAY & M. NAKATANI. 1983. Pyrimidine nucleotidase deficiency with active dephosphorylation of dTMP: evidence for existence of thymidine nucleotidase in human erythrocytes. Blood **62:** 1147.

25. PAGLIA, D. E., W. N. VALENTINE & R. A. BROCKWAY. 1985. Identification of thymidine nucleotidase and deoxyribonucleotidase activities among normal isozymes of 5'-nucleotidase in human erythrocytes. Proc. Natl. Acad. Sci. USA **81:** 588.

26. PAGLIA, D. E., W. N. VALENTINE, M. NAKATANI & B. J. RAUTH. 1983. Selective accumulation of cytosol CDP-choline as an isolated erythrocyte defect in chronic hemolysis. Proc. Natl. Acad. Sci. USA **80:** 3081.

27. SHOHET, S. B. 1972. Hemolysis and changes in erythrocyte membrane lipids. N. Engl. J. Med. **286:** 577.

28. DE VERDIER, C.-H., A. ERICSON & T. W. RUUD HANSEN. 1982. Erythrocyte nucleotide pattern in pyrimidine 5'-nucleotidase deficiency. *In* Abstracts of the Joint Meeting of the 19th Congress of the International Society of Haematology and the 17th Congress of the International Society of Blood Transfusion. P. 228. Akadémiai Nyomda. Budapest, Hungary.

29. ERICSON, A., C.-H. DE VERDIER, T. W. RUUD HANSEN & M. SEIP. 1983. Erythrocyte nucleotide pattern in two children in a Norwegian family with pyrimidine 5'-nucleotidase deficiency. Clin. Chim. Acta **134:** 25.

30. VAN ACKER, K. J., H. A. SIMMONDS, C. POTTER & J. S. CAMERON. 1977. Complete deficiency of adenine phosphoribosyltransferase. Report of a family. N. Engl. J. Med. **297:** 127.

31. KELLEY, W. N. & J. B. WYNGAARDEN. 1978. The Lesch-Nyhan syndrome. *In* The Metabolic Basis of Inherited Disease. J. B. Stanbury, J. B. Wyngaarden & D. S. Fredrickson, Eds.: 1011. McGraw-Hill. New York, N.Y.

32. WADA, Y., Y. NISHIMURA, M. TANABU, Y. YOSHIMURA, K. LINUMA, T. YOSHIDA & T. ARAKAWA. 1974. Hypouricemic, mentally retarded infant with a defect of 5-phosphoribosyl-1-pyrophosphate synthetase of erythrocytes. Tohoku J. Exp. Med. **113:** 149.

33. BECKER, M. A., P. J. KOSTEL, L. J. MEYER & J. E. SEEGMILLER. 1973. Human phosphoribosylpyrophosphate synthetase: increased enzyme-specific activity in a family with gout and excessive purine synthesis. Proc. Natl. Acad. Sci. USA **70:** 2749.

34. SPERLING, O., S. PERSKY-BROSH, P. BOER & A. DE VRIES. 1973. Human erythrocyte phosphoribosylpyrophosphate synthetase mutationally altered in regulatory properties. Biochem. Med. **7:** 389.

Cryopreservation of Human Platelets and Bone Marrow and Peripheral Blood Totipotential Mononuclear Stem Cells[a]

C. ROBERT VALERI[b]

Naval Blood Research Laboratory
Boston University School of Medicine
Boston, Massachusetts 02118

INTRODUCTION

Dr. Eugene Cronkite and his colleagues have been instrumental in establishing methods for the quantitation of platelets in blood: they documented reduced platelet count associated with hemorrhagic diathesis produced by radiation injury.[1-4] These investigators also demonstrated that fresh platelet concentrates correct the thrombocytopenic and hemorrhagic diathesis produced by radiation injury, and that fresh blood contains totipotential stem cells which restore hematopoiesis in animals exposed to total-body irradiation.[5-12]

I would like to present an update of the methods being used to isolate and cryopreserve human platelets, as well as the methods used to isolate from bone marrow and peripheral blood totipotential stem cells devoid of immunocompetent cells and methods to freeze these cells.

ISOLATION OF PLATELETS

Platelets are much more difficult to isolate and preserve than red cells: the number of platelets in one unit of blood is not sufficient for a therapeutic transfusion. Of necessity, platelets from several units of blood are pooled. This approach has been quite satisfactory, for instance, in patients who donate six to eight units of platelets

[a] The research reported here has been supported by the Office of Naval Research under Contract N00014-79-C-0168, with funds provided by the Naval Medical Research and Development Command. The opinions or assertions contained herein are those of the author, and are not to be construed as official or reflecting the views of the Navy Department or Naval Service at large.

[b] Correspondence address: Capt. C. Robert Valeri, MC, USN, Naval Blood Research Laboratory, Boston University School of Medicine, 615 Albany Street, Boston, Mass. 02118.

at times when their disease allows, for cryopreservation and subsequent autotransfusion.[13,14] However, pooled platelets for homologous transfusion increase the potential for infection and sensitization.

Plastic multiple-bag systems are now available in which platelets and plasma, as well as red cells, can be prepared from individual units of blood in a closed system, without contamination (FIGURE 1). Plateletpheresis, leukapheresis, and plasmapheresis also are being used to collect only the specific components that are needed (FIGURE 2).[15–23] The apheresis procedures are well tolerated by healthy donors, and blood products collected by these procedures have been satisfactorily preserved.[24]

Platelet transfusions have increased from fewer than 100,000 per year in 1970 to more than 1,000,000 per year today. Platelets can be stored in the liquid state at 4°C for only 2 days or at 22°C for only 5 days.[24–27] Frozen platelets, on the other hand, can be stored at −80°C for at least 2 years or at −150°C for at least 3 years with satisfactory results.[24]

Damage may occur during blood collection and platelet isolation. Platelets isolated by serial differential centrifugation may be damaged during each centrifugation step as they release ADP, calcium, and serotonin, which cause platelet aggregation. This aggregation pattern may be reversed by storing the platelets undisturbed at room temperature before resuspension: 30 min when the acid-citrate-dextrose (ACD) anticoagulant is used for blood collection, and 60 min when the citrate-phosphate-dextrose (CPD) or citrate-phosphate-dextrose-adenine (CPD-adenine) anticoagulant is used.[24,28]

Each unit of blood is collected in a multiple-bag system, usually in the ACD anticoagulant (National Institutes of Health, Formula A). Platelet isolation and resuspension are better with ACD because the lower pH of ACD is less apt to cause the platelets to aggregate.[28] The platelets are isolated by differential centrifugation, and the red cells and platelet-poor plasma are reinfused into the donor before another unit is plateletpheresed.[29] Up to eight separate units can be drawn from a single donor by this process.

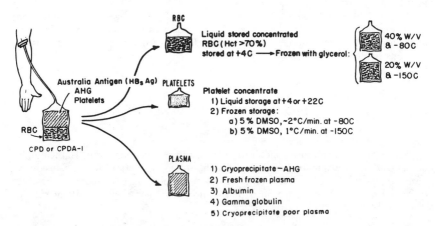

FIGURE 1. An approach to collecting 450 ml of blood and separating it into cellular components and plasma protein derivatives. Red cell and platelet concentrates and plasma protein derivatives are isolated from blood within 4 hr of collection and storage at room temperature (22 ± 2°C) and are preserved by the most appropriate method. (Reprinted with permission from: VALERI, C. R. 1976. Blood Banking and the Use of Frozen Blood Products. P. 3. CRC Press. Boca Raton, Fla.)

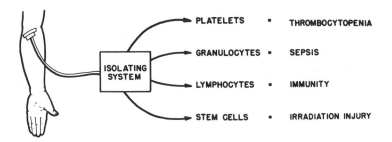

FIGURE 2. A schematic showing how platelets, phagocytic cells (granulocytes-monocytes), lymphocytes, and stem cells can be isolated from peripheral blood using mechanical cell-separating systems for treatment of the listed conditions. (Reprinted with permission from: VALERI, C. R. 1981. Critical Reviews in Clinical Laboratory Sciences **14**: 25.)

There are five cell-separating systems available commercially for platelet isolation: the IBM-Aminco Celltrifuge, the Haemonetics Blood Processor 30, the IBM Blood Processor 2997, the Fenwal CS-3000, and the Dideco Progress Cell Separator. The donor is attached to the system, and platelets from as many as eight units of blood can be isolated at a donation, a number sufficient for therapeutic effectiveness in a patient with thrombocytopenia. This procedure reduces the risk of alloimmunization of the recipient, and because only one donor is involved reduces the risk of transmission of disease.

Although usually the ACD Formula A anticoagulant is used with this cell-separating system, the ACD Formula B anticoagulant or an anticoagulant solution of 2% citrate in sodium chloride is sometimes used because it is felt that their reduced amounts of citrate will lessen the likelihood of hypocalcemia symptoms when blood is rapidly reinfused into the donor.[30] Reinfusing the citrated blood at a slower rate will also accomplish this.

INJURY TO PLATELET SURVIVAL AND FUNCTION RELATED TO ISOLATION AND PREFREEZE STORAGE

Cellular damage during platelet isolation may be related to any number of factors including: the speed and duration of centrifugation; the biocompatibility of the plastic collection container; and the biocompatibility of surfaces to which the platelets are exposed in the mechanical cell-separating systems (i.e., the reusable and disposable bowls in the IBM-Aminco Celltrifuge, the disposable bowl in the Haemonetics Blood Processor 30 or the Dideco Progress Cell Separator, the rotating single-stage channel in the IBM Blood Processor 2997, and the disposable plastic bags in the Fenwal CS-3000).[15,31,32]

Platelet isolation demands a certain technical expertise. Calibration of the centrifuge, as well as standardization of the speed and duration of centrifugation, is important in ensuring adequate recovery of platelets with minimal damage to their circulation and function.[15,33-36]

The serial differential centrifugation method involves the least risk to the donor because the 450 ml of blood taken at a time for platelet isolation amounts to only

10% of the donor's blood volume. With the mechanical cell-separating systems, there is a considerably greater risk potential for citrate toxicity, thrombocytopenia, anemia, infection, and other reactions.

In vitro tests of platelet morphology, as studied by transmission electron microscopy, and of platelet aggregation have been used to calculate the injury platelets suffer during isolation.[32,37-39] Both reversible and irreversible damage may occur during platelet isolation and preservation. The conditions of prefreeze storage that may adversely affect the viability and function of the platelets include the concentration of the platelets, the volume of plasma, the composition and thickness of the plastic freezing container, the presence or absence of agitation during storage, and the storage temperature.[15,24]

Either a polyolefin plastic bag (Fenwal Laboratories, PL-732) or a polyvinyl chloride (PVC) plastic bag containing tri(2-ethylhexyl)trimellitate (TEHTM, Cutter Laboratories) can be used for storage of a platelet concentrate isolated from a unit of blood.[25-27] Platelets stored for 5 days at 22 ± 2°C with horizontal agitation at 70 cycles/min have been found to have an *in vivo* platelet recovery value of about 40%, a life span of about 8 days, and a T_{50} (half-life) value of 4 days. In clinical studies in thrombocytopenic patients, the transfusion of a pool of six to eight units of ABO-compatible platelet concentrates produced a significant increase in platelet count and reduced the bleeding time, with no untoward effects.

CRYOPRESERVATION OF PLATELETS

There are several agents for platelet freezing: dimethyl sulfoxide (DMSO), a glycerol-glucose solution, and hydroxyethyl starch (HES). DMSO has been the most widely used. At the Naval Blood Research Laboratory, platelets have been frozen with 5% DMSO at 1°C/min and stored at −150°C and with 6% DMSO at 2-3°C/min and stored at −80°C. These frozen-thawed-washed platelets have 40 to 50% the therapeutic effectiveness of fresh platelets.[40,41]

Many investigators recommend controlling the rate of freezing to minimize platelet damage. A rate of 1°C/min has been recommended, but this requires a special programmed freezer which has been associated with some problems. Murphy *et al.*[42] reported satisfactory results when human platelets were frozen with 5% DMSO in a special programmed freezer at rates ranging from 1 to 3°C/min, but when the freezing rates were increased to greater than 5°C/min, platelet damage was observed. Lazarus *et al.*[43] reported major damage to platelets frozen with 10% DMSO at about 8°C/min in the gas phase of liquid nitrogen. However, when they froze the platelets with 10% DMSO at a controlled rate of 1°C/min and stored them in the gas phase of liquid nitrogen, survival and function of the thawed, nonwashed, previously frozen platelets were similar to those of fresh platelets. Comparable results were seen in studies at the Naval Blood Research Laboratory using 4 to 6% DMSO concentrations and freezing rates of 1-3°C/min achieved by storage of the platelets in a −80°C mechanical freezer. Our experience at the Naval Blood Research Laboratory indicates that when the volume and geometry of the freezing container are controlled, a freezing rate of 2-3°C/min can be achieved by storage in a −80°C mechanical freezer.[24]

Glycerol also has been used for platelet freezing: Dayian and co-workers[44,45] are enthusiastic about their results with platelets frozen with 5% glycerol and 4% glucose in 0.9% sodium chloride solution at 30°C/min at −150°C. The nonwashed, previously frozen platelets reportedly had recovery values *in vitro* of 90%, platelet circulation similar to that of fresh platelets, and one unit corrected an aspirin-induced prolonged bleeding time in a healthy volunteer. Our attempts to duplicate their work were disappointing, as were the attempts of Kotelba-Witkowska and Schiffer[46] and Redmond and associates.[47]

Human platelets have also been frozen with a solution of 3% glycerol in plasma by a two-step controlled-rate procedure and storage in liquid nitrogen in a polyolefin plastic bag.[48] Preliminary results with these platelets transfused to patients without washing have been encouraging.

COMPOSITION OF THE PLATELET FREEZING CONTAINER

Kim and Baldini[49] have reported that a bioriented polyolefin container produced by Union Carbide Corporation is superior to a PVC plastic container produced by Abbott Laboratories for platelet storage. Results from our studies were similar whether the platelets were frozen in polyolefin plastic bags or in PVC plastic bags.[50,51]

TEMPERATURE OF FROZEN STORAGE

Human platelets usually can be frozen either in liquid nitrogen with storage at $-150°C$, or in mechanical refrigerators with storage at $-80°C$. The proper amount of liquid nitrogen and an insulated storage container maintain the gas phase at about $-150°C$. Liquid nitrogen used with a special apparatus can also control the rate of platelet freezing. The rate of freezing in the $-80°C$ mechanical freezer is regulated by the geometry of the freezing container and the temperature of the freezer.[41]

Platelets have been satisfactorily frozen with 5% DMSO and stored in the gas phase of liquid nitrogen at $-120°C$ for 3 years,[52] and with 6% DMSO at $2-3°C/min$ and stored at $-80°C$ in a mechanical freezer for at least 2 years.[24]

POSTTHAW PROCESSING OF DMSO-FROZEN PLATELETS

DMSO-preserved platelets have been transfused without postthaw washing,[43,53–55] but platelet washing reduces the risk of toxic effects and appears to improve *in vivo* survival as well.[40] When platelets frozen with a combination of 5% DMSO and 5% dextrose were not washed before transfusion to thrombocytopenic-leukemic children, many of the recipients experienced nausea and vomiting, several developed phlebitis, and the increase in platelet count was only 30% that seen with fresh platelet transfusions.[54]

A one-dilution wash procedure removes about 95% of the DMSO and leaves about 300 mg in the unit of platelets. Platelets washed with a single dilution-centrifugation procedure were found to have better circulation than unwashed platelets,[40] and shortly after their transfusion to thrombocytopenic patients, increased platelet counts and reduced bleeding times were observed.

Before washing, the platelets are thawed without agitation in a water bath at 37°C. Kim and Baldini[49,56–58] have stressed the importance of adding the solution slowly with proper mixing to minimize osmotic swelling. The washed, resuspended platelets can be stored in plasma at 22 to 24°C for 6 to 8 hr,[58,59] but longer storage will adversely affect their circulation.

TOXICITY OF DMSO

Side effects such as local vasospasm and pain have been reported following the transfusion of platelets frozen with DMSO, but washing these platelets prevents these symptoms.[15,24] In addition, DMSO may produce an unpleasant odor in the recipient's mouth, and the patient may suffer nausea and vomiting. In animals, large doses of DMSO have been shown to produce lesions in the eye, particularly in the lens, and to potentiate the hepatic toxicity of aromatic hydrocarbons.[60–62] Careful ophthalmologic examinations and appropriate liver function studies made before and after our studies in healthy volunteers over the past 8 years showed no untoward effects of the residual DMSO in the transfused platelets. Moreover, any defect in platelet function produced by DMSO appears to be reversible.[63]

THERAPEUTIC EFFECTIVENESS OF PLATELETS FROZEN WITH DMSO

Platelets frozen with DMSO have freeze-thaw-wash recovery values of about 80%, immediate recovery values *in vivo* from 40 to 80% those of fresh platelets, normal life spans, and hemostatic effectiveness immediately or shortly after transfusion to thrombocytopenic patients.[15,24,57,59]

Because it takes about $2\frac{1}{2}$ units of cryopreserved platelets to achieve the same number of circulating platelets as 1 unit of fresh platelet concentrate, it has been necessary to pool ABO- and Rh-identical platelets obtained from several blood donors for cryopreservation.[13–15,24,52,59,64,65] Now, there is the alternative of using mechanical cell-separating systems to isolate as many as six to eight units of platelets from the blood of a single donor in 2 to 3 hr.[51,66] This reduces the risk of recipient alloimmunization and the transmission of disease.

JUSTIFICATION OF FREEZE PRESERVATION OF HUMAN PLATELETS

The hardware, software, and technical expertise for platelet cryopreservation, like those for red cell freezing, are costly, yet justified. The use of cryopreserved platelets is justified when specific platelets are needed as in the following situations:

(1) autologous platelets for patients anticipating therapeutic platelet transfusions,

(2) homologous ABO- and HLA-compatible platelets for patients with refractory thrombocytopenia,

(3) universal donor O-positive and O-negative platelets for contingency planning to support military operations, and

(4) HLA-typed platelets for use in compatibility testing of platelets *in vitro*.

Each method of platelet collection has advantages and disadvantages. Isolating platelets from a single unit of blood is the safest method for the donor, but the number obtained from one unit is not enough for a transfusion and units from different donors must be pooled. Plateletpheresis can be done using a multiple-bag system but this is time-consuming, and units from different donors might possibly be mixed during processing. Plateletpheresis using a mechanical cell-separating system (IBM-Aminco Celltrifuge, IBM Blood Processor 2997, Haemonetics Blood Processor 30, Dideco Progress Cell Separator, Fenwal CS-3000) is the easiest method, but also the most expensive. Precautions must be taken with all methods to minimize injury to the platelets during isolation, addition of the cryoprotective agent, freezing, thawing, and washing.

ISOLATION, PURIFICATION, AND CRYOPRESERVATION OF TOTIPOTENTIAL STEM CELLS

Autologous cryopreserved bone marrow has been successfully transplanted for hematopoietic reconstitution in cancer patients treated aggressively with chemotherapy or radiation therapy.[67-69] The satisfactory cryopreservation of hematopoietic stem cells depends on the concentration of cryoprotectant,[70,71] concentration of proteins,[72] rate of freezing,[73,74] temperature of storage,[75,76] thawing rate,[77] and postthaw dilution.[75-78]

Ficoll-Hypaque density gradient centrifugation is used routinely to isolate mononuclear cells from blood and to obtain bone marrow for *in vitro* tests. This technique also has been used to remove the granulocytes and red cells from bone marrow prior to cryopreservation.[70,78,79] The separation is done in centrifuge tubes, a cumbersome procedure and one which might compromise the sterility of the cells. Preliminary experiments in our laboratory have shown that mononuclear cells can be separated using a Ficoll-Hypaque procedure with a plastic bag system. This is a safe and effective way of processing bone marrow for autologous or allogeneic transplantation.

Hematopoietic stem cells, which have been frozen primarily in the vapor phase or liquid phase of nitrogen, have been stored frozen from as little as 30 min and in vials or bags for as long as 10 years.[80,81] Totipotential hematopoietic mononuclear cells can be isolated from human peripheral blood, and the purification of these cells and the cryopreservation of totipotential mononuclear stem cells devoid of immunocompetent cells are now under investigation.[82-89]

Peripheral blood stem cells have been used in combination with or as an alternative to bone marrow for hematopoietic engraftment. Autologous peripheral buffy coat cells obtained by leukapheresis have been used to reconstitute canine bone marrow,[90,91] and peripheral blood cells have been shown to produce more rapid lymphoid recovery than bone marrow cells.[92] Engraftment of transplanted bone marrow in humans appears to be enhanced when peripheral blood cells are also transfused.[93] Patients with chronic myeloid leukemia underwent successful autotransplantations after receiving previously frozen peripheral blood leukocytes.[94,95] However, bone marrow reconstitution using normal peripheral blood stem cells from an identical twin has been twice attempted unsuccessfully, although this may have been because the dose was administered in fractions over many days[96] or was very low.[97] Peripheral blood stem cells can be obtained either as a by-product of plateletpheresis using the Haemonetics Blood Processor 30,[16,98] or as the primary product of leukapheresis using the Fenwal CS-3000.[89] However, the large numbers of immunocompetent lymphocytes in the peripheral blood leukocytes should be removed to avoid graft-versus-host disease. This has been attempted with some success using immunologic techniques such as treatment with monoclonal antibodies, lectin agglutination, and rosetting with sheep erythrocytes.

Studies are in progress to simplify these procedures so that they can be used safely and effectively in clinical situations.

SUMMARY

Human platelets in sufficient numbers for a therapeutic transfusion can be collected for preservation either by pooling ABO- and Rh-compatible platelets or by apheresis procedures using mechanical cell-separating machines. Human platelets have been frozen successfully with 5 or 6% dimethyl sulfoxide (DMSO) and stored at -150 or $-80°C$, respectively. Platelets frozen with 5% DMSO have been stored at $-150°C$ for at least 3 years, and platelets frozen with 6% DMSO have been stored at $-80°C$ for at least 2 years. Approximately 95% of the DMSO usually is removed by washing the platelets after thawing, and the residual DMSO produces no untoward effects. Washed platelets resuspended in plasma can be stored at room temperature for 6 to 8 hr before transfusion.

Platelets thus frozen have freeze-thaw-wash recovery values of about 80%. *In vivo* survival values are only about 50% those seen with fresh platelets, and it is necessary to transfuse twice as many to achieve comparable results. Studies have shown that these platelets have satisfactory circulation, reduce clinical bleeding, and shorten the prolonged bleeding times associated with thrombocytopenia.

Studies are now being made on human bone marrow and peripheral blood, from which totipotential cells devoid of immunocompetent cells can be isolated and frozen.

ACKNOWLEDGMENTS

The author acknowledges the editorial assistance of Cynthia A. Valeri and the secretarial assistance of Marilyn E. Leavy.

REFERENCES

1. BRECHER, G. & E. P. CRONKITE. 1950. Morphology and enumeration of human blood platelets. J. Appl. Physiol. **3:** 365-377.
2. BRECHER, G., M. SCHNEIDERMAN & E. P. CRONKITE. 1953. The reproducibility and constancy of the platelet count. Am. J. Clin. Pathol. **23:** 15-26.

3. CRONKITE, E. P., G. J. JACOBS, G. BRECHER & G. DILLARD. 1952. The hemorrhagic phase of the acute radiation syndrome due to exposure of the whole body to penetrating ionizing radiation. Am. J. Roentgenol. Radium Ther. Nucl. Med. **67:** 796-803.

4. JACKSON, D. P., E. P. CRONKITE, G. V. LEROY & B. HALPERN. 1952. Further studies on the nature of the hemorrhagic state in radiation injury. J. Lab. Clin. Med. **39:** 449-461.

5. DILLARD, G. H. L., G. BRECHER & E. P. CRONKITE. 1951. Separation, concentration and transfusion of platelets. Proc. Soc. Exp. Biol. Med. **78:** 796-799.

6. BRECHER, G. & E. P. CRONKITE. 1953. The effects of platelet transfusions in dogs made pancytopenic by X-radiation. N.Y. State J. Med. **53:** 544-547.

7. CRONKITE, E. P., G. BRECHER & K. M. WILBUR. 1954. Development and use of a canine blood donor colony for experimental purposes. I. Leukocyte and platelet transfusions in irradiation aplasia of the dog bone marrow. Mil. Surg. **114:** 359-365.

8. FLIEDNER, T. M., D. K. SORENSEN, V. P. BOND, E. P. CRONKITE, D. P. JACKSON & E. ADAMIK. 1958. Comparative effectiveness of fresh and lyophilized platelets in controlling irradiation hemorrhage in the rat. Proc. Soc. Exp. Biol. Med. **99:** 731-733.

9. CRONKITE, E. P. & D. P. JACKSON. 1959. The use of platelet transfusions in hemorrhagic diseases. *In* Progress in Hematology. L. M. Tocantins, Ed. **II:** 239-257. Grune & Stratton. New York, N.Y.

10. JACKSON, D. P., D. K. SORENSEN, E. P. CRONKITE, V. P. BOND & T. M. FLIEDNER. 1959. Effectiveness of transfusions of fresh and lyophilized platelets in controlling bleeding due to thrombocytopenia. J. Clin. Invest. **38:** 1689-1697.

11. HJORT, P. F., V. PERMAN & E. P. CRONKITE. 1959. Fresh and disintegrated platelets in radiation thrombocytopenia: correction of prothrombin consumption without correction of bleeding. Proc. Soc. Exp. Biol. Med. **102:** 31-35.

12. SORENSEN, D. K., V. P. BOND, E. P. CRONKITE & V. PERMAN. 1960. An effective therapeutic regimen for the hemopoietic phase of the acute radiation syndrome in dogs. Radiat. Res. **13:** 669-685.

13. SCHIFFER, C. A., J. AISNER & P. H. WIERNIK. 1978. Frozen autologous platelet transfusions for patients with leukemia. N. Engl. J. Med. **299:** 7-12.

14. SCHIFFER, C. A., D. H. BUCHHOLZ, J. AISNER, J. H. WOLFF & P. H. WIERNIK. 1976. Frozen autologous platelets in the supportive care of patients with leukemia. Transfusion **16:** 321-329.

15. VALERI, C. R. 1976. Blood Banking and the Use of Frozen Blood Products. CRC Press. Boca Raton, Fla.

16. KURTZ, S. R., A. MCMICAN, R. CARCIERO, A. J. MELARAGNO, J. J. VECCHIONE & C. R. VALERI. 1981. Plateletpheresis experience with the Haemonetics Blood Processor 30, the IBM Blood Processor 2997, and the Fenwal CS-3000 Blood Processor. Vox Sang. **41:** 212-218.

17. HUNT, S. M., F. J. LIONETTI, C. R. VALERI & A. B. CALLAHAN. 1981. Cryogenic preservation of monocytes from human blood and plateletpheresis cellular residues. Blood **57:** 592-598.

18. HOGGE, D. E. & C. A. SCHIFFER. 1983. Collection of platelets depleted of red and white cells with the "surge pump" adaptation of a blood cell separator. Transfusion **23:** 177-181.

19. SCHOENDORFER, D. W., L. E. HANSEN & D. M. KENNEY. 1983. The surge technique: a method to increase purity of platelet concentrate obtained by centrifugal apheresis. Transfusion **23:** 182-189.

20. BUCHHOLZ, D. H., J. H. PORTEN, J. E. MENITOVE, L. RZAD, R. R. BUCHEYER, R. H. ASTER, A. T. LIN & J. SMITH. 1983. Description and use of the CS3000 blood cell separator for single-donor platelet collections. Transfusion **23:** 190-196.

21. KALMIN, N. D. & A. J. GRINDON. 1983. Comparison of two continuous-flow cell separators. Transfusion **23:** 197-200.

22. LOPEZ-BERESTEIN, G., J. REUBEN, E. M. HERSH, R. KILBOURN, J. P. HESTER, M. BIELSKI, M. TALPAZ & G. M. MAVLIGHT. 1983. Comparative functional analysis of lymphocytes and monocytes from plateletpheresis. Transfusion **23:** 201-206.

23. ROCK, G., R. HERZIG, N. MCCOMBIE, H. M. LAZARUS & P. TITTLEY. 1983. Automated platelet production during plasmapheresis. Transfusion **23:** 290-293.

24. VALERI, C. R. 1981. The current state of platelet and granulocyte cryopreservation. CRC Crit. Rev. Clin. Lab. Sci. **14:** 21-74.

25. MURPHY, S., R. A. KAHN, S. HOLME, G. L. PHILLIPS, W. SHERWOOD, W. DAVISSON & D. H. BUCHHOLZ. 1982. Improved storage of platelets for transfusion in a new container. Blood **60:** 194-200.

26. SIMON, T. L., E. J. NELSON, R. CARMEN & S. MURPHY. 1983. Extension of platelet concentrate storage. Transfusion **23:** 207-212.

27. LINDBERG, J. E., S. J. SLICHTER, S. MURPHY, D. D. SCHROEDER, E. J. NELSON, A. B. CHAMPION & R. A. CARMEN. 1983. In vitro function and in vivo viability of stored platelet concentrates. Effect of a secondary plasticizer component of PVC storage bags. Transfusion **23:** 294-299.

28. MOURAD, N. 1963. A simple method for obtaining platelet concentrates free of aggregates. Transfusion **8:** 48.

29. SCHIFFER, C. A., D. H. BUCHHOLZ & P. H. WIERNIK. 1974. Intensive multiunit plateletpheresis of normal donors. Transfusion **14:** 388-394.

30. HUESTIS, D. W., J. L. FLETCHER, R. F. WHITE & M. J. PRICE. 1977. Citrate anticoagulants for plateletpheresis. Transfusion **17:** 151-155.

31. BERGER, S., E. W. SALZMAN, E. W. MERRILL & P. S. L. WONG. 1974. The reaction of platelets with prosthetic surfaces. *In* Platelets: Production, Function, Transfusion, and Storage. M. G. Baldini & S. Ebbe, Eds.: 299-312. Grune & Stratton. New York, N.Y.

32. FRIEDENBERG, W. R., W. O. MYERS, E. D. PLATKA, J. N. BEATHARD, D. J. KUMMER, P. F. GATLIN, D. L. STORBER, J. R. RAY III & R. D. SAUTTER. 1978. Platelet dysfunction associated with cardiopulmonary bypass. Ann. Thorac. Surg. **25:** 298-305.

33. SLICHTER, S. J. & L. A. HARKER. 1976. Preparation and storage of platelet concentrates. I. Factors influencing the harvest of viable platelets from whole blood. Br. J. Haematol. **34:** 395-402.

34. SLICHTER, S. J. & L. A. HARKER. 1976. Preparation and storage of platelet concentrates. II. Storage variables influencing platelet viability and function. Br. J. Haematol. **34:** 403-419.

35. KAHN, R. A., I. COSSETTE & L. I. FRIEDMAN. 1976. Optimum centrifugation conditions for the preparation of platelet and plasma products. Transfusion **16:** 162-165.

36. BERSEUS, O., C. F. HÖGMAN & A. JOHANSSON. 1978. Simple method of improving the quality of platelet concentrates and the importance of production control. Transfusion **18:** 333-338.

37. MOORE, G. L., W. S. MALLIN, S. C. ROBERTS, M. L. FAILLA & J. L. GRAY. 1973. In vitro analysis of platelet function during storage of platelets from plasmapheresed donors. Transfusion **13:** 130-134.

38. WIRMAN, J. A., E. A. RUDER, R. T. SMITH & C. TS'AO. 1975. Functional and ultrastructural status of platelets prepared by the Celltrifuge. Transfusion **15:** 614-619.

39. TS'AO, C., J. A. WIRMAN & E. A. RUDER. 1975. Altered in vitro functions of platelets prepared by the Haemonetics Blood Processor. J. Lab. Clin. Med. **86:** 315-325.

40. HANDIN, R. I. & C. R. VALERI. 1972. Improved viability of previously frozen platelets. Blood **40:** 509-513.

41. VALERI, C. R., H. FEINGOLD & L. D. MARCHIONNI. 1974. A simple method for freezing human platelets using 6 percent dimethylsulfoxide and storage at −80°C. Blood **43:** 131-136.

42. MURPHY, S., S. N. SAYAR, N. L. ABDOU & F. H. GARDNER. 1974. Platelet preservation by freezing: use of dimethylsulfoxide as cryoprotective agent. Transfusion **14:** 139-144.

43. LAZARUS, H. M., E. A. KANIECKI-GREEN, S. E. WARM, M. AIKAWA & R. H. HERZIG. 1981. Therapeutic effectiveness of cryopreserved platelet concentrates for transfusion. Blood **57:** 243-249.

44. DAYIAN, G. & A. W. ROWE. 1976. Cryopreservation of human platelets for transfusion: a glycerol-glucose, moderate rate cooling procedure. Cryobiology **13:** 1-8.

45. DAYIAN, G. & J. H. PERT. 1979. A simplified method for freezing human blood platelets in glycerol-glucose using a statically controlled cooling rate device. Transfusion **19:** 255-260.

46. KOTELBA-WITKOWSKA, B. & C. A. SCHIFFER. 1982. Cryopreservation of platelet concentrates using glycerol-glucose. Transfusion **22:** 121-124.

47. REDMOND, J., II, R. B. BOLIN & B. A. CHENEY. 1983. Glycerol-glucose cryopreservation of platelets: in vivo and in vitro observations. Transfusion **23:** 213-214.

48. HERVE, P., G. POTRON, C. DROULE, M. P. BEDUCHAUD, M. MASSE, C. COFFE, J. F. BOSSET & A. PETERS. 1981. Human platelets frozen with glycerol in liquid nitrogen: biological and clinical aspects. Transfusion 21: 384-390.

49. KIM, B. K. & M. G. BALDINI. 1973. Preservation of viable platelets by freezing. Effect of plastic containers. Proc. Soc. Exp. Biol. Med. 142: 345-350.

50. VECCHIONE, J. J., A. J. MELARAGNO, A. HOLLANDER, S. DEFINA, C. P. EMERSON & C. R. VALERI. 1982. Circulation and function of human platelets isolated from units of CPDA-1, CDPA-2, and CDPA-3 anticoagulated blood and frozen with DMSO. Transfusion 22: 206-209.

51. MELARAGNO, A. J., W. A. ABDU, R. J. KATCHIS, J. J. VECCHIONE & C. R. VALERI. 1982. Cryopreservation of platelets isolated with the IBM 2997 Blood Cell Separator: a rapid and simplified approach. Vox Sang. 43: 321-326.

52. DALY, P. A., C. A. SCHIFFER, J. AISNER & P. H. WIERNIK. 1979. Successful transfusion of platelets cryopreserved for more than 3 years. Blood 54: 1023-1027.

53. DJERASSI, I. & A. ROY. 1963. A method for preservation of viable platelets: combined effects of sugars and dimethylsulfoxide. Blood 22: 703-717.

54. DJERASSI, I., S. FARBER, A. ROY & J. CAVINS. 1966. Preparation and in vivo circulation of human platelets preserved with combined dimethylsulfoxide and dextrose. Transfusion 6: 572-576.

55. WYBRAN, J., C. STACQUEZ & A. E. GOVAERTS. 1972. Storage of human platelets in liquid nitrogen—isotopic studies. Transfusion 12: 413-417.

56. KIM, B. K. & M. G. BALDINI. 1974. Biochemistry, function and hemostatic effectiveness of frozen human platelets. Proc. Soc. Exp. Biol. Med. 145: 830-835.

57. BALDINI, M. G. & B. K. KIM. 1974. Storage of human platelets by freezing. In Platelet Preservation and Transfusion. C. F. Högman, H. W. Krijnen & C. R. Valeri, Eds.: 32-35. Uppsala Offset Center AB. Uppsala, Sweden.

58. KIM, B. K., K. TANOUE & M. G. BALDINI. 1976. Storage of human platelets by freezing. Vox Sang. 30: 401-411.

59. VALERI, C. R. 1974. Therapeutic effectiveness of human platelets freeze-preserved with dimethylsulfoxide at −80 C. In Platelet Preservation and Transfusion. C. F. Högman, H. W. Krijnen & C. R. Valeri, Eds.: 41-50. Uppsala Offset Center AB. Uppsala, Sweden.

60. RUBIN, L. F. & P. A. MATTIS. 1966. Dimethylsulfoxide: lens changes in dogs during oral administration. Science 153: 83-84.

61. KOCSIS, J. J., S. HARKAWAY, M. C. SANTOYO & R. SNYDER. 1968. Dimethylsulfoxide: interactions with aromatic hydrocarbons. Science 160: 427-428.

62. HAGEMANN, R. F. 1969. Effect of dimethylsulfoxide on RNA synthesis in S-180 tumor cells. Experientia 25: 1298-1300.

63. FRATANTONI, J. C. & B. J. POINDEXTER. 1983. Dimethylsulfoxide: effects on function of fresh platelets and on the viability of platelets in storage. Transfusion 23: 109-113.

64. SCHIFFER, C. A., J. AISNER & P. H. WIERNIK. 1976. Clinical experience with transfusion of cryopreserved platelets. Br. J. Haematol. 34: 377-385.

65. ZAROULIS, C. G., J. I. SPECTOR, C. P. EMERSON & C. R. VALERI. 1979. Therapeutic effectiveness of previously frozen washed human platelets. Transfusion 19: 371-378.

66. VECCHIONE, J. J., C. M. CHOMICZ, C. P. EMERSON & C. R. VALERI. 1980. Cryopreservation of human platelets isolated by discontinuous-flow centrifugation using the Haemonetics Model 30 Blood Processor. Transfusion 20: 393-400.

67. WELLS, J. R., W. G. HO, P. GRAZE, A. SULLIVAN, R. P. GALE & M. J. CLINE. 1979. Isolation, cryopreservation, and autotransplantation of human stem cells. Exp. Hematol. 7: 12-20.

68. APPELBAUM, F. R., G. P. HERZIG, J. L. ZIEGLER, R. G. GRAW, A. S. LEVINE & A. B. DEISSEROTH. 1978. Successful engraftment of cryopreserved autologous bone marrow in patients with malignant lymphoma. Blood 52: 85-95.

69. SPITZER, D., K. A. DICKE, J. LITAM, D. S. VERMA, H. ZANDER, V. LANZOTTI, M. VALDIVIESO, K. B. McCREDIT & M. L. SAMUELS. 1980. High dose combination chemotherapy with autologous bone marrow transplantation in adult solid tumors. Cancer 45: 3075-3085.

70. Wells, J. R., A. Sullivan & M. J. Cline. 1979. A technique for the separation and cryopreservation of myeloid stem cells from human bone marrow. Cryobiology 16: 201-210.

71. Stiff, P. J., A. J. Murgo, C. G. Zaroulis, M. F. Derisi & B. D. Clarkson. 1983. Unfractionated human marrow cell cryopreservation using dimethylsulfoxide and hydroxyethyl starch. Cryobiology 20: 17-24.

72. Hill, R. S., C. A. MacKinder, B. F. Postlewaight & H. A. Blacklock. 1979. The survival of cryopreserved human bone marrow stem cells. Pathology 11: 361-367.

73. McGann, L. E., A. R. Turner, M. J. Allalunes & J. M. Turc. 1981. Cryopreservation of human peripheral blood stem cells: optimal cooling and warming conditions. Cryobiology 18: 469-472.

74. Douay, L., N. C. Gorin, R. David, J. Stachowiak, Ch. Salmon, A. Najman & G. Duhamel. 1982. Study of granulocyte-macrophage progenitor (CFU_c) preservation after slow freezing of bone marrow in the gas phase of liquid nitrogen. Exp. Hematol. 10: 360-366.

75. Grande, M. 1980. Morphology, cytochemical, and culture study of normal human bone marrow frozen at $-196°C$. Cryobiology 17: 429-438.

76. Goldman, J. M., K. H. Th'ng, D. S. Park, A. S. D. Spiers, R. M. Lowenthal & T. Ruutur. 1978. Collection, cryopreservation and subsequent viability of haemopoietic stem cells intended for treatment of chronic granulocytic leukemia in blast-cell transformation. Br. J. Haematol. 40: 185-195.

77. Parker, L. M., N. Binder, R. Gelman, C. M. Richman, R. S. Weiner & R. A. Yankee. 1981. Prolonged cryopreservation of human bone marrow. Transplantation 31: 454-457.

78. Porcellini, A., A. Manna, M. Manna, L. Moretti, F. Agostinelli & G. Lucarelli. 1981. Cryopreservation and subsequent viability of human bone marrow in hematologic malignancies: comparison of two different methods of cell reconstitution. Cryobiology 18: 541-546.

79. van de Ouweland, F., T. Dewitte, P. Geerdink & C. Haanen. 1982. Enrichment and cryopreservation of bone marrow progenitor cells for autologous reinfusion. Cryobiology 19: 292-298.

80. Rybka, W. B., K. Mittermeyer, J. W. Singer, C. D. Buckner & E. D. Thomas. 1980. Viability of human marrow after long-term preservation. Cryobiology 17: 424-428.

81. Fabian, I., D. Douer, J. R. Wells & M. J. Cline. 1982. Cryopreservation of the human multipotent stem cell. Exp. Hematol. 10: 119-122.

82. Barr, R. D., J. Whang-Peng & S. Perry. 1975. Hemopoietic stem cells in human peripheral blood. Science 190: 284-285.

83. Barr, R. D., C. A. Stevens, M. Kolkebakker & J. A. McBride. 1982. Collection of erythroid progenitor cells by cytapheresis of peripheral blood of normal donors. Transfusion 22: 388-391.

84. Fauser, A. A. & H. A. Messner. 1978. Granuloerythropoietic colonies in human bone marrow, peripheral blood and cord blood. Blood 52: 1243-1248.

85. Körbling, M., W. Ross, H. Pflieger, R. Arnold & T. M. Fliedner. 1977. Procurement of human blood stem cells by continuous-flow centrifugation—further comment. Blood 50: 753-754.

86. Weiner, R. S., C. M. Richman & R. A. Yankee. 1977. Semicontinuous flow centrifugation for the pheresis of immunocompetent cells and stem cells. Blood 49: 391-397.

87. Körbling, M., T. M. Fliedner, E. Ruber & H. Pflieger. 1980. Description of a closed plastic bag system for the collection and cryopreservation of leukapheresis-derived blood mononuclear leukocytes and CFU_c from human donors. Transfusion 20: 293-300.

88. Ash, R. C., R. A. Detrick & E. D. Zanjani. 1981. Studies of human pluripotential hemopoietic stem cells (CFU-GEMM) in vitro. Blood 58: 309-316.

89. Lasky, L. C., R. C. Ash, J. H. Kersey, E. D. Zanjani & J. McCullough. 1982. Collection of pluripotential hematopoietic stem cells by cytapheresis. Blood 59: 822-827.

90. Debelak-Fehir, K. M. & R. B. Epstein. 1975. Restoration of hematopoiesis in dogs by infusion of cryopreserved autologous peripheral white cells following busulfan-cyclophosphamide treatment. Transplantation 20: 63-67.

91. CALVO, W., T. M. FLIEDNER, E. HERBST, E. HUGL & E. BRUCH. 1976. Regeneration of blood-forming organs after autologous leukocyte transfusion in lethally irradiated dogs. II. Distribution and cellularity of the marrow in irradiated and transfused animals. Blood 47: 593-601.
92. APPELBAUM, F. R. 1979. Hemopoietic reconstitution following autologous bone marrow and peripheral blood mononuclear cell infusions. Exp. Hematol. 7: 7-11.
93. STORB, R., R. L. PRENTICE & E. D. THOMAS. 1977. Marrow transplantation for treatment of aplastic anemia. An analysis of factors associated with graft rejection. N. Engl. J. Med. 296: 61-66.
94. GOLDMAN, J. M. 1978. Modern approaches to the management of chronic granulocytic leukemia. Semin. Hematol. 15: 420-430.
95. KÖRBLING, M., P. BURKE, H. BRAINE, G. ELFENBEIN & G. SANTOS. 1981. Successful engraftment of blood derived normal hemopoietic stem cells in chronic myelogenous leukemia. Exp. Hematol. 9: 684-690.
96. HERSHKO, C., R. P. GALE, W. G. HO & M. J. CLINE. 1979. Cure of aplastic anemia in paroxysmal nocturnal haemoglobinuria by marrow transfusion from identical twins: failure of peripheral leucocyte transfusion to correct marrow aplasia. Lancet i: 945-947.
97. ABRAMS, R. A., D. GLAUBIGER, F. R. APPELBAUM & A. B. DEISSEROTH. 1980. Result of attempted hematopoietic reconstitution using isologous peripheral blood mononuclear cells: a case report. Blood 56: 516-520.
98. ABBOUD, C. N., J. K. BRENNAN, M. A. LICHTMAN & J. NUSBACHER. 1980. Quantification of erythroid and granulocytic precursor cells in plateletpheresis residues. Transfusion 20: 9-16.

DISCUSSION OF THE PAPER

E. CRONKITE (*Brookhaven National Laboratory, Upton, N.Y.*): Dr. Valeri, in his enthusiasm to give credit to Dr. Brecher and me, overstated the case. We did not, at any time, demonstrate stem cells in the peripheral blood. This was done by our friend and associate, Dr. T. Fliedner.

T. FLIEDNER (*University of Ulm, Ulm, Federal Republic of Germany*): I want to reiterate what Dr. Valeri discussed. We have developed a closed plastic bag system for collecting mononuclear cells including stem cells from human peripheral blood. In my own experiments, cells are also frozen and stored. We use the Aminco Celltrifuge and then the plastic bag system which allows us to add DMSO in a completely sterile fashion. The plasma is removed and stored separately at −20°C, whereas the cells themselves are frozen at −196°C in liquid nitrogen. We also can thaw the whole thing, add the plasma, and wash the cells so that the DMSO is removed. Using the CFU-C assay system, we get recovery rates of better than 85% of the initial numbers of CFU-C present.

I think it is very important to follow this line of investigation because although it is apparent that bone marrow is a very suitable source of stem cells, if one is thinking of establishing stem cell banks, one might as well take cells from the peripheral blood utilizing leukapheresis. It is time to consider studies in human beings along this line. I am also quite convinced (as Dr. Valeri discussed) that the removal of immunocompetent cells is quite feasible. I think that in the future we will see purified stem cells being collected from the peripheral blood.

C. R. VALERI: I agree with you Dr. Fliedner. We should also consider the ability of these cells to grow mixed colonies which can be seen in both peripheral blood and in bone marrow.

R. SHADDUCK (*Montefiore Hospital, Pittsburgh, Pa.*): I wanted to comment briefly upon the use of progenitor cell assays for estimation of stem cell content in marrows. We are involved in an autologous bone marrow transplant program in collaboration with investigators at Johns Hopkins in which we treat remission bone marrows from leukemics with a cyclophosphamide derivative. It differs from the parent compound in that it is active *in vitro*. And the intriguing observation of several years ago is that there is a near total disappearance of progenitor cells, namely, granulocyte-macrophage colony forming cells and BFU or primitive erythroid progenitor cells. Yet, these marrow suspensions are capable of repopulating these individuals after cyclophosphamide and total-body irradiation.

Dr. Porchellini, from Pasaro, Italy, also has observed in the mouse ablation of the granulocyte-macrophage cells due to this compound. So, although we have ways of measuring repopulation potential in assays and the murine system, I think we still have a long way to go in the human system.

A Normal Fixed-Loss Component of Platelet Utilization Accounting for Short Survival of Transfused Platelets[a]

N. RAPHAEL SHULMAN, JAMES V. JORDAN, JR.,
AND STEVEN FALCHUK

Clinical Hematology Branch
National Institute of Arthritis, Diabetes, and Digestive
and Kidney Diseases
National Institutes of Health
Bethesda, Maryland 20205

Disappearance patterns of ^{51}Cr-labeled autologous platelets in normal persons have been uniform in numerous laboratories (FIGURE 1).[3-8] Decay is nearly linear for approximately 8 days, with a "plateau" frequently observed on the first day and a "tailing" of the 5 to 10% of platelets surviving longer than 9 days. Inspection or analysis of the shape of platelet survival curves does not necessarily provide insight into the basic mechanisms responsible for disappearance of platelets from the circulation. Although the predominant linear decay pattern suggests that their removal is an age-dependent phenomenon, it is well recognized that a random process independent of cell age, but requiring numerous insults or "hits" to effect destruction of an individual cell, will also produce linear rather than exponential decay.[9] Conversely, when there is great variation of the intrinsic life span of individual cells, the course of age-dependent destruction can resemble an exponential function that might suggest random destruction.[9] In fact, platelet survival curves are neither purely linear nor exponential. There is no simple model that will permit precise mathematical analysis of experimental survival curves. However, the likelihood that linearity reflects primarily loss by senescence is supported by animal experiments in which artificially produced cohorts of young platelets show a significant initial plateau in survival curves and circulate for a much longer time than cohorts of old platelets.[10]

Models and formulations have been developed in attempts to closely approximate the pattern of platelet survival which appears to be a mixture of both linear and exponential components. One mathematical procedure, with no commitment to a model, involves fitting the experimental points using both a linear and a logarithmic decay function in order to estimate mean survival time.[11] A weighted mean of these two survival times is obtained, but the procedure does not predict the actual shape of the curve. Another procedure for determining mean survival is based on a model developed for red cell survival, with the assumption that platelets have a determinate life span but risk destruction by some external mechanism.[12] Age and random de-

[a] This work was presented in part in References 1 and 2.

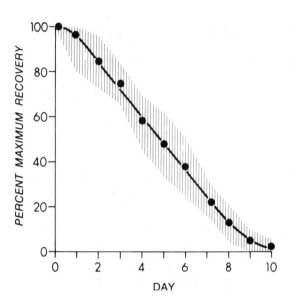

FIGURE 1. Survival of ^{51}Cr-labeled platelets in man. Points are average values obtained from 10 normal individuals expressed as percentage of maximal recovery. The boundary lines indicate the spread of values.

struction are not considered to be mutually exclusive since a cell's susceptibility to destruction might be a function of age. Methods of fitting a curve to the data, employing formulas describing this model, are iterative and require a computer for the extensive analysis. A third procedure, recommended by the International Committee for Standardization in Hematology, involves a "multiple-hit" or gamma model in which platelet destruction is considered to be due to an accumulation of insults or "hits" from the environment.[9,11] The number of "hits" before a platelet is destroyed and the waiting time between "hits" are parameters in the gamma function which are selected to minimize deviation of the fitted curve from the data points. Pure exponential or linear decay curves are special cases of the gamma function. A complicated computer program for this iterative method is available from the International Committee. Gamma curves obtained with different values for the number of "hits" closely approximate some, but not all, platelet survival data. This limited empirical agreement suggests that certain assumptions underlying the multiple-hit model are not valid.

These several mathematical analyses of platelet survival curves are empirical because the biological parameters necessary to construct an accurate model for platelet turnover are obscure. For example, the following are some fundamental unanswered questions concerning platelet utilization: (1) What function do platelets perform to support vascular integrity? (2) If their function results in destruction, is this aspect of the loss exponential, linear, or a combination of both? (3) Are there normal processes other than senescence that destroy platelets independently of their function? (4) If platelet decay is caused by multiple mechanisms, what share is attributable to each? and (5) What is the relationship between platelet age and platelet utilization? Further progress in mathematical analysis of survival curves depends upon the resolution of these uncertainties.

Insight into a possible component of platelet removal from the circulation that has not been previously considered is gained by observations on platelet transfusions in severely thrombocytopenic patients where there is no apparent basis for accelerated destruction of transfused platelets. FIGURE 2 shows the survival curves of transfused platelets in a thrombocytopenic recipient whose baseline platelet counts ranged between 6,000 and 12,000 per microliter. The initial post-transfusion platelet levels after four separate transfusions were 58,000, 105,000, 350,000, and 645,000 per microliter. Recovery of transfused platelets varied between 58 and 73%, which are normal values.[2] The noteworthy principle demonstrated here is the progressive increase in survival of transfused platelets as the initial post-transfusion platelet levels increased. Similar observations have been made on thrombocytopenic rats transfused with variable numbers of platelets, in which survival progressively lengthened as circulating platelets were elevated from sub- to supranormal levels (FIGURE 3).[13]

In the usual clinical platelet transfusion (equivalent to platelets from four to six units of blood), for example in conjunction with thrombocytopenia induced by chemotherapy, increments in the recipient most often are in the range of 40,000 to 60,000 per microliter, and therapeutic post-transfusion platelet levels rarely exceed 100,000 per microliter (see FIGURE 2). Transfused platelets in nonalloimmunized thrombocytopenic patients with impaired production characteristically survive for only 3 to 5 days compared to the approximate 10-day survival of platelets in nonthrombocytopenic individuals. Short survival times in thrombocytopenic patients have been interpreted

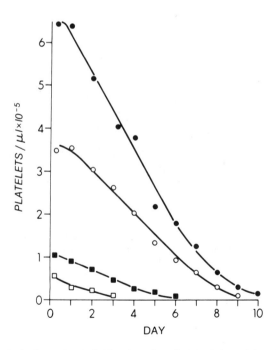

FIGURE 2. Survival of transfused platelets in a thrombocytopenic recipient. The patient had Wiskott-Aldrich syndrome. Four transfusions were given therapeutically on different occasions; the transfusion that elevated platelets to 645,000 per microliter was the last of the series. Survival was determined by platelet counts.

as reflecting increased platelet utilization in thrombocytopenic states. This concept is based on tenuous evidence that platelets interact with endothelium, and that, in thrombocytopenia, a deficit must be compensated for by increased utilization of transfused platelets.

Because intravascular retention of red cells is dependent on adequate platelets, it is likely that some type of platelet-endothelium interaction takes place. However, studies designed to evaluate platelet interaction with endothelium[14,15] have been inconclusive because: (1) possible autoradiographic artifacts may have accounted for apparent deposit of platelets on endothelium of thrombocytopenic animals, (2) dilution

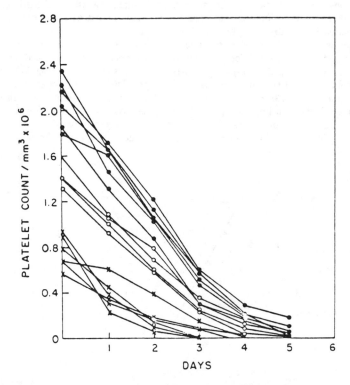

FIGURE 3. Platelet survival in thrombocytopenic rats transfused to differing levels of circulating platelets. Rats were made thrombocytopenic by whole-body irradiation and were transfused with platelet concentrates prepared using acidified ACD anticoagulant. (Reprinted with permission from Reference 13.)

of labeled platelets by the unlabeled pool in normal animals may have prevented accumulation of endothelial-associated radioactivity, and (3) radioactivity that was apparently associated with endothelium in thrombocytopenic animals might have been due to substances derived from platelets rather than actual cells.[14] Although platelets may interact with endothelium, the reaction has not been documented as yet, and notions concerning the mechanism and extent of interaction remain conjectural. If platelets do interact with endothelium, it seems evident from the following interrelated observations that the short life span of platelets transfused into thrombocytopenic recipients is not caused by increased platelet utilization. When radiolabeled platelets are infused into thrombocytopenic animals, endothelial-associated radioactivity accumulates maximally in 30 min to 1 hr.[14,15] However, the recovery of transfused platelets in the circulation 2 to 6 hr after transfusion in thrombocytopenic recipients is usually the same as that in nonthrombocytopenic recipients.[2,16,17] Normal recovery is not compatible with immediate increased utilization. If, for whatever reason, utilization were a more gradual process, survival would be prolonged after correction of a supposed deficit in thrombocytopenic recipients and a bimodal survival curve would be expected; but this does not occur. Moreover, the proportion of infused platelets that terminates in the spleen and liver of thrombocytopenic recipients with production defects[6,17,18] is the same as that in normal individuals[3,6,19] regardless of the degree of thrombocytopenia before transfusion. Therefore, in both the normal and thrombocytopenic states, most platelets are apparently removed by reticuloendothelial phagocytosis as a result of senescence and/or injury. These various findings indicate that platelets are not utilized to a greater extent in the thrombocytopenic, than in the normal, state.

How could thrombocytopenia per se, without excess platelet utilization, lead to short survival of transfused platelets? It is apparent that if a fixed amount of platelets (say as little as 10,000 per microliter) were lost from the circulation each day (by some unspecified process) under both normal and thrombocytopenic conditions, then a normal individual with 200,000 platelets per microliter could lose only 5% per day by this process, but a thrombocytopenic individual with 20,000 platelets per microliter would lose 50% per day. Thus, loss per day of a fixed amount of platelets, in addition to other losses involving a fixed percentage of the population attributable to senescence and a possible exponential component of unknown cause, would result in shorter survival as fewer platelets were transfused into thrombocytopenic recipients. Theoretical curves based on a model incorporating a fixed loss plus senescence, with or without exponential destruction, closely approximate those of transfused platelets in thrombocytopenic recipients with production defects, as well as normal survival curves obtained with ^{51}Cr (FIGURE 4). The basic formula used to generate the curves of FIGURE 4 is

$$n_t = n_0(1 - kt) - \alpha t,$$

where t is the time in days after transfusion, n_t is the concentration of cells at time t, n_0 is the immediate post-transfusion concentration, k is the rate constant for senescent loss (the reciprocal of cell life span in days), and α is the constant for the fixed quantity lost per day.

The first part of the equation, $n_t = n_0(1 - kt)$, is the well-known description of senescent decay which appears to be the major component of platelet survival. Assuming that platelets have an inherent finite life span of 10 days, the rate constant, k, would be 0.1. To account for an additional fixed loss per day, the term $-\alpha t$ is added. The fixed quantity lost per day, α, is assumed to be approximately 10,000 platelets per microliter. At near normal or greater values for n_0, the value for α would not greatly decrease n_t, the number of cells remaining at time t; but at low values for n_0, the effect would be marked. As shown in FIGURE 4, a fixed loss of 10,000 platelets per microliter per day, plus a 10% loss of initial platelets per day by senescence, would result in a survival of 9 days when starting at a circulating level of 250,000 platelets per microliter; 7 days when starting at 100,000 per microliter; and 4 days when starting at 50,000 per microliter. The fixed loss would have progressively less effect on survival as initial platelet levels exceeded normal values. At an initial level of 600,000 platelets per microliter, the disappearance time by these same calculations would be just under 10 days, in keeping with the observation that platelets of patients with thrombocytosis survive normally. Thus, a normal fixed loss of approximately

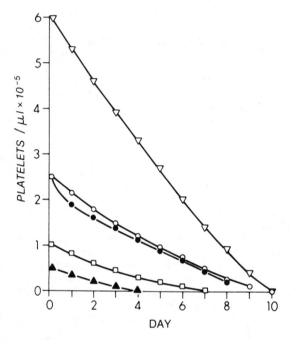

FIGURE 4. Theoretical platelet survival curves calculated to include a fixed-loss component. The normal life span for senescent decay was assumed to be 10 days, making $k = 0.1$. The value for α was assumed to be 10,000 platelets per microliter per day. Point-to-point corrections have been made for the decrease in cells available for loss by senescence, owing to their removal in the fixed-loss component. Superimposed on these linear losses may be a component of exponential loss in which cells are destroyed at a constant rate independent of their age. Point-to-point calculations of a 10% per day exponential loss superimposed on senescent and fixed losses are shown as solid circles for survival of platelets at an initial concentration of 250,000 per microliter (●). Points for the other curves at $n_0 = 600,000$ (▽), 250,000 (○), 100,000 (□), and 50,000 (▲) platelets per microliter were calculated assuming only senescent and fixed losses. Corrections of loss by senescence for that portion of cells lost by other assumed mechanisms would be greater for decay of transfused platelets in thrombocytopenic recipients than in the steady state, wherein all lost cells would be replenished.

10,000 platelets per microliter per day would have a significant effect in shortening survival if few platelets were transfused, but would have relatively little effect if large amounts of platelets were transfused.

Although an additional normal component of random or exponential loss of platelets has been postulated, the basis for and the amount of this component have not been established. By superimposing a random loss of as much as 10% per day on decreases due to senescence plus a fixed loss, only slightly accelerated decay occurs, as shown by the solid-circle curve of FIGURE 4 compared to the open-circle curve for a post-transfusion level of 250,000 platelets per microliter.

Thus, a model for normal platelet destruction incorporating a fixed loss, plus senescence, with or without an exponential component, generates curves that closely approximate those of transfused platelets in thrombocytopenic recipients with impaired production, as well as those obtained by labeling techniques in individuals with normal platelet levels. Since a fixed-loss component of platelet utilization reasonably explains heretofore obscure platelet survival observations, experimental evaluation of mechanisms that might cause this type of cell loss is warranted.

REFERENCES

1. SHULMAN, N. R. & J. V. JORDAN. 1981. A fixed-loss component of platelet utilization accounting for short survival of transfused platelets. Clin. Res. 29(2): 572a. (Abstract.)
2. SHULMAN, N. R. & J. V. JORDAN. 1982. Platelet dynamics. *In* Hemostasis and Thrombosis. R. Colman, J. Hirsh, V. Marder & E. Salzman, Eds.: 237–258. Lippincott. Philadelphia, Pa.
3. ASTER, R. H. & J. H. JANDL. 1964. Platelet sequestration in man. I. Methods. J. Clin. Invest. 43: 843.
4. AAS, K. A. & F. H. GARDNER. 1958. Survival of blood platelets labeled with chromium[51]. J. Clin. Invest. 37: 1257.
5. ABRAHAMSEN, A. F. 1965. The effect of EDTA and ACD on the recovery and survival of Cr[51]-labelled blood platelets. Scand. J. Haematol. 2: 52.
6. SHULMAN, N. R., V. J. MARDER & R. S. WEINRACH. 1965. Similarities between known antiplatelet antibodies and the factor responsible for thrombocytopenia in idiopathic purpura. Physiologic, serologic, and isotope studies. Ann. N.Y. Acad. Sci. 124: 499.
7. KOTILAINEN, M. 1969. Platelet kinetics in normal subjects and in haematological disorders. Scand. J. Haematol. Suppl. 5: 32.
8. O'NEILL, B. & B. FIRKIN. 1964. Platelet survival studies in coagulation disorders, thrombocythemia, and conditions associated with atherosclerosis. J. Lab. Clin. Med. 64: 188.
9. MURPHY, E. A. & J. F. MUSTARD. 1971. Studies of platelet economy. *In* Platelet Kinetics. J. M. Paulus, Ed.: 24. North-Holland. Amsterdam, the Netherlands.
10. GINSBURG, A. D. & R. H. ASTER. 1969. Kinetic studies with [51]chromium-labeled platelet cohorts in rats. J. Lab. Clin. Med. 74: 138.
11. INTERNATIONAL COMMITTEE FOR STANDARDIZATION IN HEMATOLOGY. 1977. Recommended methods for radioisotope platelet survival studies. Blood 50: 1137.
12. DORNHORST, A. C. 1951. The interpretation of red cell survival curves. Blood 6: 1284.
13. HEYSSEL, R. M., L. J. SILVER, M. WASSON & A. B. BRILL. 1967. The relation of blood platelet survival and distribution to ^{14}C-serotonin distribution and excretion. Blood 29: 341.
14. CRONKITE, E. P., V. P. BOND, T. M. FLIEDNER, D. A. PAGLIA & E. R. ADAMIK. 1961. Studies on the origin, production and destruction of platelets. *In* The Blood Platelet. S. A. Johnson, R. W. Monto, J. W. Rebuck & R. C. Horn, Eds.: 595. Little, Brown. Boston, Mass.
15. WOJCIK, J. D., D. L. VAN HORN, A. J. WEBBER & S. A. JOHNSON. 1969. Mechanism whereby platelets support the endothelium. Transfusion 9(6): 324.
16. HIRSCH, E. O. & F. H. GARDNER. 1952. The transfusion of human blood platelets. With a note on the transfusion of granulocytes. J. Lab. Clin. Med. 39: 556.
17. ASTER, R. H. 1967. Studies of the mechanism of "hypersplenic" thrombocytopenia in rats. J. Lab. Clin. Med. 70: 736.
18. ASTER, R. H. & J. H. JANDL. 1964. Platelet sequestration in man. II. Immunological and clinical studies. J. Clin. Invest. 43: 856.
19. ASTER, R. H. 1969. Studies of the fate of platelets in rats and man. Blood 34: 117.

DISCUSSION OF THE PAPER

K. BRINKHAUS (*University of North Carolina Medical School, Chapel Hill, N.C.*): When you look at the insides of the plastic materials such as catheters, etc., used in infusions, the scanning electron microscope shows platelets are stuck there. There is some difference between the biomaterials from which these catheters are made. Even heparin-bonded catheters do not prevent adherence of platelets. I wonder if it is possible to do some theoretical calculations taking into account the surface area of the catheter material to which platelets are exposed which may explain the fixed loss reported by Dr. Shulman.

Clinical Applications of Measurement of Serum Immunoreactive Levels of Erythropoietin[a]

MARILYN E. MILLER

Division of Hematologic Research
The Memorial Hospital
Pawtucket, Rhode Island 02860

MANJU CHANDRA

Division of Pediatric Nephrology
North Shore University Hospital
Manhasset, New York 11030

JOSEPH F. GARCIA[b]

Division of Biology and Medicine
Lawrence Berkeley Laboratory
University of California
Berkeley, California 94704

The purification of erythropoietin (Ep) by Miyake *et al.*[1] in 1977 enabled investigators to more clearly define the role of this hormone in erythropoiesis in man. Radioimmunoassays were rapidly developed by Garcia *et al.*[2] and Sherwood and Goldwasser.[3] Undoubtedly differences between levels of immunoreactive and biologically active Ep will be found but the resolution of these discrepancies will expand our understanding of the erythron. Recently Weiss *et al.*[4] described a monoclonal antibody against Ep. Because of this breakthrough, large quantities of pure hormone should soon be available to a larger number of investigators than currently have access to it. The major clinical use of this hormone will probably be in the treatment of the anemia of chronic renal disease. In the relatively few years since the radioimmunoassay (RIA) was developed, measurements of the levels of this hormone have been made in several disease states as well as in normal man. Most of the findings to date confirm the predictions that

[a] Supported in part by National Institutes of Health Grant HL 31936-01.
[b] Deceased.

have been made over the years based on studies done using the rather crude bioassay for Ep. In the present study we shall review and expand on what is known about subjects with chronic lung and renal disease.

METHODS

Sera or plasma for erythropoietin measurements were separated within 1 hr of collection and maintained at 4°C until assayed. Ep was measured by RIA using a technique previously described.[5] Pure human EP was used for iodination (kindly supplied by Dr. Eugene Goldwasser, University of Chicago, Chicago, Ill.). It was extracted from the urine of severely anemic human beings and had a specific activity of 70,400 units/mg of protein. The standard reference Ep preparation was the second International Reference Preparation (IRP) of human urine Ep (obtained from the National Institute for Medical Research, London, England). Antisera to Ep were produced in rabbits immunized with human urinary Ep. The intraassay coefficient of variation of Ep values was 8.4% and the interassay coefficient of variation was 9.7% in a normal human serum pool.

All human studies were done after approval by the Human Subjects Review Committee at Brookhaven National Laboratory, Upton, New York. Informed consent was obtained prior to each investigation.

Eighteen hematologically normal, nonsmoking males were randomly assigned to receive either 19-nortestosterone decanoate (Deca-Durabolin) or saline intramuscularly (i.m.) in a double blind study. Serum Ep levels were measured on three occasions prior to injection and at 2, 4, 6, 24, 48, and 72 hr postinjection. The data were statistically analyzed using analyses of variance and covariance with repeated measures.[6]

Five hematologically normal men and women who smoked at least one package of cigarettes per day and whose pulmonary function studies and arterial blood gases were at least 80% of predicted values had carboxyhemoglobin and Ep levels measured at 0900, 1200, 1600, 2000, and 2400 hr for 2 consecutive days while they continued smoking cigarettes. Cigarette smoking was discontinued on the third day of study and levels of carboxyhemoglobin and Ep were measured at 24 and 48 hr after the cessation of smoking and thrice weekly thereafter for 2 weeks. One of the five subjects was unable to remain off cigarettes.

RESULTS

Levels of immunoreactive Ep in a normal working population on no medications are presented in TABLE 1. In this limited population ($n = 187$) there was no difference in Ep levels between men and women, smokers and nonsmokers, or age groups. In earlier studies we did not detect a diurnal variation in Ep levels in normal men and women who were nonsmokers.[7] Blood loss of 3, 10, or 50 ml between 0830 and 0900 hr for 5 consecutive days did not increase Ep levels on subsequent days (TABLE 2). A single phlebotomy of 50 or 100 ml did not increase Ep levels while a 450-ml phlebotomy was followed by an increase in Ep levels.[8] The Ep response to a 200-ml phlebotomy was equivocal.

The effect of administration of androgen (Deca-Durabolin) on Ep levels is presented in FIGURE 1. Statistical analysis of the data using the repeated-measures model demonstrated that there was no significant effect of the androgen on Ep levels.

Of the five cigarette-smoking subjects (three male and two female) one male was unable to continue the study and resumed cigarette smoking 24 hr after cigarettes were discontinued. The data from the remaining two male subjects are presented in FIGURE 2. Decreasing the level of carboxyhemoglobin from a maximum of 8% to 1% was not associated with any dramatic changes in Ep levels.

DISCUSSION

The measurement of immunoreactive Ep levels in a variety of clinical conditions has already been reported. It seems clear that one of the major diagnostic clinical

TABLE 1. Immunoreactive Erythropoietin Levels (mU/ml) in a Working Population

	Males		Females		Total Number of Subjects
Age Range	Smokers	Nonsmokers	Smokers	Nonsmokers	
18-30	16.5 ± 1.3 (16)[a]	15.7 ± 0.9 (25)	16.7 ± 1.5 (10)	15.4 ± 1.4 (14)	65
31-40	17.7 ± 2.1 (15)	16.4 ± 0.9 (23)	16.2 ± 2.0 (8)	17.1 ± 1.7 (11)	57
41-50	18.5 ± 2.2 (10)	18.7 ± 1.9 (10)	17.5 ± 2.0 (5)	17.6 ± 1.3 (6)	31
51-64	15.8 ± 1.4 (14)	19.9 ± 1.8 (8)	16.2 ± 2.2 (3)	18.7 ± 1.8 (9)	34

[a] $\bar{x}$ ± SEM (n).

applications of this test will be in the differentiation of primary versus secondary polycythemia. Koeffler and Goldwasser[9] and Garcia *et al.*[5] have reported on the differences in Ep response between the two conditions. Levels of Ep are lower than normal in patients with untreated polycythemia vera, similar to normal in treated polycythemia vera patients, and considerably higher than normal in patients with secondary polycythemia. This finding should considerably shorten the time that is oftentimes required to diagnose polycythemia vera. Erslev *et al.*[10] found Ep levels of less than 5 mU/ml in patients with polycythemia vera with bioassay. In their study they concentrated the plasma from a 450-ml phlebotomy for biologic assay. Obviously, this cannot be done in all patients with polycythemia but it is supportive of the data derived from the RIA.

Patients with chronic lung disease are a group that fails to be easily categorized. Relatively few of these patients develop true increases in red cell mass despite significant hypoxemia. Vanier *et al.*[11] reported that infection could not be the sole explanation. In a study of noninfected subjects with chronic lung disease of moderate severity, Miller *et al.*[7] demonstrated that they had diurnal variations of Ep levels with peak levels observed at midnight. This would be expected in cigarette smokers since the level of carboxyhemoglobin generally increases as the day progresses, and in fact, in

TABLE 2. The Effect of Daily Blood Loss on Serum Levels of Immunoreactive Erythropoietin

Volume Phlebotomized Daily (ml)	Erythropoietin Levels (mU/ml)				
	Day 1	Day 2	Day 3	Day 4	Day 5
3	30 ± 4[a]	27 ± 3	26 ± 5	28 ± 3	27 ± 4
10	17 ± 2	22 ± 3	21 ± 2	21 ± 4	23 ± 3
50	26 ± 4	27 ± 5	19 ± 4	28 ± 4	23 ± 3

[a] $\bar{x}$ ± SEM; n = 5-6.

their study the carboxyhemoglobin level was the only variable measured that correlated with the serum Ep level. This was not the sole explanation for their findings since similar patterns were observed in nonsmokers. Despite this small increase in Ep levels at midnight the red cell mass was normal. In the present study four subjects (cigarette smokers) with normal lung function failed to have detectable differences in Ep levels when carboxyhemoglobin levels fluctuated between 8 and 1%. It is likely that small increases in carboxyhemoglobin are not sufficient to trigger an Ep response in persons with normal lung function and probably assume importance only when superimposed on pulmonary disease which has already led to arterial hypoxemia or when carboxyhemoglobin levels are markedly increased. In patients with impaired pulmonary function the added insult of further impairing the ability of the hemoglobin molecule to transport oxygen is likely to result in tissue hypoxia. In those patients with significant pulmonary damage resulting in arterial hypoxemia, further studies are needed to explain the lack of polycythemia in the vast majority. There are several potential mechanisms. First there must be accurate quantitation of the degree of hypoxemia required to trigger an Ep response in normal man. If in fact subjects with the same degree of arterial hypoxemia do not show similar increments in Ep, more investigative effort should be directed toward elucidating the role of the lung in Ep production. If the contrary is true, i.e., the Ep response is normal, then the mechanism of Ep action

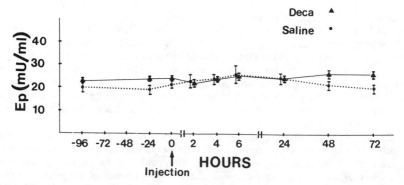

FIGURE 1. Comparison of the effects of Deca-Durabolin (▲——▲; 100 mg i.m.; n = 10) and saline (●···●; 2 ml i.m.; n = 9) on serum levels of immunoreactive Ep in normal male nonsmokers.

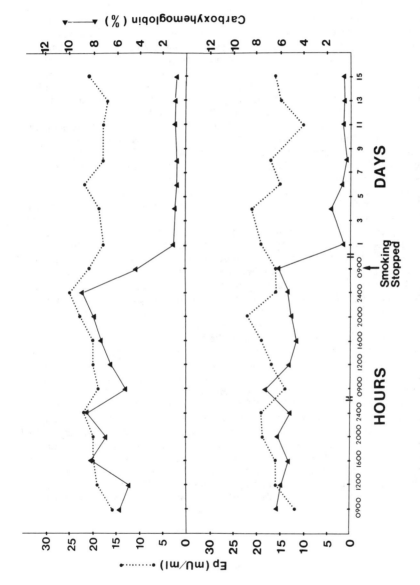

FIGURE 2. Measurements of serum immunoreactive Ep (● · · · ●) and carboxyhemoglobin (▲——▲) in two male smokers during cigarette smoking and for 2 weeks following cessation of cigarette smoking.

on erythroid progenitor cells would warrant further investigation. The purification of Ep makes these studies tenable in the not too distant future.

Several investigators have raised the possibility that uremic patients have serum inhibitors to Ep.[12,13] If in fact this is validated, the use of Ep to correct the anemia of chronic renal failure may prove to be untenable. Chandra et al. have provided two cogent examples of the potential therapeutic effectiveness of Ep in the treatment of the anemia of chronic renal failure.[14,15] In the first instance a renal transplant patient clearly maintained a normal hematocrit when the renal graft failed. Coincident with the graft failure the hematocrit rose to normal, transfusions were not required, and the Ep level was 77 mU/ml. In the second study Chandra et al.[15] demonstrated that patients with chronic renal failure secondary to polycystic kidney disease (PKD) maintained significantly higher hematocrits with markedly reduced transfusion requirements when compared to patients with chronic renal failure resultant from other etiologies (OKD). Serum Ep levels were 22.6 ± 2.4 mU/ml in PKD patients and 12.4 ± 0.7 mU/ml in OKD patients. Although the Ep levels were inappropriately low for the degree of anemia in both groups, the twofold difference in Ep level was associated with a sixfold reduction in transfusion requirement in patients with PKD. These data are compatible with the notion that Ep will probably be a useful therapeutic agent for the treatment of the anemia of chronic renal failure. In this study there was no difference in Ep levels in patients who were on androgen therapy when compared to those who were not. In the present study a single injection of Deca-Durabolin did not influence Ep levels in normal nonsmoking males at the time intervals studied. These data would support the hypothesis that the mechanism of the androgen effect involves more than Ep levels and the most likely explanation is the hypothesis of Jepson and Lowenstein[16] that the effect is a direct stem cell effect. One fact which has never been explained is why some patients with the anemia of chronic renal failure fail to respond to androgens. Perhaps there is a subgroup of patients with an inhibitor to erythropoiesis and these are the patients who may not respond to erythropoietin. Clearly more work is required in this area of erythropoiesis.

We have just begun to unravel some of the heretofore unexplained phenomena in Ep production. Several major clinical conditions remain unexplained such as the anemia associated with chronic inflammatory disease and malignant disease. Compensated hemolytic anemias are also poorly understood. The mechanism by which Ep exerts its action on the erythroid progenitor cell will undoubtedly be unraveled now that a monoclonal antibody to Ep has been described. When larger amounts of Ep are produced, perhaps by genetic engineering as suggested by Nathan and Sytkowski[17] in a recent editorial, the RIA for Ep will be a frequently used clinical tool in the differential diagnoses of disorders of red cell production. Elucidation of the role of Ep in red cell production will further extend our understanding of non-Ep regulators of red cell production. The correlation between in vivo and in vitro erythropoiesis will also be clarified. We have arrived at a major milestone in Ep research and studies of the mechanism of Ep action on the erythroid progenitor cell will undoubtedly be forthcoming.

REFERENCES

1. MIYAKE, T., C. K. H. KUNG & E. GOLDWASSER. 1977. J. Biol. Chem. 252: 5558-5564.
2. GARCIA, J. F., J. B. SHERWOOD & E. GOLDWASSER. 1979. Blood Cells 5: 405-419.
3. SHERWOOD, J. B. & E. GOLDWASSER. 1979. Blood 54: 885-893.

4. WEISS, T. L., C. J. KAVINSKY & E. GOLDWASSER. 1982. Proc. Natl. Acad. Sci. USA **79:** 5465-5469.
5. GARCIA, J. F., S. N. EBBE, L. HOLLANDER, H. O. CUTTING, M. E. MILLER & E. P. CRONKITE. 1982. J. Lab. Clin. Med. **99:** 624-635.
6. WINER, B. J. 1971. Statistical Principles in Experimental Design. 2nd edit. McGraw-Hill Book Co. New York, N.Y.
7. MILLER, M. E., J. F. GARCIA, R. A. COHEN, E. P. CRONKITE, G. MOCCIA & J. ACEVEDO. 1981. Br. J. Haematol. **49:** 189-200.
8. MILLER, M. E., E. P. CRONKITE & J. F. GARCIA. 1982. Br. J. Haematol. **52:** 545-549.
9. KOEFFLER, H. P. & E. GOLDWASSER. 1981. Ann. Intern. Med. **94:** 44-47.
10. ERSLEY, A. J., J. CARO, E. KANSU, O. MILLER & E. COBBS. 1979. Am. J. Med. **66:** 243-247.
11. VANIER, T., M. J. DULFANO, C. WU & J. F. DESFORGES. 1963. N. Engl. J. Med.: 169-178.
12. ERSLEV, A. J., L. A. KAZAL & O. P. MILLER. 1971. Proc. Soc. Exp. Biol. Med. **138:** 1025-1029.
13. MORIYAMA, Y., A. REGE & J. W. FISHER. 1971. Proc. Soc. Exp. Biol. Med. **148:** 94-97.
14. CHANDRA, M., J. F. GARCIA, M. E. MILLER, R. S. WALDBAUM, P. A. BLUESTONE & M. MCVICAR. 1983. J. Pediatr. **103:** 80-83.
15. CHANDRA, M., M. E. MILLER, J. F. GARCIA, R. T. MOSEY & M. MCVICAR. 1981. Kidney Int. **21:** 228.
16. JEPSON, J. L. & L. LOWENSTEIN. 1964. Blood **24:** 726.
17. NATHAN, D. & A. SYTKOWSKI. 1983. N. Engl. J. Med. **308:** 520-522.

DISCUSSION OF THE PAPER

P. VINCENT (*Kanematsu Research Laboratories, Royal Prince Alfred Hospital, Camperdown, Australia*): In one of the earlier papers in which Dr. Eugene Cronkite is a coauthor there is a comment on erythropoietic factor. That paper is in Spanish and, therefore, is perhaps a bit obscure. However, those studies were done utilizing a biologic test. Since the biologic tests are different from the radioimmunoassay, I wonder if you have done both these tests to see if there are differences.

M. E. MILLER: We have done a number of biological assays on the same samples that Dr. Garcia, and now Dr. Gisela Clemons, have assayed. We have found a striking correlation between the biological assay and the radioimmunoassay in levels where we can detect activity (50 mU/ml and above). Dr. Cronkite and I have reviewed the last series of experiments that we did in an animal system and found that the only time there was a discrepancy was when we attempted to measure plasma clearance of erythropoietin in mice. There was far more immunoreactive erythropoietin than bioreactive erythropoietin in these studies. Wherever else we have done the same determinations, we have had no disagreements.

R. SHADDUCK (*Montefiore Hospital, Pittsburgh, Pa.*): Do you believe that there is a local production of erythropoietin in the bone marrow in response to certain kinds of stimuli?

MILLER: There is some evidence to suggest that this may be true. Drs. Ivan Rich and Bernard Kubanek have shown that macrophages produce erythropoietin. I have not seen any other group reproduce that work so I am hesitant to say that it is a potential mechanism.

Radiation Sensitivity and Cancer in Ataxia-Telangiectasia[a]

ROBERT B. PAINTER

Laboratory of Radiobiology and Environmental Health
University of California
San Francisco, California 94143

Ataxia-telangiectasia (A-T) is a human autosomal recessive disease of relatively high frequency, afflicting about one person in 40,000 in the United States. In addition to the clinical symptoms inherent in its name, A-T is characterized by immunodeficiencies and a high incidence of neoplasms. Its interest to radiobiology was kindled first by reports that A-T patients with tumors were extraordinarily sensitive to standard radiotherapeutic regimes[1-3] and then by the demonstration that fibroblasts from A-T patients were hypersensitive to the killing effects of ionizing radiation.[4,5] This radiosensitivity of A-T fibroblasts is invariant, and A-T is the only human clinical syndrome thus far described that is always accompanied by sensitivity to ionizing radiation.

It has been tempting to attribute the radiosensitivity of A-T patients to a DNA repair deficiency and then to ascribe the clinical abnormalities of the disease to this putative defect in DNA repair. Because cancer in another human autosomal disease, xeroderma pigmentosum (XP), is almost certainly due to a defect in the repair of ultraviolet-light-induced DNA damage, A-T has been perceived as the "ionizing-radiation analogue" of XP. However, complications have arisen that cast doubt on this idea. After the first report that cells from A-T patients were defective in excision repair of ionizing-radiation-induced DNA base damage,[6] it was found that cells from other A-T patients, equally radiosensitive in terms of reproductive integrity, were normal in excision repair.[7] The repair of single-strand breaks,[8-10] double-strand breaks,[11] thymine damage,[12] and other less well defined kinds of ionizing-radiation-induced DNA damage[13] is normal in A-T cells; thus, there is no known correlation between defective DNA repair and the abnormal radiosensitivity in A-T.

In the past few years, however, it has been consistently shown that A-T cells do exhibit an abnormality in DNA synthesis; normal semiconservative DNA synthesis in A-T cells is, paradoxically, *resistant* to ionizing radiation. The typical two-component curve observed when the DNA synthesis rate in normal cells is plotted against dose is not found for A-T cells (FIGURE 1). Instead, a single-component curve is generated, lacking the initial steep, low-dose component observed for normal cells. This result has been found by many workers throughout the world[14-17] and appears to be an intrinsic feature of A-T.[18] A resistant DNA synthesis is also observed after treatment of A-T cells with those chemical DNA-damaging agents, such as bleomycin[19]

[a]This work was supported by the U.S. Department of Energy under Contract DE-AC03-76-SF01012.

and neocarzinostatin,[20] that directly produce DNA strand breaks, but it is not seen after treatment with alkylating agents or other DNA-damaging agents that do not directly break DNA.[19]

A second unexpected response of A-T cells to ionizing radiation is their reduced mitotic delay compared to normal cells.[21,22] Not only is the time period during which mitotic activity is reduced shorter in A-T cells, but also the percentage of cells in mitosis does not drop as low in A-T cells as in normal cells (FIGURE 2). Because the frequency of chromosome aberrations induced in A-T cells irradiated in G_2 is much higher than that in normal cells, it was proposed that the defect in A-T cells is one that causes the irradiated G_2 cells to enter mitosis precociously, thereby expressing aberrational damage that in normal cells is repaired during their longer mitotic delay.[16] Similarly, in cells in DNA synthesis, the delays that inhibit the rate of DNA synthesis in normal cells do not occur in A-T cells, thus possibly permitting the copying of radiation-induced DNA damage.

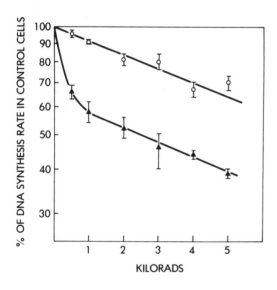

FIGURE 1. Rate of DNA synthesis as a function of X-radiation dose in human cells. ▲, Normal fibroblasts; ○, AT3BI fibroblasts. Reprinted from Reference 16.

What, if any, causal relationships exist between these abnormal radiobiological end points and the clinical symptoms observed in A-T? Although this question cannot be definitively answered, some speculation may be of value. First, it is possible that radioresistant DNA synthesis and reduced radiation-induced mitotic delay reflect a defective damage-recognition system that plays a role in the increased cancer incidence among A-T patients. Intracellular metabolism constantly generates free radicals similar to those responsible for the indirect effects of ionizing radiation. The occasional DNA strand break that is induced by these radicals in normal cells is handled by normal mechanisms, including possibly a delay to allow time for repair. In A-T cells, the failure to delay may occasionally cause the fixation of this damage, either by replication or by precocious entry into mitosis. If this damage is manifested as an aberration, there will be, over time, many more opportunities for formation of abnormal, stable

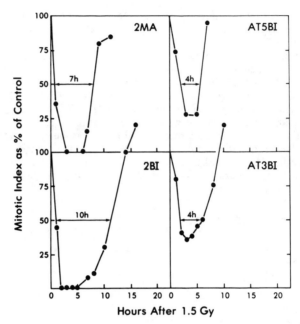

FIGURE 2. Mitotic index in normal human fibroblasts (2MA and 2BI) and in A-T fibroblasts (AT5BI and AT3BI) after exposure to 1.5 Gy of X radiation. Redrawn from References 21 and 22 with permission of the authors.

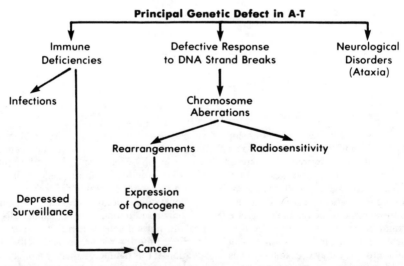

FIGURE 3. Scheme whereby symptoms of A-T, except for cancer, arise directly from the principal genetic defect and are not the result of faulty DNA replication or repair.

chromosomal rearrangements. It is possible that occasionally (but much more frequently than in normal cells) such a rearrangement will cause an endogenous oncogene to be stably integrated next to an active promoter, thus initiating the first step in carcinogenesis.

In contrast, it does not seem to me that the defect in recognition of DNA damage is responsible for the immunological and neurological anomalies of A-T. These are manifested early in life; indeed, the continued production of α-fetoprotein found in A-T patients[23] suggests that some step(s) in differentiation is at fault. This abnormal differentiation seems to be an intrinsic feature that is a direct result of the principal defect per se (FIGURE 3). Another possibility, of course, is that the principal genetic defect causes the chromosomal aberrations and that these aberrations are responsible for all the other symptoms of A-T (FIGURE 4). This seems unlikely because (1) other diseases that show chromosomal aberrations, e.g., Fanconi's anemia, are not accom-

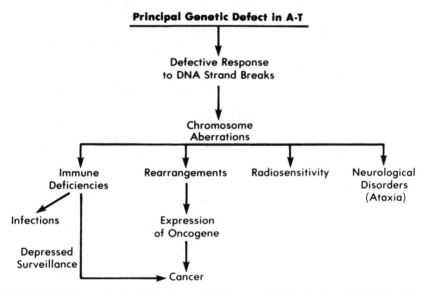

FIGURE 4. Scheme whereby all symptoms of A-T are mediated by the defect in DNA metabolism that causes chromosome aberrations.

panied by neurological or immunological abnormalities, and (2) some immunodeficiency and neurological diseases show no indication of defective DNA repair or DNA synthesis. In contrast, chromosomal changes are almost always associated with neoplastic disease and in many cases seem to play a role in its etiology.[24]

REFERENCES

1. GOTOFF, S. P., E. AMIRMOKRI & E. J. LIEBNER. 1967. Ataxia telangiectasia. Neoplasia, untoward response to x-irradiation, and tuberous sclerosis. Am. J. Dis. Child. **114:** 617-625.

2. MORGAN, J. L., T. M. HOLCOMB & R. W. MORRISSEY. 1968. Radiation reaction in ataxia telangiectasia. Am. J. Dis. Child. **116:** 557-558.
3. CUNLIFFE, P. N., J. R. MANN, A. H. CAMERON, K. D. ROBERTS & H. W. C. WARD. 1975. Radiosensitivity in ataxia-telangiectasia. Br. J. Radiol. **48:** 374-376.
4. TAYLOR, A. M. R., D. G. HARNDEN, C. F. ARLETT, S. A. HARCOURT, A. R. LEHMANN, S. STEVENS & B. A. BRIDGES. 1975. Ataxia telangiectasia: a human mutation with abnormal radiation sensitivity. Nature **258:** 427-429.
5. COX, R. & W. K. MASSON. 1980. Radiosensitivity in cultured human fibroblasts. Int. J. Radiat. Biol. **38:** 575-576.
6. PATERSON, M. C., B. P. SMITH, P. H. M. LOHMAN, A. K. ANDERSON & L. FISHMAN. 1976. Defective excision repair of γ ray-damaged DNA in human (ataxia telangiectasia) fibroblasts. Nature **260:** 444-446.
7. PATERSON, M. C. & P. J. SMITH. 1979. Ataxia telangiectasia: an inherited human disorder involving hypersensitivity to ionizing radiation and related DNA-damaging chemicals. Annu. Rev. Genet. **13:** 291-318.
8. SHERIDAN, R. B., III & P. C. HUANG. 1979. Ataxia telangiectasia: further considerations of the evidence for single strand break repair. Mutat. Res. **61:** 415-417.
9. FORNACE, A. J., JR. & J. B. LITTLE. 1980. Normal repair of DNA single-strand breaks in patients with ataxia telangiectasia. Biochim. Biophys. Acta **607:** 432-437.
10. HARIHARAN, P. V., S. ELECZKO, B. P. SMITH & M. C. PATERSON. 1981. Normal rejoining of DNA strand breaks in ataxia telangiectasia fibroblast lines after low X-ray exposure. Radiat. Res. **86:** 589-597.
11. LEHMANN, A. R. & S. STEVENS. 1977. The production and repair of double strand breaks in cells from normal humans and from patients with ataxia telangiectasia. Biochim. Biophys. Acta **474:** 49-60.
12. REMSEN, J. F. & P. A. CERUTTI. 1977. Excision of gamma-ray induced thymine lesions by preparations from ataxia telangiectasia fibroblasts. Mutat. Res. **43:** 139-146.
13. PATERSON, M. C. 1978. Ataxia telangiectasia: a model inherited disease linking deficient DNA repair with radiosensitivity and cancer proneness. *In* DNA Repair Mechanisms. P. C. Hanawalt, E. C. Friedberg & C. F. Fox, Eds.: 637-650. Academic Press, Inc. New York, N.Y.
14. HOULDSWORTH, J. & M. F. LAVIN. 1980. Effect of ionizing radiation on DNA synthesis in ataxia telangiectasia cells. Nucleic Acids Res. **8:** 3709-3720.
15. EDWARDS, M. J. & A. M. R. TAYLOR. 1980. Unusual levels of (ADP-ribose)$_n$ and DNA synthesis in ataxia telangiectasia cells following γ-ray irradiation. Nature **287:** 745-747.
16. PAINTER, R. B. & B. R. YOUNG. 1980. Radiosensitivity in ataxia-telangiectasia: a new explanation. Proc. Natl. Acad. Sci. USA **77:** 7315-7317.
17. DE WIT, J., N. G. J. JASPERS & D. BOOTSMA. 1981. The rate of DNA synthesis in normal human and ataxia telangiectasia cells after exposure to X-irradiation. Mutat. Res. **80:** 221-226.
18. PAINTER, R. B. 1981. Radioresistant DNA synthesis: an intrinsic feature of ataxia telangiectasia. Mutat. Res. **84:** 183-190.
19. CRAMER, P. & R. B. PAINTER. 1981. Bleomycin-resistant DNA synthesis in ataxia telangiectasia cells. Nature **291:** 671-672.
20. SHILOH, Y., E. TABOR & Y. BECKER. 1982. Cellular hypersensitivity to neocarzinostatin in ataxia-telangiectasia skin fibroblasts. Cancer Res. **42:** 2247-2249.
21. ZAMPETTI-BOSSELER, F. & D. SCOTT. 1981. Cell death, chromosome damage and mitotic delay in normal human, ataxia telangiectasia and retinoblastoma fibroblasts after X-irradiation. Int. J. Radiat. Biol. **39:** 547-558.
22. SCOTT, D. & F. ZAMPETTI-BOSSELER. 1982. Cell cycle dependence of mitotic delay in X-irradiated normal and ataxia-telangiectasia fibroblasts. Int. J. Radiat. Biol. **42:** 679-683.
23. WALDMANN, T. A. & K. R. MCINTIRE. 1972. Serum-alpha-fetoprotein levels in patients with ataxia telangiectasia. Lancet **ii:** 1112-1115.
24. GERMAN, J. (Ed.). 1983. Chromosome Mutation and Neoplasia. Alan R. Liss. New York, N.Y.

Some Reflections on Scientific Research

MARCEL BESSIS

Institut de Pathologie Cellulaire
I.N.S.E.R.M. Unité 48
Hôpital de Bicêtre
Paris, France

It is a pleasure to have an opportunity to evoke the memories of the scientific discussions that have linked us to Gene Cronkite for the past thirty years. Over the past few months, I have read and reread with admiration and astonishment, the long list of Gene's contributions to science from which I have chosen two scientific subjects, the possibility of transfusing platelets and the use of extracorporeal irradiation of blood cells, with which to illustrate some of my favorite philosophical preoccupations:

(1) Who deserves the credit for a discovery?
(2) Why do scientists want to make discoveries?
(3) Are there recipes for making discoveries?

The first publication about platelet transfusion was "Separation, concentration, and transfusion of platelets" by G. H. L. Dillard, G. Brecher, and E. P. Cronkite. This fundamental article, published in 1951, is only two and a half pages long.

The first publication on white cell transfusion was "Transfusion of separated leukocytes into irradiated dogs with aplastic marrows" by G. Brecher, K. M. Wilbur, and E. P. Cronkite.

Needless to say, both operations have saved the lives of many patients. Still, these discoveries are either attributed to investigators who have only repeated or improved the method—or, surprisingly, to no one in particular.

We read in the highly respected and highly respectable book, "History of Hematology," which was recently published (that is, 35 years after the original article): "Selective transfusion of platelets has emerged from the growing field of blood banking." For the historian, the author of the discovery that blood platelets can be transfused was "the growing field of blood banking." This quotation gives me the first opportunity to make an excursion into philosophy:

Who really deserves the credit for a discovery?

In 1951, there were only a few people who somehow got the credit for a discovery. Here are some dictionary definitions of these people:

OBSERVER: one engaged in the methods of close observations.
DISCOVERER: one who first finds out something hitherto unknown.
INVESTIGATOR: one who conducts systematic enquiries.
FORERUNNER: one who suggests a proposition for which he has no proof.

In fact, each discovery is due to several contributors, but some are greater contributors than others. . . .

I will come back later to this subject, since I would first like to make a few remarks about what is called a "forerunner" or "pioneer."

Scientists of the time reported observations and developed hypotheses with no way of determining who was correct. Much later when the truth was discovered, it happened that only one of them had been right. He is the one who is called a forerunner; but, usually, he is no more deserving of praise than any of the others whose theories were wrong! Somehow, as the great writer Jorge Luis Borges said: "The fact is, each discovery creates its own forerunners. Each discovery modifies our conception of the past as well as of the future." The fact is that forerunners exist only *after* the discovery has been made and, as Borges remarked, a discovery modifies the historian's concept of the past.

Today those involved in the process of a discovery are much more numerous:

Observers	Writers
Discoverers	Lecturers
Investigators	Editors
Technicians	Censors
Statisticians	Administrators

One of my colleagues assesses the contribution made by joint authors of a paper by what he calls a "delta coefficient," a figure which measures the percentage contribution. Perhaps this idea should be adopted generally and the "delta" incorporated in the author line of each paper:

Title of Paper

Author 1 (97%), Author 2 (2%), and Author 3 (1%)

Using this approach, small fractions of Nobel prizes could be awarded to large numbers of scientists as an incentive to work harder and publish more joint papers.

A scientific discovery is no longer the work of an individual or that of a small group; it is the work of a scientific community. After all, if you think about it from a certain perspective, this applies to artists also. Who knows the names of the Egyptian artists who built the Pyramids? Who knows the names of those who built the cathedrals?

But then, why is it so important to identify the author of an article? Why identify a discovery with a name?

Why do scientists want to make discoveries?

I can offer a range of reasons:

INSECURITY,	desire to be acknowledged.
VANITY,	to obtain notoriety—to be a star.
POWER,	to direct the course of science.
CURIOSITY,	intellectual pleasure.
ALTRUISM,	to do good for mankind.

This list is certainly not complete, but perhaps two of these motivations, which have emerged only recently, are now the most powerful:

(1) the star system established during the second part of the twentieth century, with its prizes which are a fascination to all scientists; and

(2) the fact that research is no longer a game for amateurs. It is a way to make a living, to have a career. This has pushed research into a new era, the era of research entrepreneurs.

These are the actual motivations of today's professional researchers: to become famous, to publish or perish.

But in 1951, for Gene Cronkite and his associates, the main motivation was the same as that of the genuine scientist Robert Hooke who, in 1665, charmingly wrote:

ſo great is the ſatisfaꞔion *of* finding *out* new things,

that I dare compare the contentment *which they will injoy,*

not only to that of contemplation, *but even to that which*

moſt men prefer of the very Senſes themſelves.

Hooke states that the deepest motivation of those who discover a secret of Nature springs from a very special kind of satisfaction, a satisfaction which transcends intellectual—and even sensual—pleasure.

At the end of the twentieth century, is there still room in research for this sort of motivation or will medical research become an industry? Can we still experience this fleeting and delicious sensation that scientists such as Gene Cronkite pursued all their lives?

I would now like to discuss Gene's work on the extracorporeal irradiation of the blood. This technique has been used to investigate crucial problems in hemopoiesis, immunology, and cancer research.

"The role of extracorporeal irradiation of blood in treatment of leukemia" was one of the first papers written by Gene and his collaborators, Arjun D. Chanana and Kanti R. Rai. The technique of extracorporeal irradiation of the blood was the source of many original observations and, above all, of new conceptual thinking. Today, hematologists think in terms of cell physiology and try to follow the creative imagination of Gene Cronkite.

In a recent paper on leukemia ("Leukemia revisited"), Gene stated: "In neoplastic tissue, Virchow considered the body 'a cell-state in which every cell is a citizen' and disease is merely a conflict of citizens. When I first read Virchow's notions, I applauded his imagination and considered his thoughts rather naive. Today, the metaphor is clear. We have killer cells, managerial cells, suppressor cells, helper cells, inductive microenvironments, and more certainly to come."

Over the years, an immense number of facts have accumulated in the field of cancer. Facts but not ideas. What we need is new metaphors, new ideas.

But how does one get new ideas? How can one break free from the tyranny of accepted ideas?

Are there any recipes to make discoveries?

It seems evident to me that poets, artists, and scientists create in much the same way. They need metaphors and dreams. Like artists, researchers see in their dreams the realities they wish to create. Images and emotions are subconsciously rearranged in a thousand ways. From these vague outlines, a miracle is born: the miracle of a new idea.

It has occurred to certain philosophers that if scientific creativity needs dreams, then the research industry should incorporate such elements into the system. If dreams are essential components of creation, then why not use the new discoveries in dream physiology to develop industrialized dreaming? This consists of:

    (1) generation of the dream (good wine, pharmacology),
    (2) detection of the dream (electrophysiology),
    (3) recording of the dream (dream censor),
    (4) selection of ideas (head of department).

Physiologists have observed periods of intense electrical activity in the brain which indicate when dreams are occurring. Sleepers awakened during these periods can readily recall the content of their dreams. One may easily imagine a device that would automatically rouse sleepers when they are dreaming and they could then dictate their dreams to a tape recorder.

Chemists now have at their disposal a large pharmacopoeia. After taking a dream-inducing tablet at dinner time, our researcher of the future will, with breakfast, swallow a tablet that will help him evaluate his night production and perk up his writing style.

Many books have recently been devoted to this approach and these techniques have now been developed into a team approach. In order to give the dreams direction, a group "dream leader" ensures that certain rules are followed. Words are played with their meaning transformed, irrational approaches considered, and unusual incidents provoked. Then, the group leader sorts out any new idea from the tapes of the dreams and the ramblings. He reports his selections to the science entrepreneur who decides which ones to retain and develop.

However, to quote Gene Cronkite again, "No amount of planning will ever replace dumb luck."

This conference has been superb. It has shown us the way that Gene Cronkite has inspired not only his pupils but his peers and his friends.

We all admire Gene Cronkite because he is one of the most distinguished scientists, known everywhere in the world and, more important, we love and respect him because he is a member of a rather rare species: the gentleman-scientist.

I know I speak for all of us in expressing our affection to Gene and Betty Cronkite and in saying how delighted we are that Gene continues to share with us his knowledge, his wisdom, his new ideas, and, above all, the special generosity of his friendship.

Index of Contributors

(Italicized page numbers refer to comments made in discussion.)